Emergency Orthopedics Handbook

Daniel Purcell
Sneha A. Chinai
Brandon R. Allen
Moira Davenport
Editors

Emergency Orthopedics Handbook

Springer

Editors
Daniel Purcell
Emergency Department
New York University Langone
Medical Center
Brooklyn, NY
USA

Brandon R. Allen
Department of Emergency
Medicine
University of Florida
Newberry, FL
USA

Sneha A. Chinai
Department of Emergency
Medicine
University of Massachusetts
Medical School
Worchester, MA
USA

Moira Davenport
Allegheny General Hospital
Temple University
Pittsburgh, PA
USA

ISBN 978-3-030-00706-5 ISBN 978-3-030-00707-2 (eBook)
https://doi.org/10.1007/978-3-030-00707-2

Library of Congress Control Number: 2018964429

This Springer imprint is published by the registered company Springer Nature Switzerland AG
The registered company address is: Gewerbestrasse 11, 6330 Cham, Switzerland

Dedication

Daniel Purcell

Success is not the key to happiness. Happiness is the key to success. If you love what you are doing, you will be successful.

–Albert Schweitzer

This book is dedicated to all those involved in creating the ultimate reference manual depicting management of select musculoskeletal/orthopedic conditions in the emergency department. Without the sacrifice and tireless efforts of so many, this would not have been possible. Rejoice and celebrate, as we have created a masterpiece to be implemented by so many, fostering education and enhancing patient care for years to come. Special thanks to my wife Carmen, and my four children Cory, Miley, Aubrey, and Haley, who allowed me to follow my dreams and make this project a reality – I love you guys!

Sneha A. Chinai

This book is dedicated to all the providers who will use this guide to take better care of their patients with orthopedic complaints.

Brandon R. Allen
For my children, Nila and Owen, who continue to remind me what is important in life

Moira Davenport
Nobody said it's going to be easy. You have to dig into yourself. Think about your family. Think about the journey itself. THINK IN THE MOMENT.

–Meb Keflezighi

4× USA Olympic team member
2004 Olympic marathon silver medalist
2009 NYC Marathon Champion
2014 Boston Marathon Champion
This book is dedicated to those who care for musculoskeletal conditions in the emergency department and on the sidelines. It goes without saying that this work is also dedicated to those who sustain orthopedic injuries in the pursuit of better health and competitive aspirations. Lastly, huge thanks to my family for putting up with me on this crazy journey and for supporting me every step of the way! I would not be where I am today without JD, PD, MG, JJG, CPG, MAG, SMG, RE, and EDE. I think you have all earned honorary medical degrees by this point.

Foreword

It might be cliché, but it is true that Emergency Medicine providers are a "Jack of All Trades" and are required to know how to diagnose life- and limb-threatening diseases that cross all specialties. With the wide breadth of knowledge that Emergency Medicine providers must know, there is an increased need for textbooks that specifically address the needs of Emergency Medicine providers. Reading other specialty textbooks can lead to frustration as one tries to find the few nuggets of information that are pertinent to the emergency department. Ideally, Emergency Medicine textbooks are designed for quick reference, have great illustrations to be able to walk a provider through a rarely done procedure, and are focused on the life and limb threats.

Orthopedics is one area that many Emergency Medicine providers do not have a specialist readily available to take over the case, and there can be considerable sequalae if fractures, dislocations, and infections are not diagnosed and treated quickly. In fact, though missing an acute myocardial infarction is associated with large malpractice payouts, orthopedic injuries account for more medicolegal cases overall. It is imperative that Emergency Medicine providers have a good systematic approach to orthopedic cases to ensure good outcomes, and they must be familiar with multiple different reduction techniques in order to ensure a successful reduction.

This book, *Emergency Orthopedics Handbook*, ideally fits the needs of the busy Emergency Medicine provider. The text quickly gets to the pertinent information that is needed on a busy shift, while having great illustrations that can help ensure a successful joint reduction, arthrocentesis, or application of a splint. Unsure how to measure compartment pressures, or what pressure is consistent with acute compartment pressure see Chap. 3, need help reducing a nursemaid's elbow see Chap. 5, and if you are worried about a septic ankle see Chap. 4 for detailed illustrations on how to approach the joint. This textbook will quickly become your handy resource for orthopedic emergencies and to confirm your treatment of the more common cases.

Wishing you all the best in your care of patients with orthopedic emergencies.

Michael C. Bond, MD, FACEP, FAAEM
Department of Emergency Medicine
University of Maryland School of Medicine,
Baltimore, MD, USA

Preface

Musculoskeletal disorders are among the most common presenting complaints to the emergency department. Pathology may encompass acute traumatic injury, exacerbation of a chronic condition, and in extreme instances, limb and/or life threatening events. Knowledge of their management not only directly impacts results of immediate care, but also long-term patient outcomes. Preparation for success involves a favorable combination of advanced education, skillful experience, and associated technical expertise. Creation of a reference source that combines scholarly activity and innovative visual demonstration would thus be an invaluable tool to facilitate this effect.

The purpose of this publication was to formulate a comprehensive, yet pertinent compilation of various musculoskeletal conditions evaluated and remedied by assorted "emergency care" providers. It is intended to educate the novice practitioner in an expedient and adept manner, while also communicating advanced instruction to the isolated community provider. Our goal is to support enhanced recognition, as well as implementation of expert care for a multitude of receiving musculoskeletal conditions.

This anthology resulted from collaboration among multiple contributors and is directly reflected within its organization and content. We suspect Emergency Medicine Orthopedics will have an immediate and extensive impact upon the care of countless patient circumstances, immeasurably heightening the functional quality of their lives.

The authors would like to extend a sincere appreciation regarding consideration of this resource within your respective treatment domains and are confident its delineated content will categorically optimize future musculoskeletal patient encounters. Thank you for your support and please contact us with any questions and/or feedback. Good luck!

New York, NY, USA — Daniel Purcell, MD
Worcester, MA, USA — Sneha A. Chinai, MD
Gainesville, FL, USA — Brandon R. Allen, MD
Pittsburgh, PA, USA — Moira Davenport, MD

Contents

Contributors

Brandon R. Allen, MD Department of Emergency Medicine, University of Florida Health, University of Florida, Gainesville, FL, USA

Justin Chapman, MD Department of Emergency Medicine, UMass Memorial Medical Center, Worcester, MA, USA

Sneha A. Chinai, MD Department of Emergency Medicine, University of Massachusetts Medical School, Worcester, MA, USA

Moira Davenport, MD Allegheny General Hospital, Temple University, Pittsburgh, PA, USA

Salvador Forte, DO Department of Orthopedic Surgery, Philadelphia College of Osteopathic Medicine, Philadelphia, PA, USA

Daniel Purcell, MD Emergency Department, New York University Langone Medical Center Brooklyn, New York, NY, USA

Matthew R. Rebesco, MD Department of Emergency Medicine, UMass Memorial Medical Center, Worcester, MA, USA

Brian R. Sharp, MD, FACEP BerbeeWalsh Department of Emergency Medicine, University of Wisconsin School of Medicine and Public Health, Madison, WI, USA

Eric M. Steinberg, DO, FACEP Department of Emergency Medicine, Mount Sinai Beth Israel, New York, NY, USA

Bryan A. Terry, MD The Brooklyn Hospital Center, Brooklyn, NY, USA

Laura Walker, MD Department of Emergency Medicine, Mayo Clinic, Rochester, MN, USA

Chapter 1
Key Motor and Sensory Exam

Eric M. Steinberg, Salvador Forte, Bryan A. Terry, and Daniel Purcell

E. M. Steinberg
Department of Emergency Medicine, Mount Sinai Beth Israel, New York, NY, USA

S. Forte
Department of Orthopedic Surgery, Philadelphia College of Osteopathic Medicine, Philadelphia, PA, USA

B. A. Terry
The Brooklyn Hospital Center, Brooklyn, NY, USA

D. Purcell (✉)
Emergency Department, New York University Langone Medical Center Brooklyn, New York, NY, USA
e-mail: daniel.purcell@nyumc.org

D. Purcell et al. (eds.), *Emergency Orthopedics Handbook*,
https://doi.org/10.1007/978-3-030-00707-2_1

Table 1.1 Key physical exam findings: upper extremity

Nerve lesion	Mechanism of injury	Sensory deficit(s)	Motor deficit(s)	Classic presentation
Axillary (C5, C6)	Humeral head dislocation (anterior MC) Proximal humerus fracture (surgical neck-head/shaft transition) Quadrilateral space syndrome (axillary nerve/posterior humeral circumflex artery)	Superolateral upper arm (area over deltoid insertion)	Active abduction of the shoulder >20° (supraspinatus initiates abduction ~0–20°)	Acute: anterior dislocation-"squared off" shoulder Chronic: deltoid muscle atrophy
Radial (C5, C6, C7, C8)	Mid-shaft humerus fracture Compression in axilla crutch usage, arm draped over couch/bench ("Saturday night palsy") Radial head dislocation/subluxation (Monteggia fracture, "Nursemaid's" elbow)	**Superficial branch:** anatomic snuffbox Dorsal 1st web space Lateral 1/2 dorsum hand, up to level of proximal phalanx (median nerve innervates distal region)	**Radial nerve (proper)/deep branch:** forearm extension (triceps) **PIN:** forearm supination (supinator muscle), extension of wrist and fingers at MCP joints PIN-only motor component, no sensory component ("PIN = no pain")	**Radial**: inability to extend forearm against gravity Absent/decreased triceps reflex **PIN:** wrist drop No extensor pollicis longus function ("Thumbs up") Absent/decreased brachioradialis reflex Ulnar deviation of wrist (See Fig.1.1)

Nerve lesion	Mechanism of injury	Sensory deficit(s)	Motor deficit(s)	Classic presentation
Median (C6, C7, C8, T1)	**Proximal injury**: supracondylar humerus fracture	Thenar eminence. Lateral 3.5 digits	"OK" sign Flexion of wrist Flexion of thumb (FPL), 2nd/3rd digit DIPJ (FDP). **Anterior Interosseous nerve**: forearm pronation	"Hand of benediction"/"Pope's blessing" Absent function of lateral ½ FDP/lumbricals with unopposed digital extensor function: cannot close index/middle fingers when make fist Ulnar deviation of wrist (unopposed FCU) (See Fig. 1.2)
	Distal injury: carpal tunnel syndrome/acute CTS (radio-carpal dislocation/distal radius fracture) Lunate/peri-lunate dislocation	Lateral 3.5 digits	Thumb opposition	"Ape" hand/"simian" hand Thumb/index finger paralyzed in adduction and hyperextension Carpal tunnel syndrome: thenar muscle atrophy ("wasting") ** ***ACTS requires immediate surgical decompression*** **

(continued)

Table 1.1 (continued)

Nerve lesion	Mechanism of injury	Sensory deficit(s)	Motor deficit(s)	Classic presentation
Ulnar (C8, T1)	**Proximal injury**: Humeral medial epicondyle fracture Clavicle fracture Cubital tunnel syndrome Supracondylar humeral fracture (peds)	Medial forearm (medial antebrachial cutaneous nerve) Hypothenar eminence Medial 1.5 digits	Flexion of medial fingers Flexion/ulnar deviation at wrist	Radial deviation of the wrist Volkmann's ischemic contracture (forearm compartment syndrome post-supracondylar humeral fracture)
	Distal injury: Hook of hamate fracture Entrapment in Guyon's canal Ulnar artery thrombosis	Medial 1.5 digits	Adduction/abduction fingers (interosseus muscles) Adduction of thumb (adductor pollicis) Extension of fingers (lumbricals)	"Claw" hand-hyperextension MCPJ/flexion PIPJ, DIPJ of ring/little fingers (See Fig. 1.3). Dorsal IO atrophy (permanent atrophy between the thumb and forefinger)
Musculocutaneous (C5, C6, C7)	Brachial plexus upper trunk/lateral cord injury Bicipital aponeurosis (lacertus fibrosus) compression	Lateral forearm (lateral antebrachial cutaneous nerve)	Forearm flexion/supination	Absent/decreased biceps reflex Decreased flexion and/or supination strength (latter more affected)

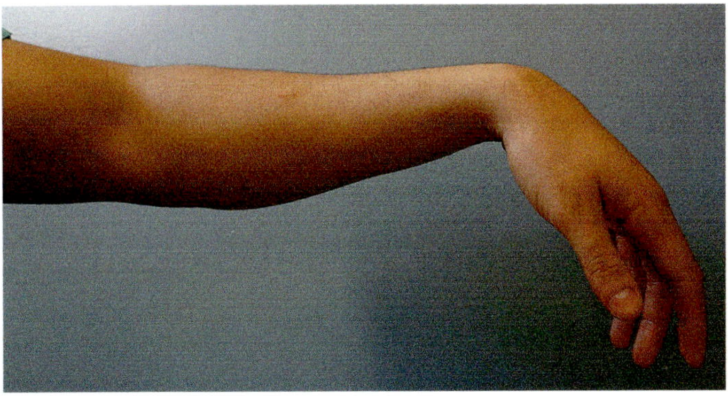

FIGURE 1.1 Wrist drop

FIGURE 1.2 Proximal median nerve injury – cannot flex second and third fingers

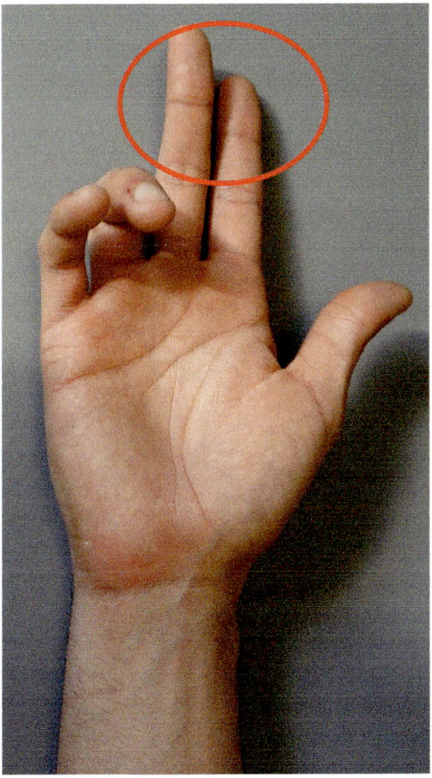

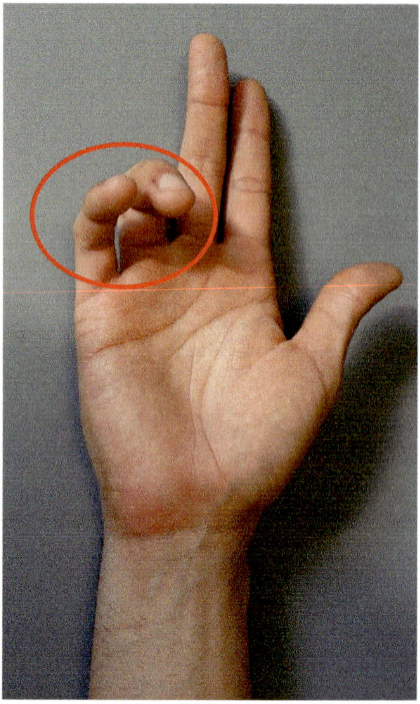

FIGURE 1.3 Distal ulnar nerve injury – cannot extend fourth and fifth digits

Figure 1.4

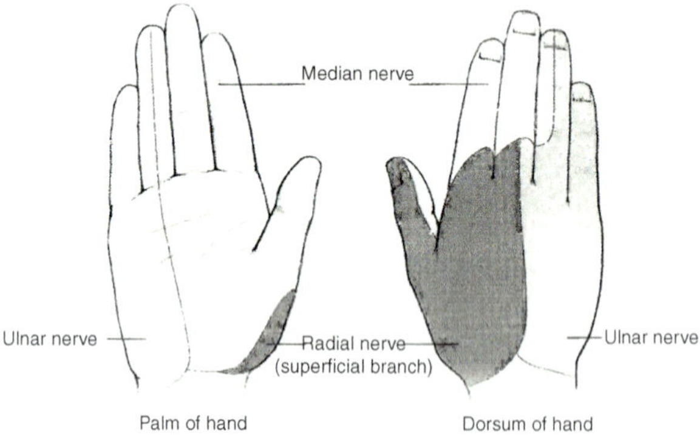

FIGURE 1.4 Cutaneous Innervation of Hand. (Reprinted with permission from White J. USMLE road map: gross anatomy. McGraw-Hill: Appleton & Lange; 2003. ©McGraw-Hill Education)

Figure 1.5

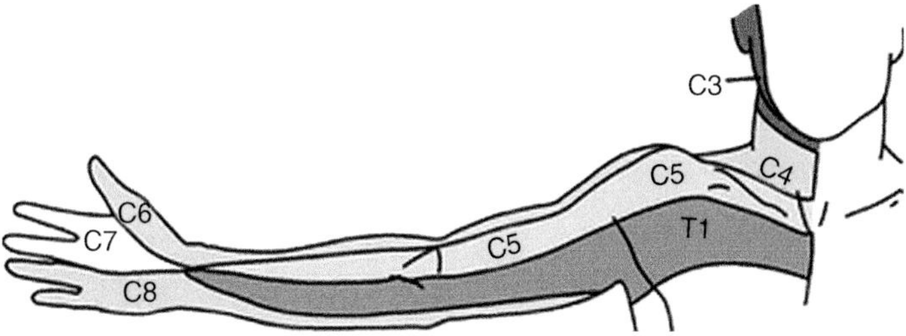

FIGURE 1.5 Dermatomes of upper extremity – anterior. (Reprinted from Keegan JJ, Garrett FD. The segmental distribution of the cutaneous nerves in the limbs of man. Anat Rec. 1948;102:409–37. With permission from John Wiley and Sons)

Figure 1.6

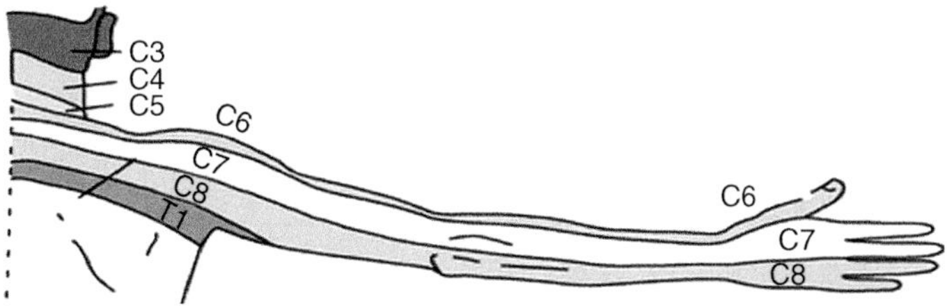

FIGURE 1.6 Dermatomes of upper extremity – posterior. (Reprinted from Keegan JJ, Garrett FD. The segmental distribution of the cutaneous nerves in the limbs of man. Anat Rec. 1948;102:409–37. With permission from John Wiley and Sons)

TABLE 1.2 Specialized testing: shoulder

Test	What it's testing	How to do it	Positive test
Hyper-adduction (crossed-arm adduction)	AC joint pathology	Hand on affected side contacts contralateral shoulder.	Pain at AC joint as acromion contacts lateral end of clavicle.
Neer's sign	Subacromial impingement	Forward flexion and internal rotation (thumb points down); stabilize scapula throughout ROM. (See Figs. 1.7 and 1.8)	Pain at subacromial space at >90° flexion as posterior rotator cuff tendons pinched against coracoacromial arch. **Positive Neer's test: inject 10 ml 1% lidocaine and repeat testing-pain relieved following injection**
"Scaption"/"empty beer can" sign	Supraspinatus pathology	Humerus flexed 90 degrees, 30 degrees adduction, forearm extended/pronated (scapular plane)-patient points thumb down-apply downward pressure (See Fig. 1.9).	Pain/inability to resist downward pressure

Test	What it's testing	How to do it	Positive test
Apprehension/ relocation	Glenohumeral anterior instability	Apprehension: patient supine/upright with shoulder abducted 90°/maximal external rotation. Support patient elbow while applying anterior-directed pressure to proximal humerus.	Pain, apprehension.
		Relocation: apply a posterior force	Relief of above
O'Brien's	Labral pathology (SLAP lesion)	Humerus: 90° forward flexion, 10° adduction, forearm pronation; apply inferior directed force	Positive test: pain that is relieved with the same movement repeated with forearm supination
Drop arm	Rotator cuff tear (supraspinatus dysfunction)	Passively abduct humerus and instruct patient to lower arm in controlled fashion.	Patient may be able to resist gravity initially due to intact deltoid, but eventually fails to control descent.
Spurling's sign	Cervical disc disease/root disorder	Head rotated to affected side-radicular symptoms reproduced with axial loading (See Fig. 1.10).	Radiation below elbow cervical spine pathology versus above elbow commonly rotator cuff pathology

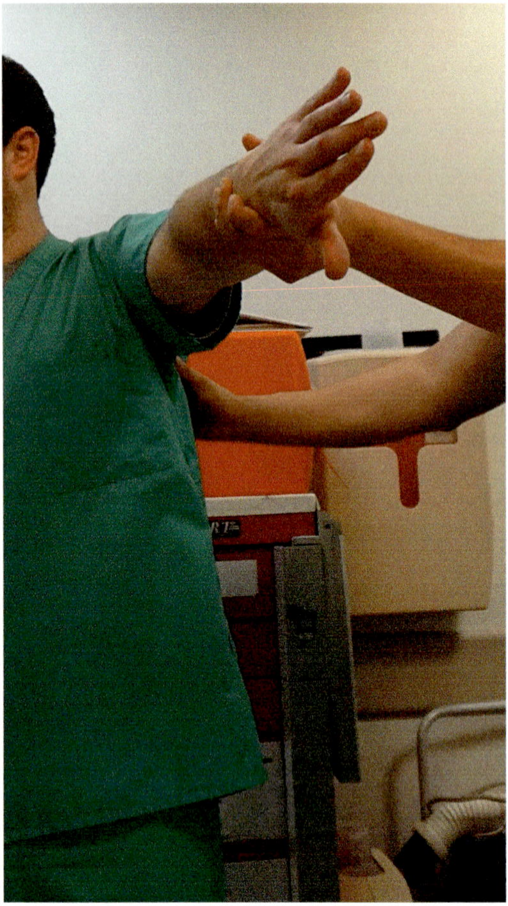

FIGURE 1.7 Neer's maneuver setup

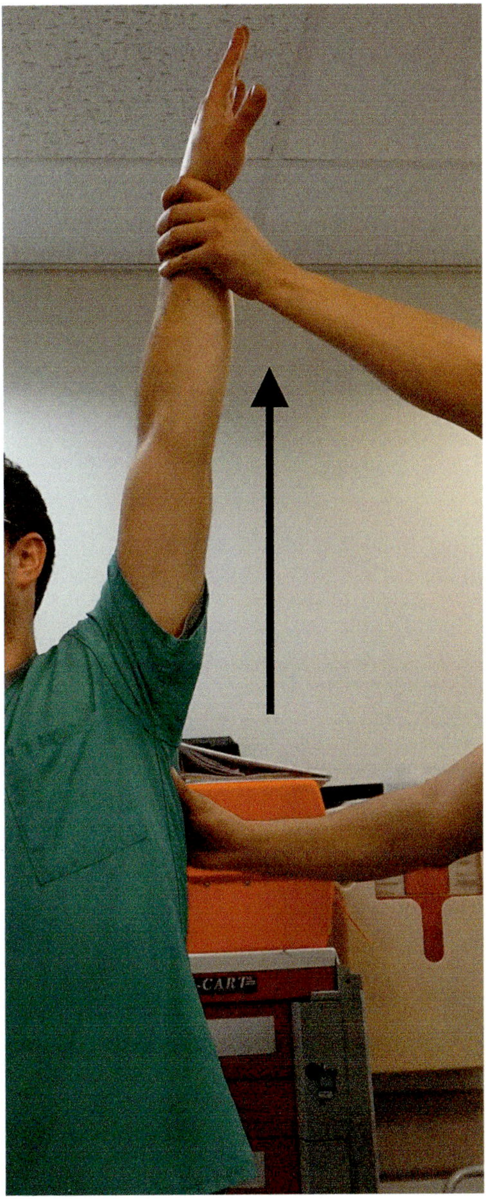

FIGURE 1.8 Neer's maneuver

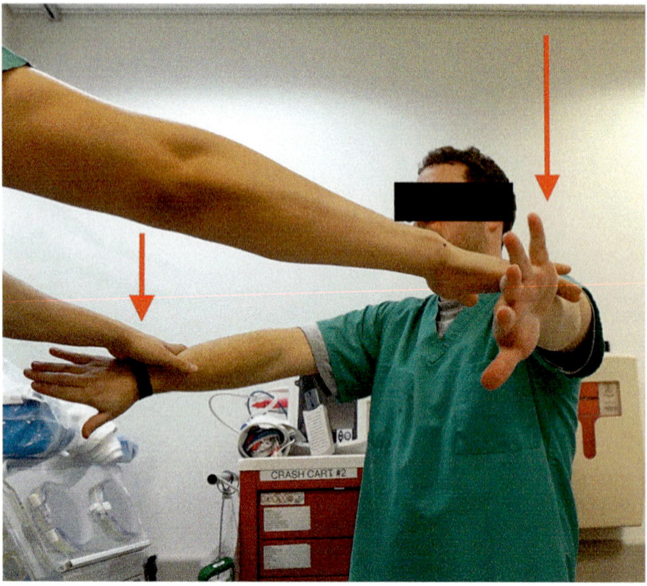

FIGURE 1.9 "Empty beer can" test/"Scaption"

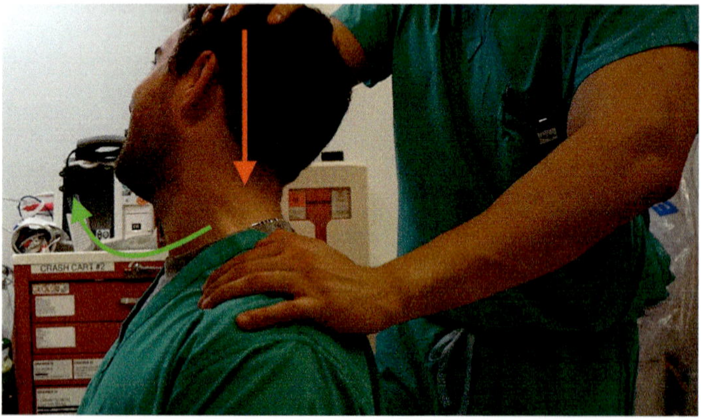

FIGURE 1.10 Spurling's maneuver performed on the patient's right side. Reproduction of symptoms is a positive sign

Pearls (Upper Extremity)

- Assessment of vascular status: palpate distal pulses, measure capillary refill, and qualify temperature and color (compare versus unaffected extremity).
- ***Indications for emergent reduction: neurovascular deficit*** (e.g., radial nerve neuropraxia with mid-shaft humeral fracture) and/or ***tenting of skin from bony deformity*** (e.g., superiorly displaced clavicle fracture can lead to skin/tissue necrosis).
- Must have multi-planar imaging of shoulder (axillary lateral, velpeau axillary view, or CT) if concern exists for shoulder dislocation.

Shoulder X-Ray (See Figs. 1.11, 1.12, 1.13, and 1.14)

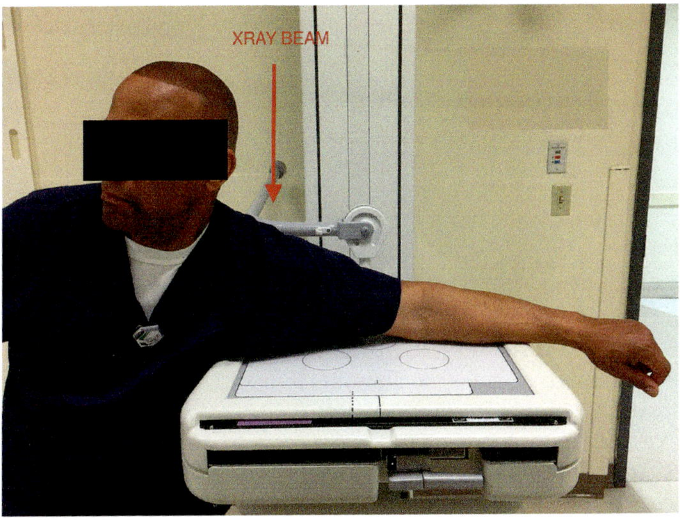

FIGURE 1.11 Axillary view radiograph setup

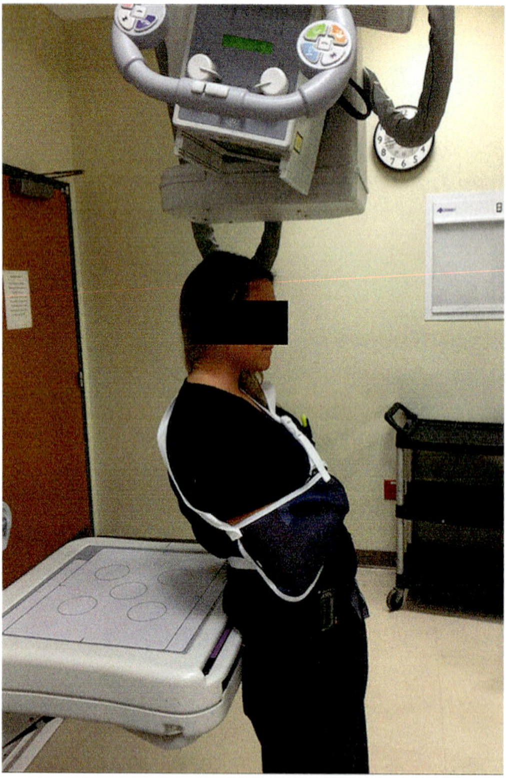

FIGURE 1.12 Velpeau view setup

Pearls (Upper Extremity) Continued

- Decreased ER (external rotation) shoulder: osteoarthritis, adhesive capsulitis, and/or posterior dislocation (electrocution, seizures).
- Adhesive capsulitis ("frozen shoulder"): **decreased *active* ROM versus *passive* ROM** (decreased ER most common).
- Diabetic patient with an infected shoulder-suspect syrinx (Charcot shoulder).

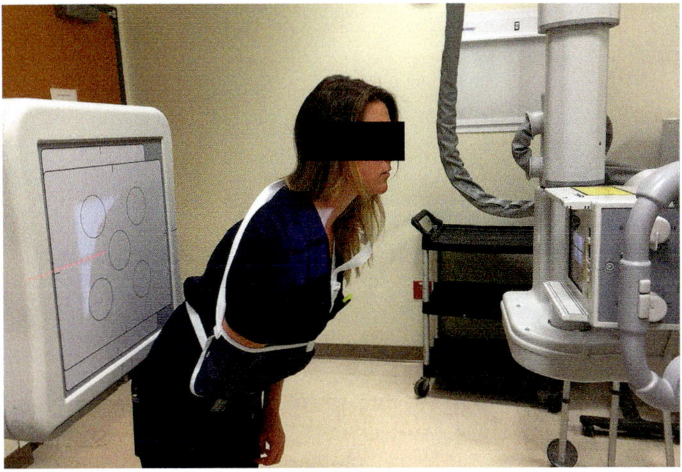

FIGURE 1.13 Modified Velpeau view setup

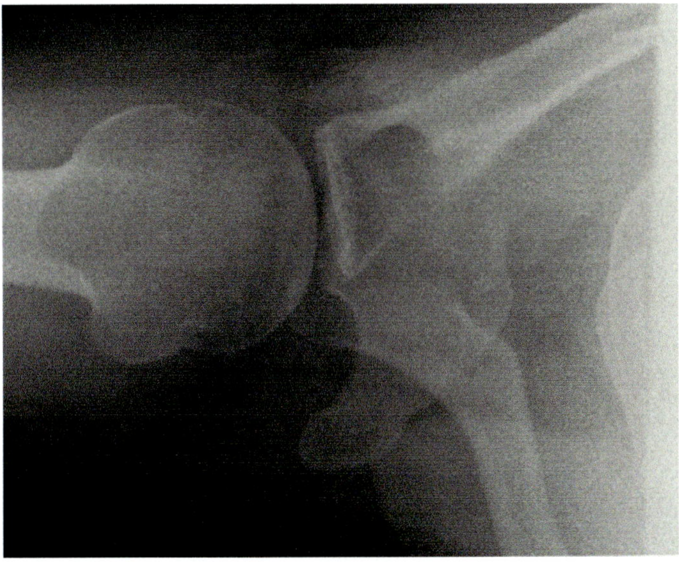

FIGURE 1.14 Axillary view radiograph. (Reprinted from http://eorif.com/shoulder-dislocation-images. With permission from eORIF, LLC)

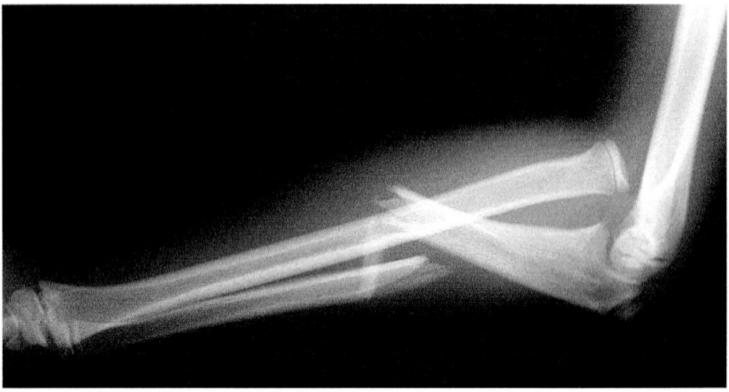

FIGURE 1.15 Monteggia fracture: proximal ulna fracture/radial head dislocation. (Image reprinted with permission from Medscape Drugs & Diseases (http://emedicine.medscape.com/), 2017, available at: http://emedicine.medscape.com/article/1231438-overview)

- **"Terrible triad" injury**: elbow dislocation, radial head fracture, and coronoid process fracture.
- Radial head/neck occult fracture: check for **"sail sign"** (posterior fat pad elevation), assess for block to elbow motion (+/− local anesthetic injection to decrease pain) (See Fig. 1.17).
- Educate patient regarding signs of acute carpal tunnel syndrome (ACTS) following radio-carpal dislocation/displaced distal radius fractures (median nerve can be stretched/tethered).
- Not all distal radius fractures are "Colles'" fractures (apex volar (palmar)/dorsal displacement of distal fracture fragment) versus opposite pattern (Smith fracture = reverse Colles' fracture).
- Flexor tenosynovitis: ***KANAVEL signs*** – flexed posture finger(s), fusiform swelling, pain with passive extension of the affected finger(s), and associated tenderness along the flexor tendon sheath.
- Snuff box tenderness and/or pain with axial loading of the thumb (FOOSH injury): treat for **presumed** scaphoid fracture (thumb spica immobilization even with initial negative imaging to decrease risk of nonunion/AVN *(distal → proximal blood supply)*

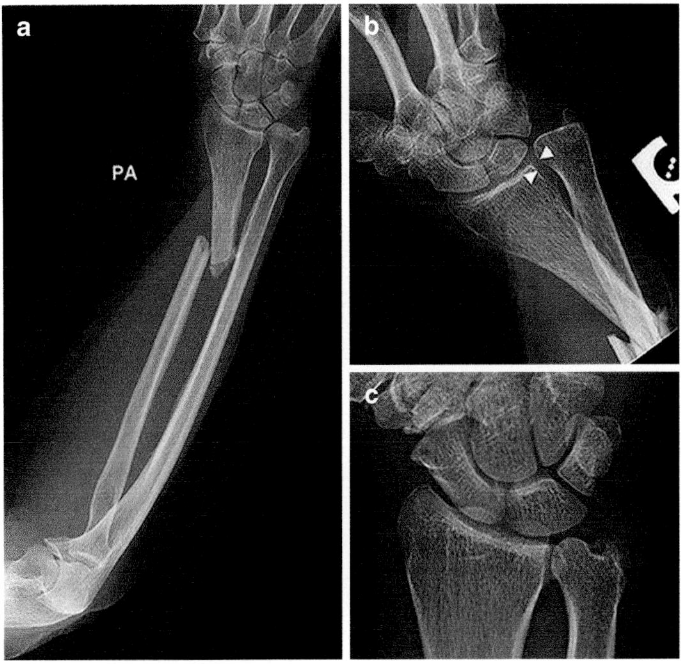

FIGURE 1.16 Galeazzi fracture. (**a**) PA forearm radiograph with displaced fracture of the distal one third of the radial shaft. (**b**) Wrist radiograph in the same patient demonstrates subluxation of the distal radioulnar joint (DRUJ), with mild DRUJ widening, measuring 5 mm (arrowheads), and mild radial foreshortening. (**c**) Comparison normal wrist radiograph. Notice the small caliber of a normal, tight DRUJ. (Reprinted from Wong PK-W, Hanna TN, Shuaib W, Sanders SM, Khosa F. What's in a name? Upper extremity fracture eponyms (Part 1). Int J Emerg Med. 2015;8(1):27. With permission from Creative Commons License 4.0: https://creativecommons.org/licenses/by/4.0/)

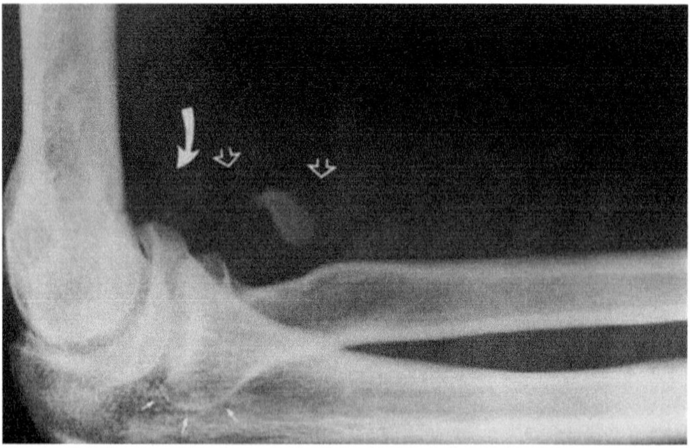

FIGURE 1.17 Anterior Fat Pad Sign may also indicate an occult fracture. (Reprinted from Palmié S, Heller M. Elbow. In: Heller M, Fink A, editors. Radiology of trauma. Medical radiology (Diagnostic imaging and radiation oncology – softcover edition). Berlin/Heidelberg: Springer Verlag; 2000: p. 227–50. With permission from Springer Nature)

Pearls (Lower Extremity)

- Sciatic nerve dysfunction (tibial/peroneal divisions): must first rule out lumbosacral spinal pathology.
- Hip dislocations: most common posterior (perform neurovascular exam ***before and after*** reduction).
  Orthopedic Emergency: Native hip dislocation.
- Risk of AVN increases proportionately with dislocation time.
- "Trendelenburg gait" (gluteus medius lurch): patient displaces center of gravity laterally over the opposite side pelvis to compensate for loss of ipsilateral pelvic stabilization based upon poorly functioning gluteus medius muscle (See Fig.1.21a, b).
- Obturator nerve (cutaneous innervation) can be responsible for "knee pain" with actual hip joint pathology ***(always perform a full hip examination on every patient that presents with knee pain)***.

Table 1.3 Key physical exam findings: lower extremity

Nerve lesion	Mechanism of injury	Sensory deficit(s)	Motor deficit(s)	Classic presentation
Obturator (L2-L4)	Pelvic trauma (hematoma). Pelvic neoplasm (compression). Gynecologic surgery. Pregnancy	Medial thigh	Hip adduction	Decreased/absent adductor reflex
Femoral (L2-L4)	Hip arthroplasty (anterior approach). Psoas abscess. Pelvic neoplasm. Aortic/iliac artery aneurysm. Diabetic amyotrophy (inflammatory vasculitis)	Anterior thigh/ Medial lower leg → medial malleolus (greater saphenous-terminal branch)	Hip flexion (iliopsoas). Extension of the lower leg at the knee joint	Decreased/absent knee (quadriceps reflex)-predominately L4 innervation

(continued)

TABLE 1.3 (continued)

Nerve lesion	Mechanism of injury	Sensory deficit(s)	Motor deficit(s)	Classic presentation
Sciatic: peroneal (fibular) division(L4-S2)	Hip arthroplasty (posterior approach). Hip fracture/dislocation (posterior). Piriformis syndrome. Knee dislocation (crosses popliteal space). Compression fibular head/neck (tethered), direct injury (ankle ORIF-lateral approach-superficial peroneal nerve injury)	Anterior leg (deep peroneal). Lateral leg (lesser saphenous). Lateral dorsum of foot	Anterolateral compartments: Ankle dorsiflexion. Foot eversion (superficial peroneal nerve: peroneus longus, brevis, and tertius muscles)	***"Foot drop"*** ("Steppage" gait): Deep peroneal nerve injury → tibialis anterior muscle dysfunction (loss of ankle dorsiflexion) (See Fig. 1.18).

Nerve lesion	Mechanism of injury	Sensory deficit(s)	Motor deficit(s)	Classic presentation
Sciatic: tibial division (L4-S3)	**Proximal tibial nerve injury rare** Hip arthroplasty (posterior approach). Hip fracture/dislocation (posterior) Knee dislocation (crosses popliteal space). Compartment syndrome. Tarsal tunnel syndrome (tibial nerve entrapment by ankle flexor retinaculum). Morton's neuroma: interdigital nerves become compressed by their adjacent metatarsal heads and/or stretched as they cross the deep metatarsal ligament	Posterior leg. Medial 3.5 toes (medial plantar nerve)/lateral 1.5 toes (lateral plantar nerve)	Posterior compartment (superficial and deep): ankle/toe plantar flexion. Foot inversion (tibial nerve: tibialis anterior and posterior muscles)	Decreased/absent ankle (Achilles) reflex. Cannot perform heel rise (single leg raise). Tarsal tunnel syndrome: pain/ sensory disturbance of plantar aspect of foot. Sural nerve entrapment (neuropathy) Morton's neuroma: Localized pain/ discomfort. Worse when toe box compressed (e.g., tight-fitting shoes)

(continued)

TABLE 1.3 (continued)

Nerve lesion	Mechanism of injury	Sensory deficit(s)	Motor deficit(s)	Classic presentation
Superior gluteal (L4-S1)	Misplaced gluteal injection. Muscular dystrophies	No sensory component	Hip abduction/ medial rotation thigh (gluteus medius/minimus/ TFL)	Trendelenburg gait: unilateral loss of hip abductor function (core center of gravity shifted, trunk cannot be supported on affected side). Waddling gait: bilateral loss of hip abductor function
Inferior gluteal (L5, S1, S2)	Hip arthroplasty (posterior approach). Pelvic neoplasm	No sensory component	Hip extension/ lateral rotation of thigh (gluteus maximus)	Difficulty rising from a seated position, climbing stairs, jumping, incline level walking

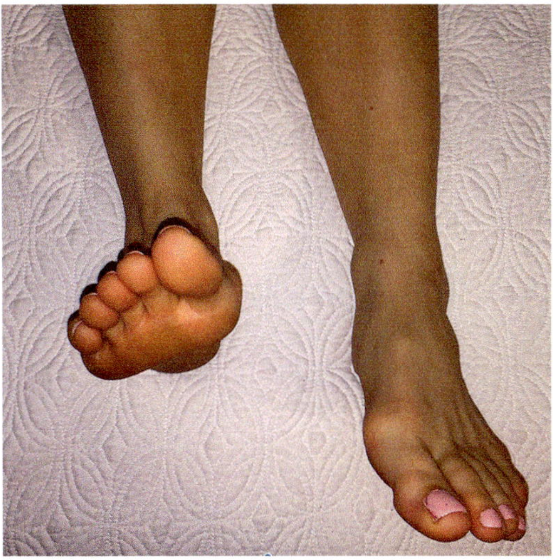

FIGURE 1.18 Left foot drop

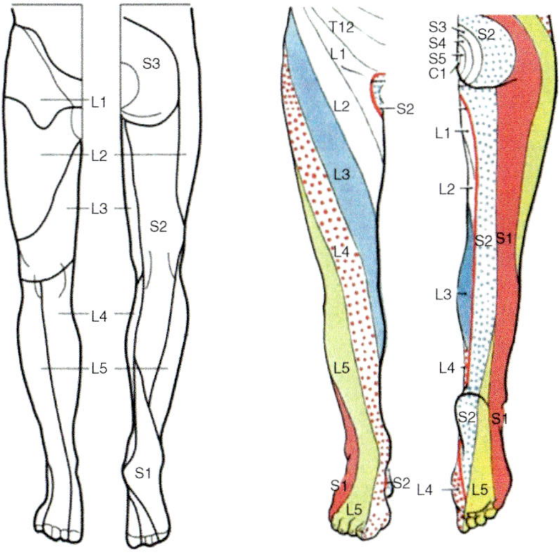

FIGURE 1.19 Dermatomes of lower extremity. (Reprinted from Wong YM. Commentary: differential cerebral response to somatosensory stimulation of an acupuncture point vs. two non-acupuncture points measured with EEG and fMRI. Front Hum Neurosci. 2016;10:63. With permission from Creative Commons License 4.0: https://creativecommons.org/licenses/by/4.0/)

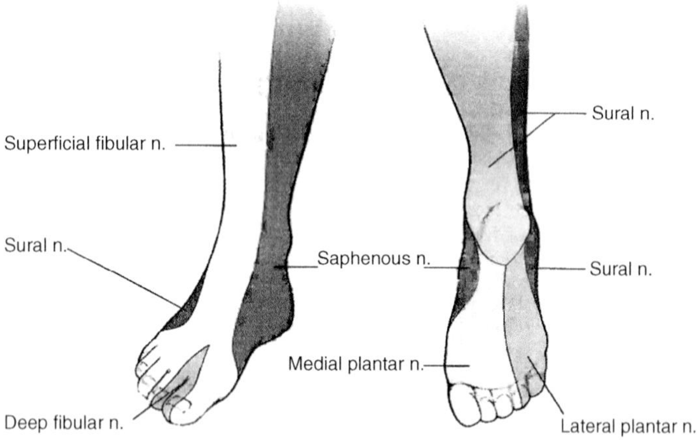

FIGURE 1.20 Cutaneous innervation of lower leg/foot. (Reprinted with permission from White J. USMLE road map: gross anatomy. McGraw-Hill: Appleton & Lange; 2003 ©McGraw-Hill Education)

- Meralgia paresthetica: entrapment of the lateral femoral cutaneous nerve – most commonly occurs as it travels under the inguinal ligament. Patient will experience +/– pain, altered sensation in lateral/superolateral thigh (suspect in obese individuals +/– tight-fitting belts).

  ****Orthopedic Emergency: Knee Dislocation – Beware of "spontaneous" relocation.****

  - Requires disruption of at least three of four major knee ligaments.
  - Ankle/brachial index <0.9 needs vascular consult +/– CT angiogram (See Fig. 1.22).

- Peroneal nerve division dysfunction more common versus tibial division pathology (more superficial anatomic location/greater amount of structural tethering).

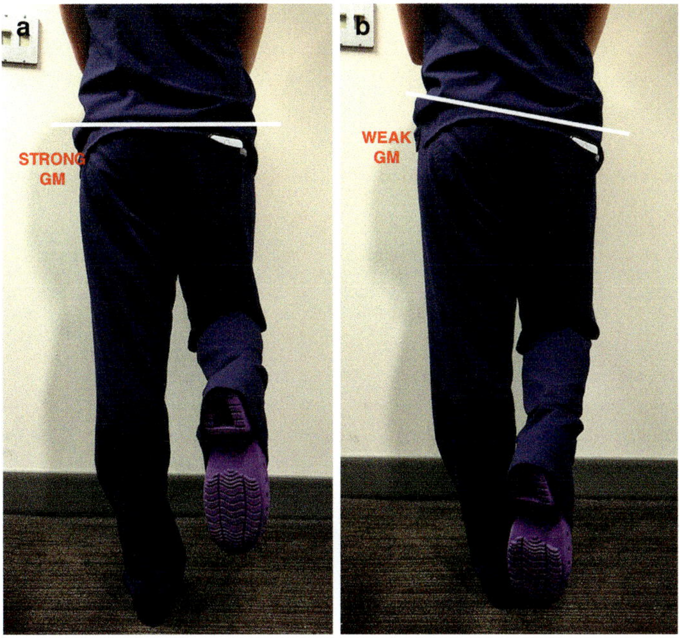

FIGURE 1.21 Superior Gluteal nerve injury: (**a**) Normal pelvic stabilization; (**b**) Weakness of the left-side gluteus medius muscle causes the right-side pelvis/hip to drop

Ottawa Knee Rules

Imaging required if patient fulfills one of the following: >55 years, TTP patella/fibula head, cannot flex knee to 90°, inability to bear weight *immediately and not able to walk four steps in ED.*

- Noncontact/change of direction/deceleration injury, hear "pop," inability to bear weight, joint hemarthrosis-ACL injury until proven otherwise.

- MVC/"dashboard injury" (possible PCL injury): examine for bruising over anterior leg, + posterior drawer testing, posterior tibial sag (Godfrey sign), and/or tibial spine avulsion on imaging.
- TTP medial/lateral joint line, +/– effusion, absence of other findings-consider medial/lateral meniscus injury (See Table 1.3).

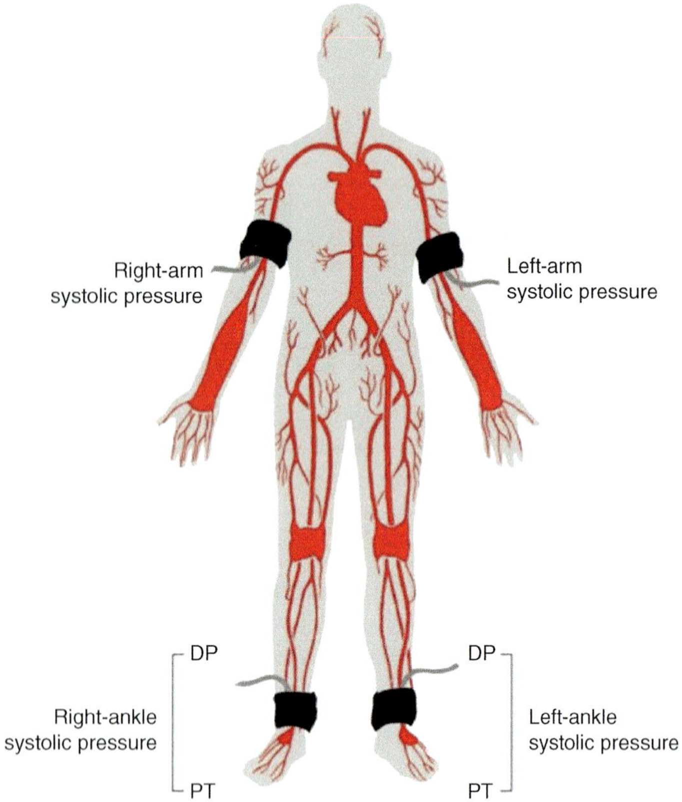

FIGURE 1.22 Ankle-Brachial index cuff locations. (Reprinted from Petznick AM, Shubrook JH. Treatment of specific macrovascular beds in patients with diabetes mellitus. Osteopath Med Prim Care. 2010;4:5. With permission from Creative Commons License 2.0: https://creativecommons.org/licenses/by/2.0/)

TABLE 1.4 Specialized testing: knee

Test	What it's testing	How to do it	Positive test
Valgus/varus stress	MCL/LCL stability	Patient supine, knee placed in 30° of flexion. Stabilize thigh and apply valgus (lateral) and varus (medial) stress to lower leg (See Figs. 1.23 and 1.24).	Laxity with valgus stress = MCL injury. Laxity with varus stress = LCL injury
Lachman	ACL integrity ***(most specific for ACL injury)***	Patient supine, knee placed in 30° flexion. Lateral hand stabilizes femur, while medial hand applies anterior force to tibia (See Fig. 1.25).	Absent/increased endpoint translation versus uninjured side
Anterior/posterior drawer	ACL/PCL ***(most specific for PCL injury)***	Patient supine, knee flexed to 90°, foot flat/stabilized. Apply anterior and posterior force to proximal tibia (See Figs. 1.26 and 1.27).	Absent/increased endpoint translation versus uninjured side
Godfrey's sign Posterior Sag test/ modified Posterior Sag test	PCL injury	Patient supine, knee flexed to 90°, foot either flat or stabilized by hand. Observe whether gravity displaces proximal tibia in relation to distal femur (See Figs. 1.28 and 1.29).	Evidence of posterior tibial displacement with gravity compared to contralateral side

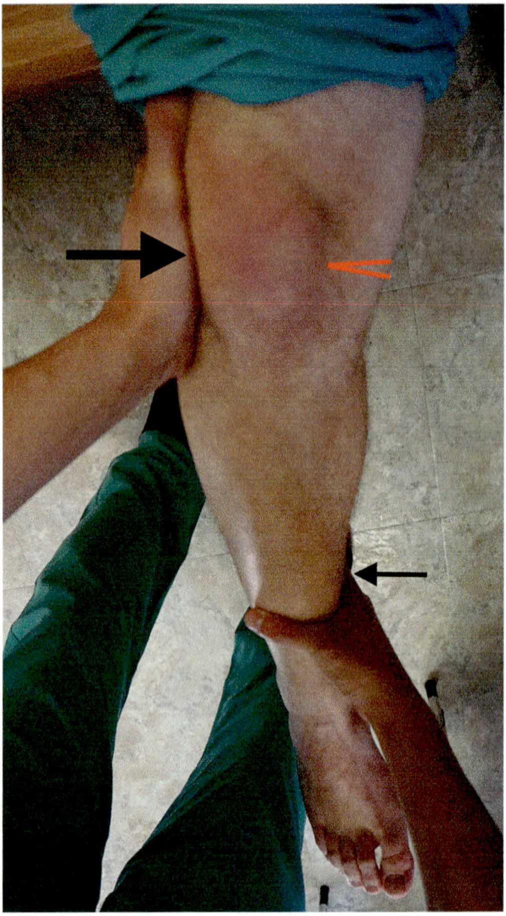

FIGURE 1.23 Valgus stress of the right leg

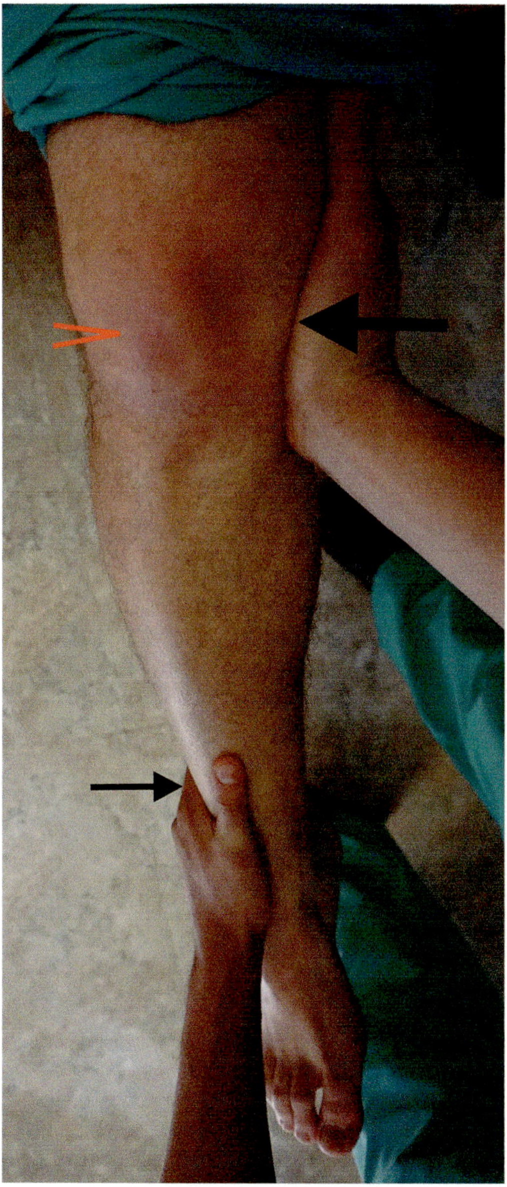

FIGURE 1.24 Varus stress of the right leg

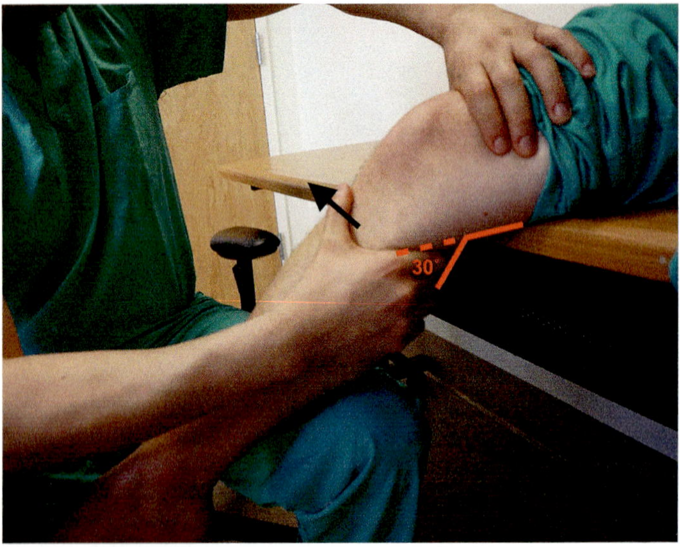

FIGURE 1.25 Lachman test

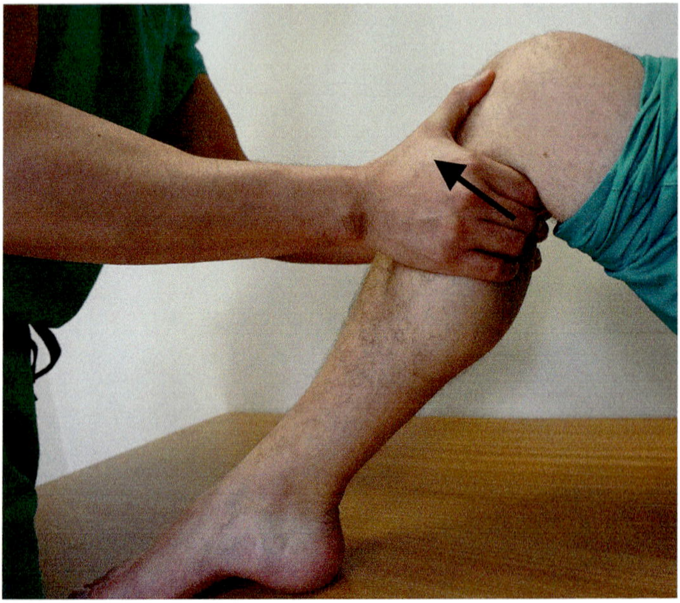

FIGURE 1.26 Anterior drawer test

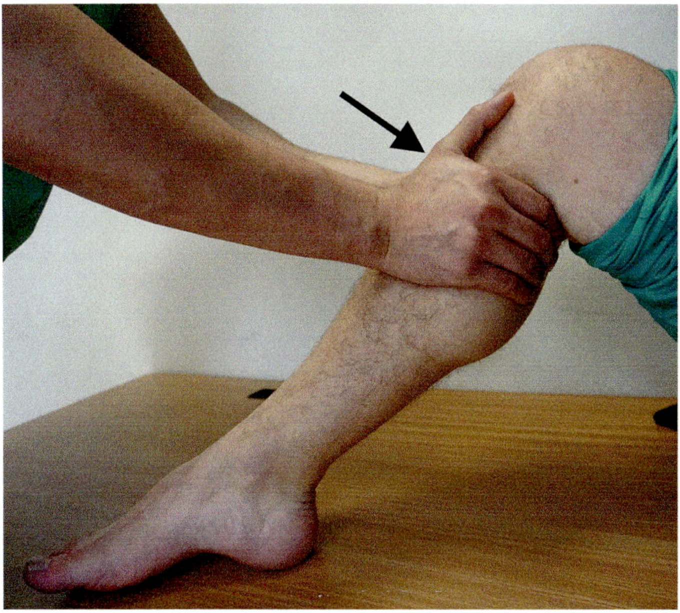

FIGURE 1.27 Posterior drawer

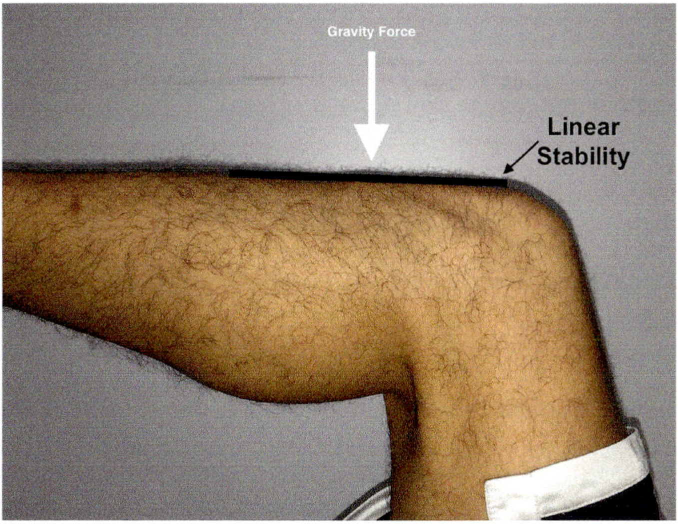

FIGURE 1.28 Negative Godfrey's sign (posterior sag test): no evidence of posterior tibial displacement with gravity (PCL Intact)

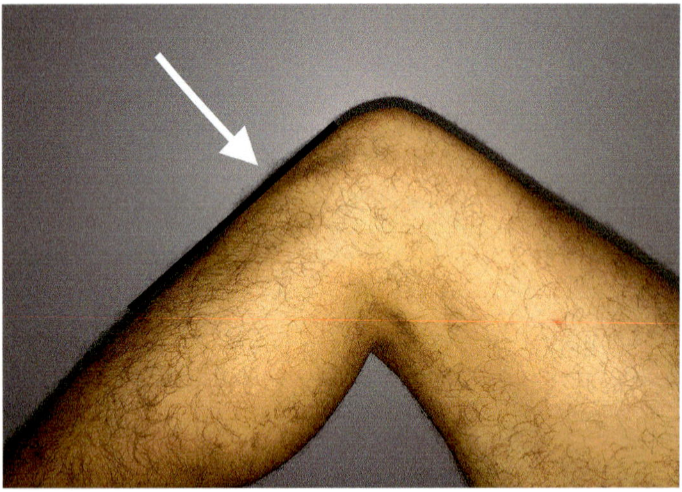

FIGURE 1.29 Posterior sag test modified (PCL Intact)

Ottawa Ankle Rules

Imaging required if:
Pain in malleolar zone and/or any of the following:

- Bony tenderness along distal 6 cm of posterior edge of tibia or tip of medial malleolus
- Bony tenderness along distal 6 cm of posterior edge of fibula or tip of lateral malleolus
- Inability to bear weight *both immediately and in ED for four steps*

Ottawa Foot Rules

Imaging required if:
Pain in the mid-foot zone and any one of the following:

- Bony tenderness at base of fifth metatarsal
- Bony tenderness at the navicular bone
- Inability to bear weight *both immediately and in ED for four steps*

Table 1.5 Specialized testing: ankle

Test	What it's testing	How to do it	Positive test
Anterior drawer	ATFL (anterior talo-fibular) ligament stability	Place foot in slight plantar flexion, stabilize distal leg, and apply an anterior force to the heel (attempt to subluxate talus anteriorly) (See Fig. 1.30).	Weak endpoint/increased laxity versus contralateral side; +/– audible, palpable "clunk" with subluxation/relocation
Talar tilt	ATFL and CFL (calcaneo-fibular) ligament stability	Stabilize medial aspect of distal leg (just proximal to medial malleolus) and apply inversion force to the hindfoot (See Fig. 1.31).	Pain/increased laxity (tilt of lateral aspect of talus) versus contralateral side
External rotation stress	Evaluation of supination-external rotation (SER) injuries. **Deltoid ligament integrity** *(major structural stabilizer of ankle joint)*	1. Manual: knee bent to 90° to relax gastrocnemius muscle; lower leg stabilized and external rotation force applied to foot (See Fig. 1.32). 2. Gravity stress view: position affected extremity with lateral side foot facing down, ankle is dorsiflexed to neutral (See Fig. 1.33).	1. Pain/increased laxity with movement. 2. Imaging demonstrates disrupted syndesmosis and/or medial clear space widening

(continued)

Table 1.5 (continued)

Test	What it's testing	How to do it	Positive test
Squeeze	Syndesmotic injury/"high-ankle" sprain	Squeeze anterior tibia/fibula together just above ankle joint	Pain in ankle and/or distal lower leg secondary to syndesmotic ligament(s) (interosseous membrane) and/or bony disruption
Thompson	Achilles tendon rupture	Patient prone, squeeze calf and observe for active foot plantar flexion (See Fig. 1.34a, b).	Absence of ankle plantar flexion likely indicates tear (intact plantaris/associated foot plantar flexor musculature can sometimes yields false results). Palpable defect usually present just proximal to tendinous insertion; can assist in confirming diagnosis

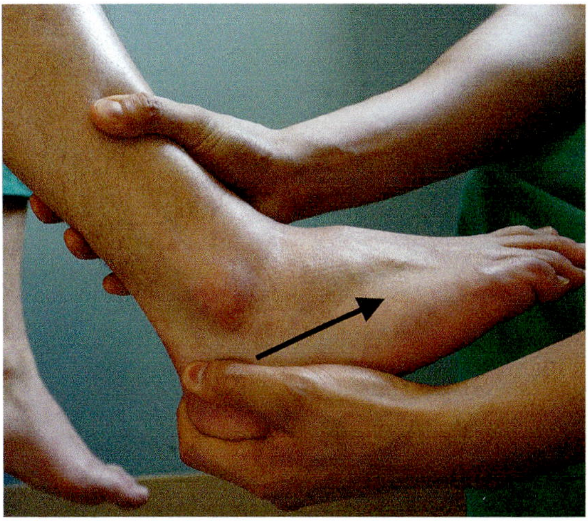

Figure 1.30 Anterior drawer test

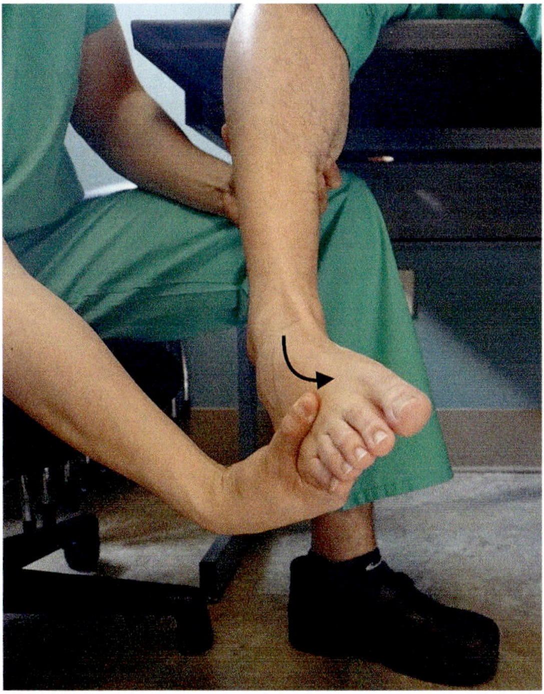

Figure 1.31 Talar tilt test

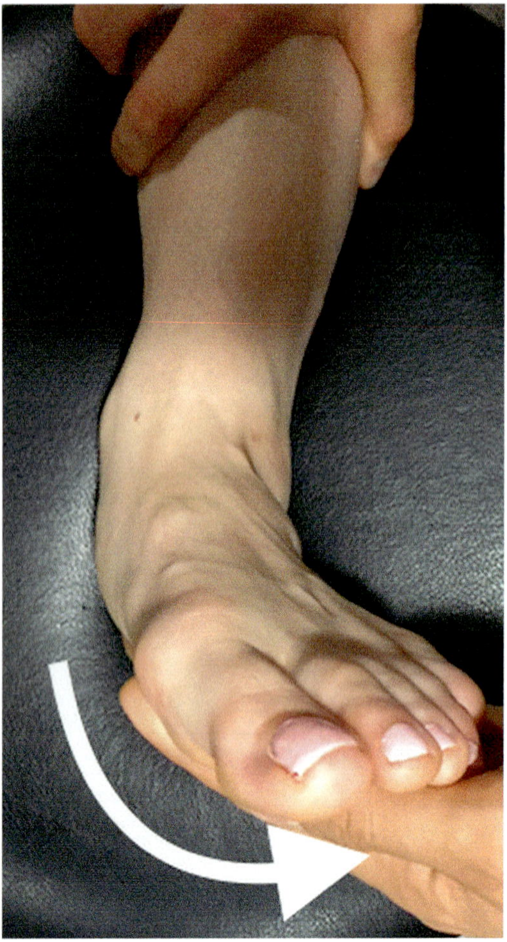

FIGURE 1.32 External rotation manual stress view

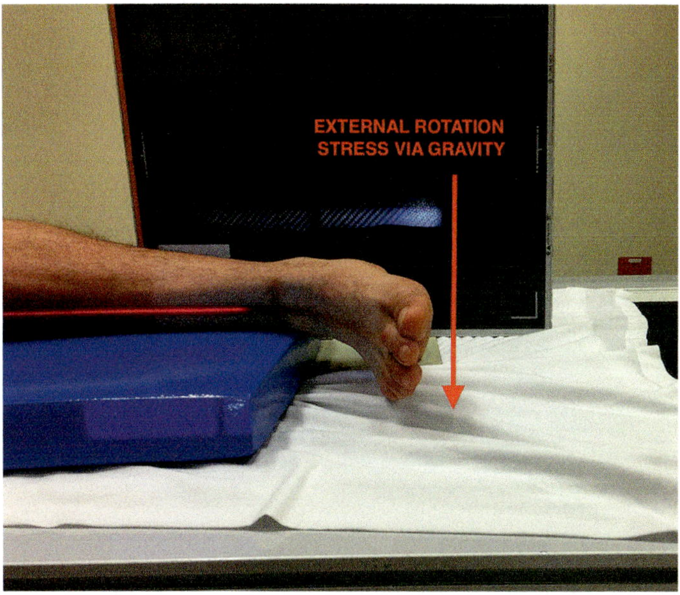

FIGURE 1.33 Gravity stress view

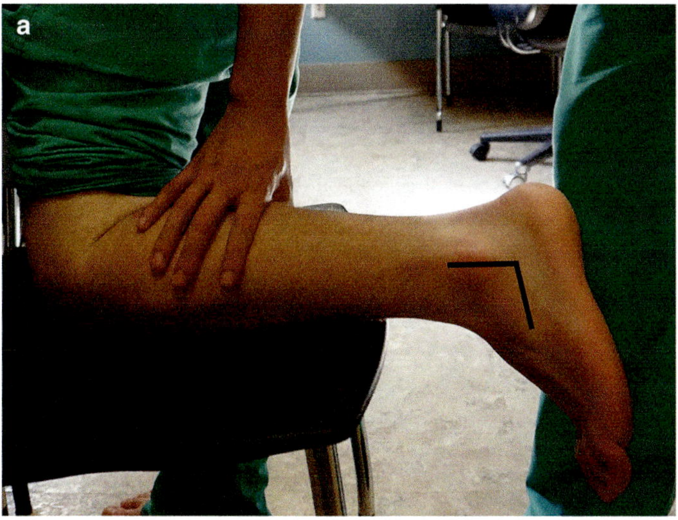

FIGURE 1.34 (**a**, **b**) Thompson squeeze test: patients prone or placed backwards on chair with knee flexed 90 degrees. Negative test indicates active ankle plantarflexion with calf squeeze

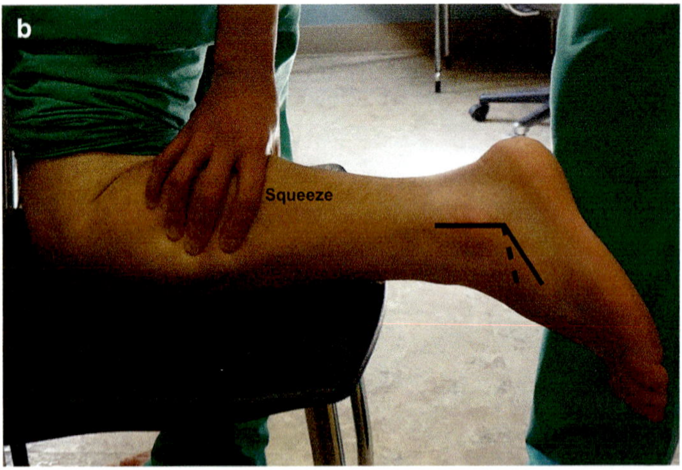

FIGURE 1.34 (continued)

Suggested Reading

1. Asbury AK. Chapter 23. Numbness, tingling, and sensory loss. In: Longo DL, Fauci AS, Kasper DL, Hauser SL, Jameson JL, Loscalzo J, editors. Harrison's principles of internal medicine. 18th ed. New York: McGraw-Hill; 2012. http://www.accessmedicine.com.
2. Brukner P, Khan KM. Acute ankle injuries. In: Clinical sports medicine. 3rd ed. San Francisco: McGraw-Hill; 2006.
3. Burbank K, et al. Chronic shoulder pain: part I. Evaluation & diagnosis. Am Fam Phys. 2008;77(4):453–60.
4. Clegg TE, Roberts CS, Greene JW, Prather BA. Hip dislocations–epidemiology, treatment, and outcomes. Injury. 2010;41(4):329–34.
5. Cosgarea AJ, Jay PR. Posterior cruciate ligament injuries: evaluation and management. J Am Acad Orthop Surg. 2001;9(5):297–307.
6. DeLee JC. Fracture and dislocation of the hip. In: Rockwood CA, Green DP, Bucholz RW, et al., editors. Fractures in adults. 4th ed. Philadelphia: Lippincott Williams & Wilkins; 1996. p. 1756–803.

7. DeLee J, Drez D, Miller MD. DeLee and Drez's orthopaedic sports medicine. 2nd ed. Philadelphia: Elsevier Science; 2002. p. 1038–40.
8. Dodson CC, Cordasco FA. Anterior glenohumeral joint dislocations. Orthop Clin North Am. 2008;39(4):507–18.
9. Eachempati KK, Dua A, Malhotra R, Bhan S, Bera JR. The external rotation method for reduction of acute anterior dislocations and fracture-dislocations of the shoulder. J Bone Joint Surg Am. 2004;86-A(11):2431–4.
10. Gottsegen C, et al. Avulsion fractures of the knee: imaging findings and clinical significance. Radiographics. 2008;28:1755–70.
11. Hillyard RF, Fox J. Sciatic nerve injuries associated with traumatic posterior hip dislocations. Am J Emerg Med. 2003;21(7):545–8.
12. Johnson MW, et al. Acute knee effusions: a systematic approach to diagnosis. Am Fam Phys. 2000;61(8):2391–400.
13. Kothari RU, Dronen SC. Prospective evaluation of the scapular manipulation technique in reducing anterior shoulder dislocations. Ann Emerg Med. 1992;21(11):1349–52.
14. Lee BK, Nam SW. Rupture of posterior cruciate ligament: diagnosis and treatment principles. Knee Surg Relat Res. 2011;23(3):135–41.
15. Magee D. Lower leg, ankle, and foot. In: Orthopedic physical assessment. 4th ed. St. Louis: Elsevier Sciences; 2006.

Chapter 2
Anesthesia

Daniel Purcell, Eric M. Steinberg, and Bryan A. Terry

General

- Means of inducing local, reversible anesthesia with loss of nociception.
- Indications:
  - Fracture/dislocation reduction, laceration repair, I&D/FB removal, assessment of potential block to motion (e.g., evaluation of elbow ROM in radial head/neck fracture)
  - Pain control: pre-/post-procedure (e.g., shoulder dislocation reduction), hip fracture (e.g., femoral nerve block), knee osteoarthritis (e.g., steroid injection)
  - Diagnostic/therapeutic: assessment of injury (e.g., quadricep/patellar tendon tear +/– gravity), carpal tunnel/"trigger finger" (e.g., steroid injection), sub-

D. Purcell (✉)
Emergency Department, New York University Langone Medical Center Brooklyn, New York, NY, USA
e-mail: daniel.purcell@nyumc.org

E. M. Steinberg
Department of Emergency Medicine, Mount Sinai Beth Israel, New York, NY, USA

B. A. Terry
The Brooklyn Hospital Center, Brooklyn, NY, USA

D. Purcell et al. (eds.), *Emergency Orthopedics Handbook*,
https://doi.org/10.1007/978-3-030-00707-2_2

acromial impingement (e.g., Neer's sign), arthrocentesis (e.g., RA/gout versus septic arthritis)

- Advantages of nerve blocks over local infiltration:
  - Local infiltration may cause unwanted tissue swelling, increased tissue tension, and impair wound closure.
  - Local infiltration may also cause increased pressure within confined spaces (fingers, toes, etc.) leading to an increased risk of compartment syndrome.

- Always use sterile technique and discard sharps in appropriate containers when task is completed.
- Perform and document full neurovascular exam *prior* to anesthetic block placement.
- Use larger gauge (e.g., 18 G) needles to draw up anesthetic and smaller gauge needles (e.g., 25 G) for delivery; smaller gauges lower the potential incidence of nerve damage, can minimize pain, and possibly diminish patient anxiety/apprehension.
- Before injecting anesthetic, always aspirate to confirm needle has not entered a vascular structure (artery/vein) and unimpeded flow is obtained (decreased risk of having violated a soft-tissue structure (e.g., tendon).
- Most commonly used regional anesthetics.
  - ***Lidocaine/Xylocaine (1–2%):*** alters signal conduction in neurons by blocking fast voltage-gated sodium channels responsible for signal propagation; thus it does not merely prevent pain signal propagation, but also eliminates initial generation.
  - ***Toxic dose without epinephrine is 4 mg/kg and 7mg/kg with epinephrine***.
  - When implemented with epinephrine, it induces vasoconstriction to generate higher local tissue concentrations, resulting in longer duration of blockade.
  - Rapid onset (<2 min), high tissue penetration.
  - Peak effect may take ~20–30 min.
  - Duration of action ~1–2 hrs.
  - *Note*: use of epinephrine was previously considered contraindicated in ears, nose, penis, fingers, and toes as they are supplied by "terminal" vessels with a theoretical potential for vasospasm and associated

infarction/necrosis; this belief is currently debated in the literature.

- ***Bupivacaine/Marcaine (0.25–0.5%):*** binds to intracellular portion of sodium channels and blocks sodium influx into nerve cells preventing depolarization.
- ***Toxic dose without epinephrine is 2 mg/kg and 3 mg/kg with epinephrine***.
- Slower onset (~5 min), longer lasting (~2–4 hrs).
- Some prefer lidocaine/bupivicaine combinations; however, studies are inconclusive regarding reported advantages.
- Overall adverse effects depend on anesthetic agent implemented, method and site of administration.
- Potential side effects: localized prolonged anesthesia/paresthesias, hematoma formation, excessive pressure within a confined cavity, severing of nerves and/or surrounding soft tissue structures during injection.
- Systemic reactions such as depressed/altered CNS syndromes (nystagmus, dizziness and seizures), allergic reactions, vasovagal episodes and cyanosis can also occur.
- Anesthetic penetration is limited in infected tissue (e.g., abscess) and may require higher doses to achieve desired concentration.
- Relative contraindications: infection/associated skin changes overlying potential injection site, anesthetic allergy, existing neurologic injury, etc.

Regional Blocks

Upper Extremity

A. ***Digital nerve block:***

- There are two main digital nerves, accompanied by digital vessels on the ventrolateral aspects of each finger/toe, while two smaller dorsal digital nerves navigate the dorsolateral aspect (See Figs. 2.1, 2.2 and 2.3).

– Utilization: fracture/dislocation, laceration repair, felon/paronychia drainage, subungual hematoma trephination, etc.
Prior to implementation: assess capillary refill, radial/ulnar border sensation, muscle function +/– 2-point discrimination

Technique:

- ***Positioning:***
  - Stabilize wrist in prone (palm down) position.
  - Sterile surgical field should be prepared as close as possible to the MCP joint. Generally performed on dorsal aspect because it is considered less painful and also affords potential for greater anesthesia.
  - Direct the needle perpendicular on each side of the MCPJ web space, and inject ~1 ml of anesthetic to reach the volar digital nerve and an additional ~1 ml while withdrawing to anesthetize the dorsal digital nerve.
- ***Potential modifications:***

  (a) ***"Fan" technique:*** needle inserted down to the bone, midway between palmar/dorsal surfaces of the digit,

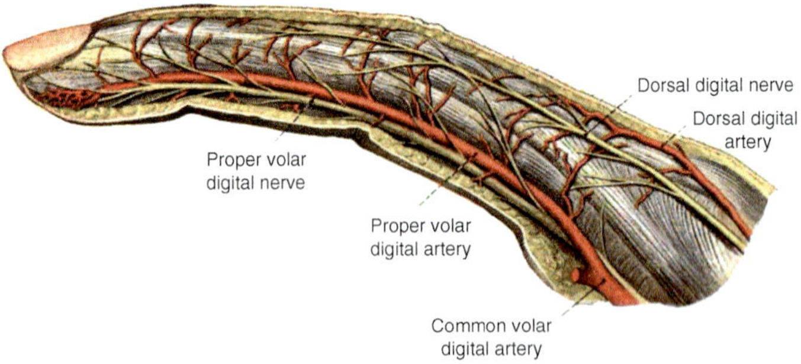

FIGURE 2.1 Digital nerve anatomy. (Reprinted from Wikipedia https://commons.wikimedia.org/wiki/File:Sobo_1909_723.png)

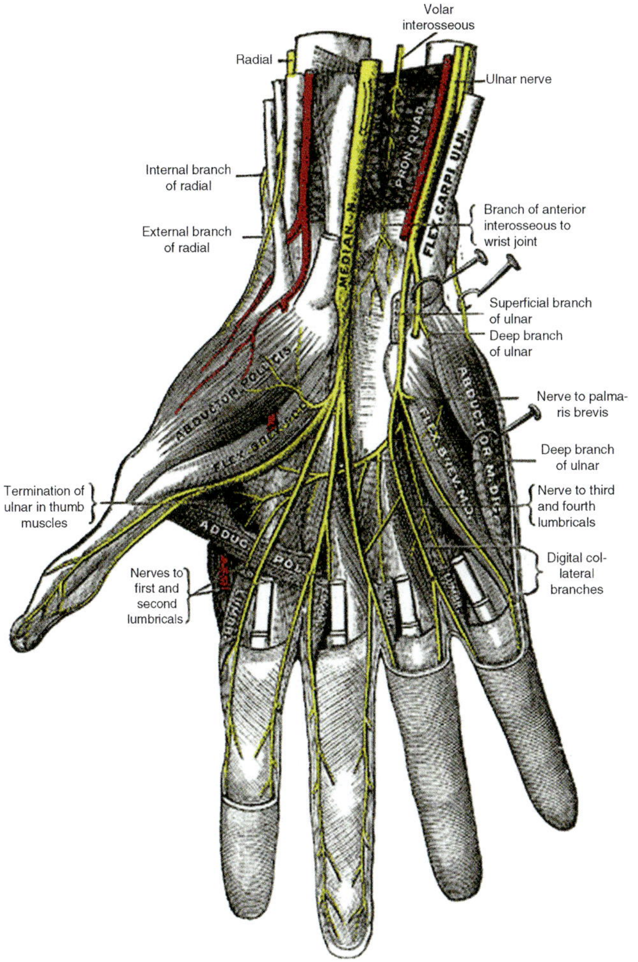

FIGURE 2.2 Hand nerve anatomy: volar branches correspond to dermatomal distribution. (Reprinted from: https://commons.wikimedia.org/wiki/Gray%27s_Anatomy_plates#/media/File:Gray817.png)

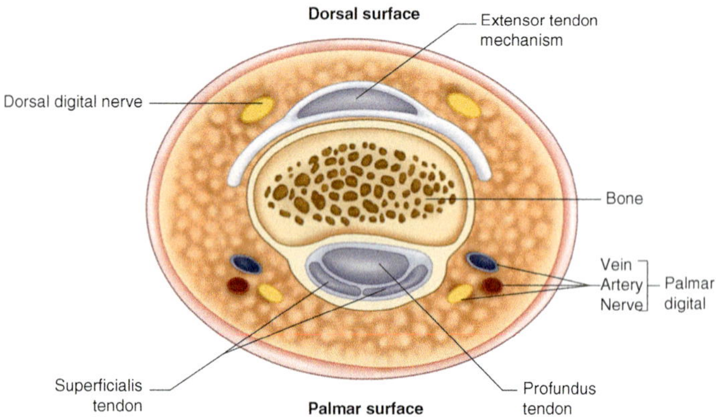

FIGURE 2.3 Cross section of finger

~1–2 cm distal to the web space. Anesthetic is delivered initially with the needle perpendicular to the digit and then angled slightly toward the palmar and dorsal surfaces as additional solution is injected.

(b) ***"Ring" block:*** involves insertion of needle at ventrolateral aspect of the digit, which is then advanced medially.

**Allow ~5 min for full anesthesia with lidocaine and ~15 min with bupivacaine. If complete anesthesia is not obtained, additional anesthetic and/or modification of technique should be considered (See Figs. 2.4, 2.5 and 2.6).

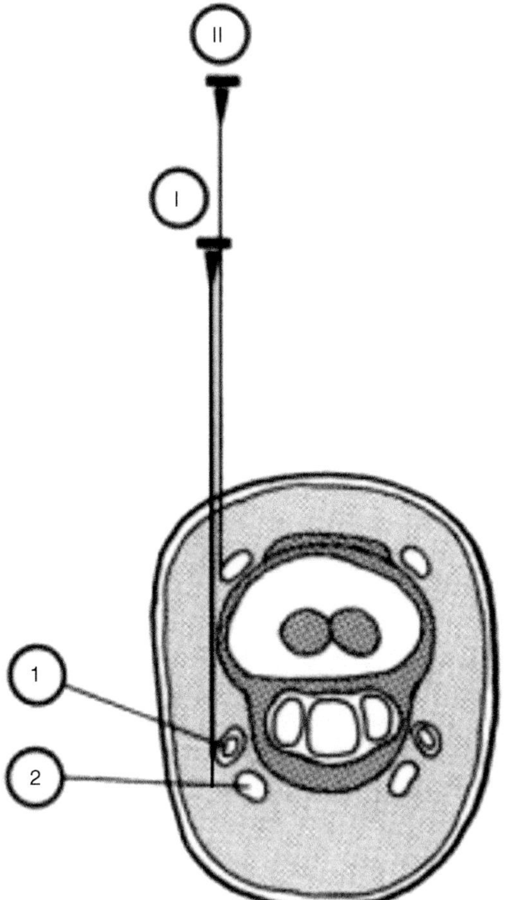

FIGURE 2.4 Digital block: anatomy and insertion sites (I. needle on palmar digital nerve, II. (1) needle on dorsal digital nerve, (1) common palmar artery, (2) dorsal branch of ulnar nerve). (Reprinted from Raj P, Nolte H, Stanton-Hicks M. Upper-extremity blocks. In: Illustrated manual of regional anesthesia. Berlin/Heidelberg: Springer; 1988. p. 35–46. With permission from Springer Nature)

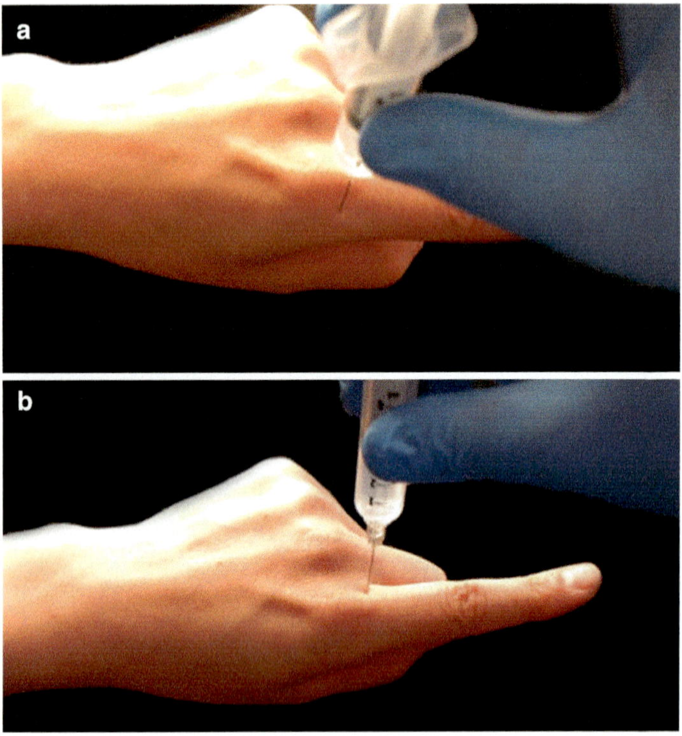

FIGURE 2.5 Digital block: (**a**) lateral and (**b**) medial insertions

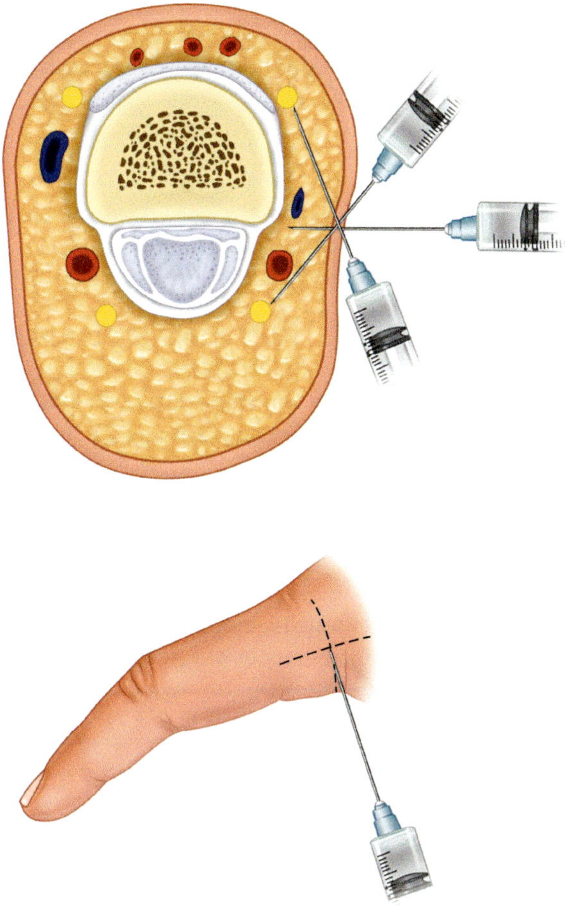

FIGURE 2.6 "Fan" technique

B. ***Flexor tendon sheath block (transthecal block):*** addition/alternative to the digital nerve block.

- Utilizes FTS to anesthetize the digital nerves.
- Advantage is provision of anesthesia to the entire digit with single injection.

Technique:

- ***Positioning:***
  - Place hand/wrist in supine (palm up) position.
  - Have patient flex their finger to better visualize the underlying tendon, and also identify the distal palmar crease (intended injection site is just distal to this landmark).
  - Hold needle at 45° angle to this landmark, and direct it distally; once "pop" is felt/heard, FTS has been penetrated.
  - Aspirate and inject ~2–3 ml of anesthetic.
    ****Intra-neural injection can generate significant discomfort; if encountered, withdraw needle slightly before administration****
  - ***Modified version:*** identify metacarpal crease (volar base of finger), configure needle perpendicular, and insert until the bone is encountered; aspirate/inject as needle is slowly withdrawn (See Fig. 2.7).

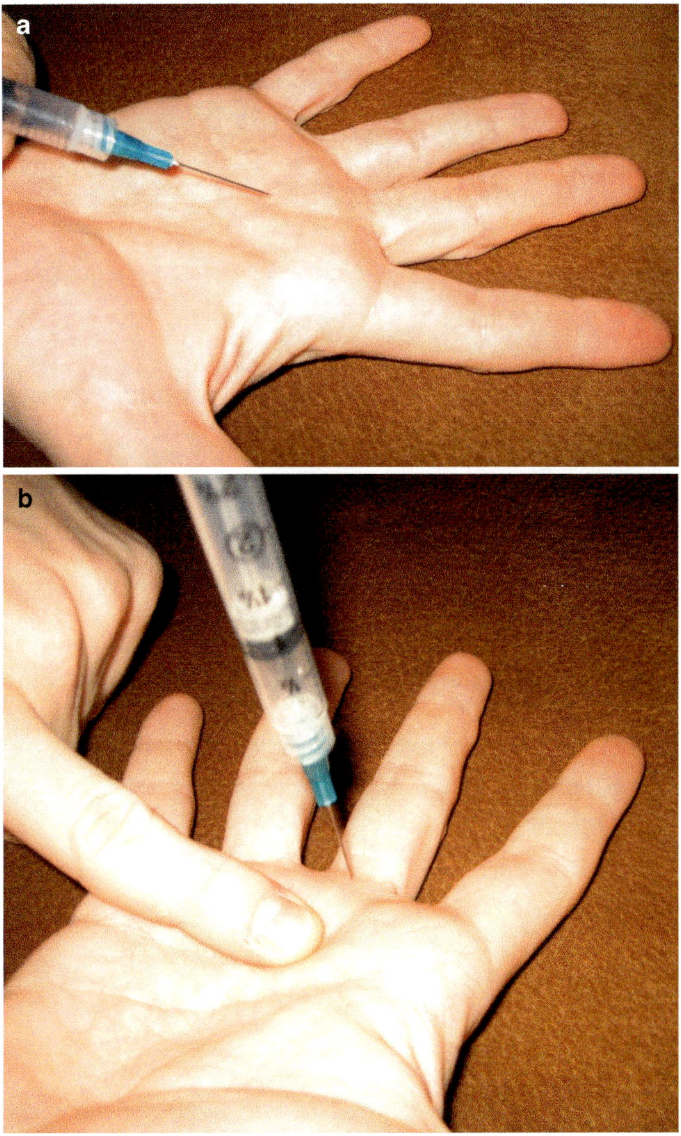

FIGURE 2.7 Transthecal block: (**a**) traditional approach and (**b**) modified approach. (**a**, **b**: Images reprinted with permission from Medscape Drugs & Diseases (http://emedicine.medscape.com/), 2016, available at: http://emedicine.medscape.com/article/80887-overview)

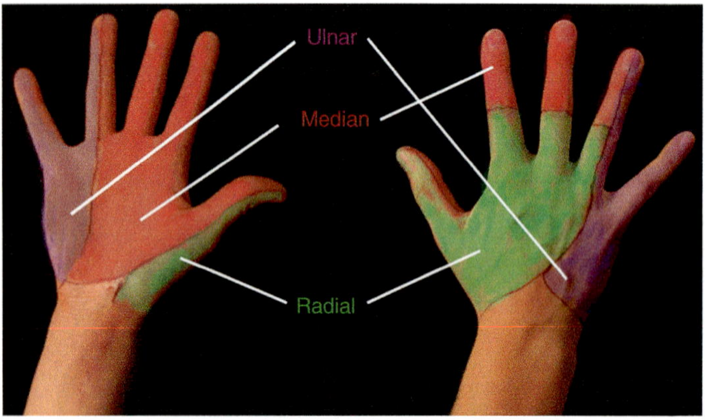

Figure 2.8 Cutaneous hand sensation. (Adapted from Ailes D, Waseem M. Regional anesthesia (nerve blocks). In: Ganti L, editors. Atlas of emergency medicine procedures. New York: Springer; 2016. p. 511–23. With permission from Springer Nature)

C. ***Wrist blocks*** (See Fig. 2.8):

1. ***Median nerve block:***

   - Provides nociception to volar aspect of lateral 3.5 digits (thumb, index, middle, and radial aspect of ring finger) and dorsal aspect of index, middle, and radial half of ring finger distal to PIPJ.

Technique:

- ***Positioning:***
  - Supinate forearm (palm up position); place small roll under wrist to slightly extend wrist.
  - Have patient flex wrist and oppose thumb and little finger to visualize palmaris longus tendon (if present).
  - Insert needle at 45° angle just lateral this region, ~2 cm proximal to wrist flexion crease.
    If individual lacks PL tendon, initiate ~5 mm ulnar (medial) to the FCR tendon or midpoint of wrist just proximal to wrist crease
  - Needle first pierces flexor retinaculum, and then a lack of resistance is encountered; aspirate and inject ~3–5 cc anesthetic.

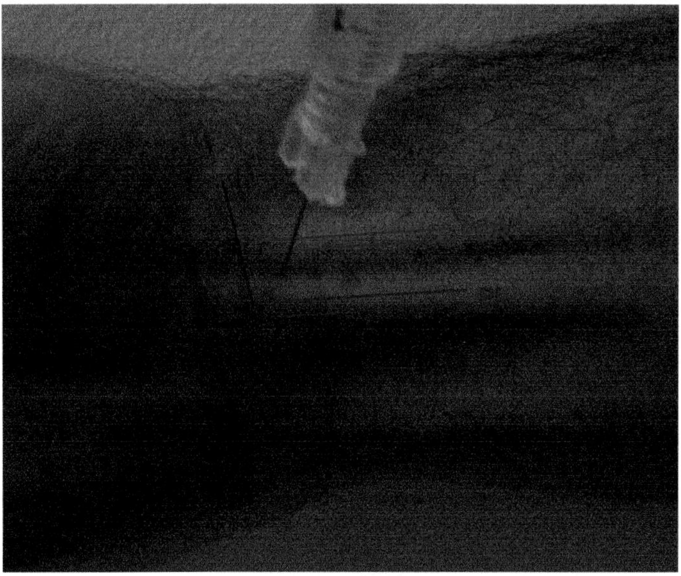

FIGURE 2.9 Flexor tendon anatomy/injection site. (Image reprinted with permission from Medscape Drugs & Diseases (http://emedicine.medscape.com/), 2016, available at: http://emedicine.medscape.com/article/1369028-overview)

  - If pain/paresthesias elicited, withdraw needle slightly to avoid intraneural injection.
    Palmar branch of median nerve is more superficial, thus also infiltrate with ~2 cc anesthetic as needle withdrawn (See Fig. 2.9).

2. ***Radial nerve block:***

   - Provides anesthesia to dorsal thumb web space and associated dorsolateral aspect of hand proximal to DIPJ of index, middle +/– medial aspect of the ring finger (superficial branch radial nerve).

Technique:

- ***Positioning:***

  - Pronate forearm (palm down position) and locate radial styloid and "anatomic snuffbox."

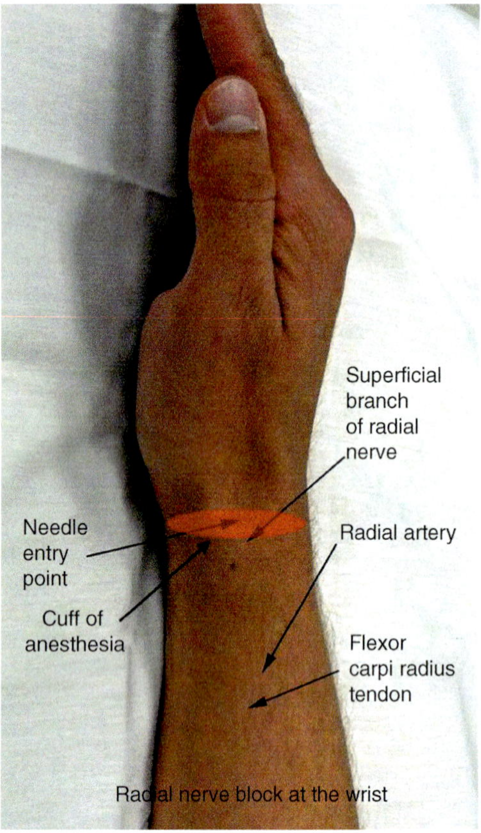

FIGURE 2.10 Radial wrist landmarks: cuff of anesthesia in red. (Image reprinted with permission from Medscape Drugs & Diseases (http://emedicine.medscape.com/), 2016, available at: http://emedicine.medscape.com/article/1361691-overview)

– Inject skin wheal proximal to "snuffbox," just distal to radial styloid, aiming medially toward middle of dorsal wrist; inject another ~3–5 cc aiming laterally in "cuff-like" fashion.

  Radial artery traverses the "snuffbox"; thus be sure to aspirate prior to injection (See Figs. 2.10, 2.11 and 2.12).

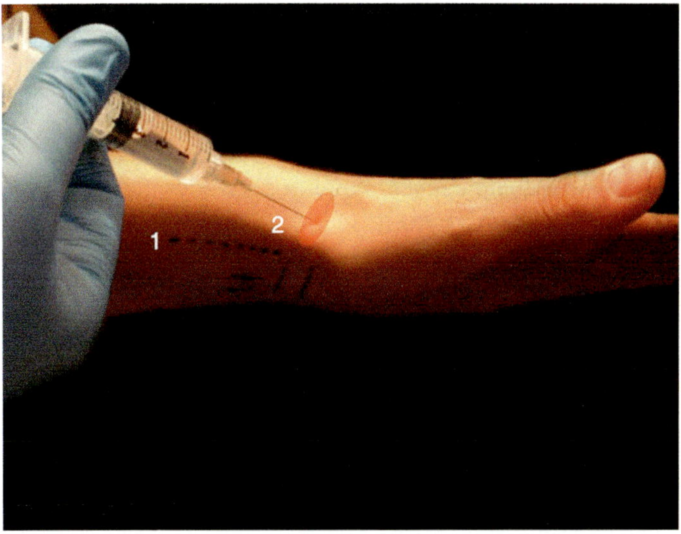

FIGURE 2.11 Radial nerve block at the wrist, lateral view: (1) radial artery, (2) anatomical snuffbox, with injection area shaded

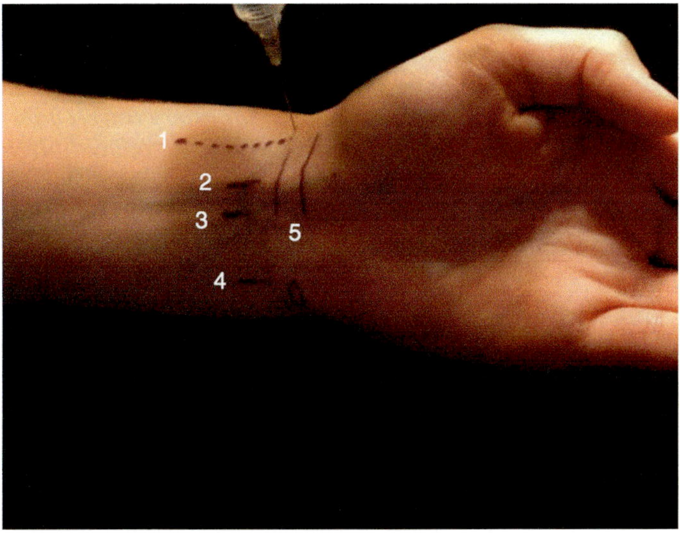

FIGURE 2.12 Radial nerve block at the wrist, anterior view: (1) radial artery, (2) flexor carpi radialis tendon, (3) palmaris longus tendon, (4) ulnar artery, (5) proximal and distal wrist creases

3. ***Ulnar nerve block:***

  - Provides anesthesia to medial 1.5 digits (ulnar aspect of ring finger and entire little finger). There are two branches that comprise its sensory function that must be accounted for:
    - ***Palmar branch:*** supplies cutaneous innervation to the anterior skin and nails.
    - ***Dorsal sensory branch:*** supplies cutaneous innervation to the posterior skin (except the nail beds).

Technique:

- ***Positioning:***
  - ***Palmar branch:*** supinate patient forearm (palm up position); place small roll under wrist to slightly extend wrist.
  - ***Dorsal sensory branch:*** pronate patient forearm (hand down position).

- ***Palmar branch:*** have patient make fist and attempt to visualize FCU tendon. Orient needle horizontally ~5 cm proximal to wrist crease, and advance it beneath the tendon to depth of ~5–10 mm past the tendon edge. *****Aspirate prior to injection as ulnar artery travels adjacent to the nerve (artery is more superficial and radial)*****
- ***Dorsal sensory branch:*** pass needle subcutaneously, and direct dorsally toward base of fifth metacarpal at the level of the ulnar styloid (See Figs. 2.13 and 2.14).

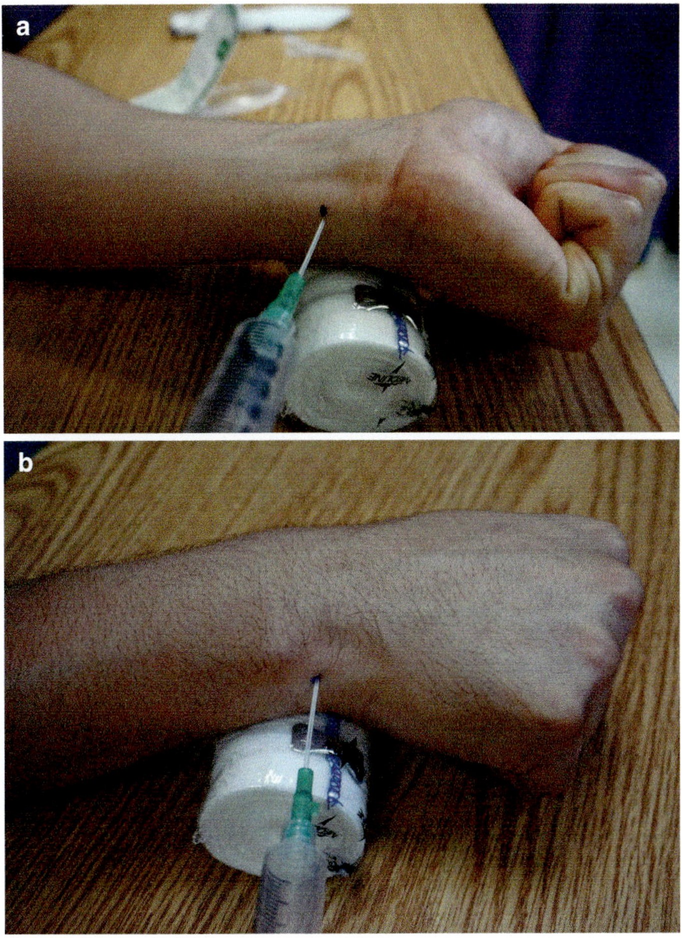

FIGURE 2.13 Ulnar nerve block: (**a**) needle placement for palmar branch and (**b**) needle placement for dorsal branch

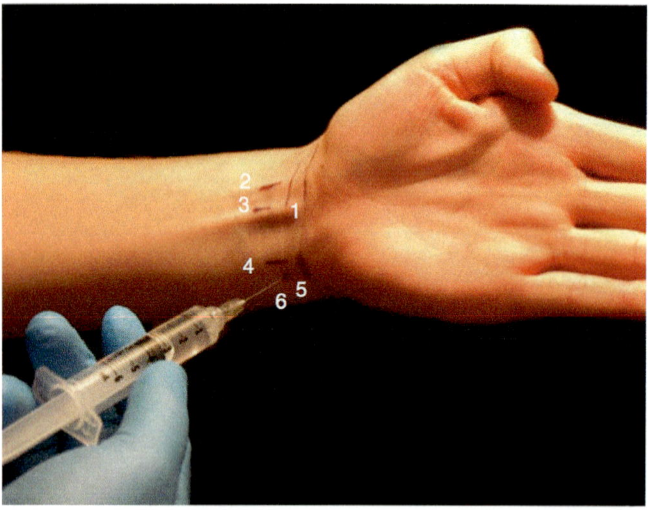

FIGURE 2.14 Ulnar nerve block for palmar branch, anterior approach: (1) proximal and distal wrist creases, (2) flexor carpi radialis tendon, (3) palmaris longus tendon, (4) ulnar artery, (5) styloid process, (6) flexor carpi ulnaris

Lower Extremity *(See Fig. 2.15)*

Complete foot/ankle nociception requires anesthesia of five individual nerves classified according to anatomic location: (See Figs. 2.16–2.19)

- ***Anterior ankle block:*** superficial/deep peroneal and saphenous nerves.
- ***Posterior ankle block:*** tibial and sural nerves.

Anterior Block

A. ***Superficial peroneal nerve:***

- Provides anesthesia to dorsum of foot (See Fig. 2.20).

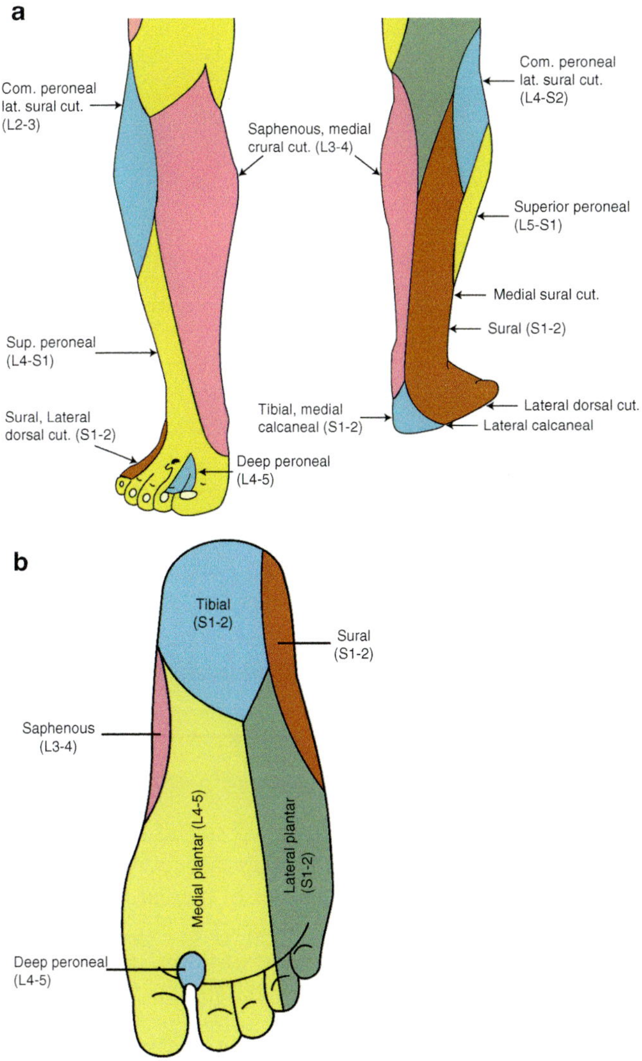

FIGURE 2.15 Dermatome distribution: (**a**) lower extremity and (**b**) dorsum of foot (Note: majority of sole innervated by tibial nerve and it's medial and lateral plantar branches). (**a**: Adapted from: https://commons.wikimedia.org/wiki/File:Gray826and831.svg. **b**: Adapted from: https://commons.wikimedia.org/wiki/File:Gray834.svg)

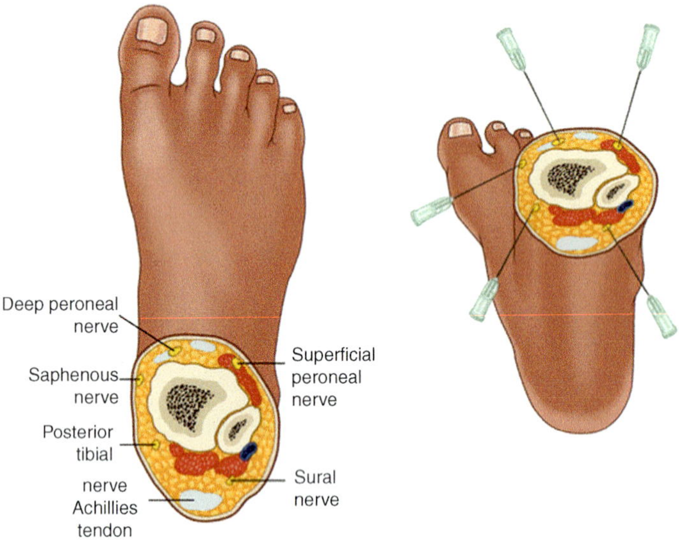

FIGURE 2.16 Ankle anatomy and insertion points. (Reprinted from Tom M, Halaszynski TM. Peripheral nerve blocks. In: Sikka P, Beaman S, Street J, editors. Basic clinical anesthesia. New York: Springer; 2015. p. 233–51. With permission from Springer Nature)

Technique:

- ***Positioning:***
  - Supine with foot in neutral versus internal rotation.
  - Draw line from distal anterior aspect of lateral malleolus to the anterior border of medial malleolus.
  - Inject ~5–10 cc starting anterior to lateral malleolus, and continue in transverse fashion until reaching medial malleolus (See Fig. 2.21).

B. ***Deep peroneal nerve:***

- Provides anesthesia to web space between first and second toes.

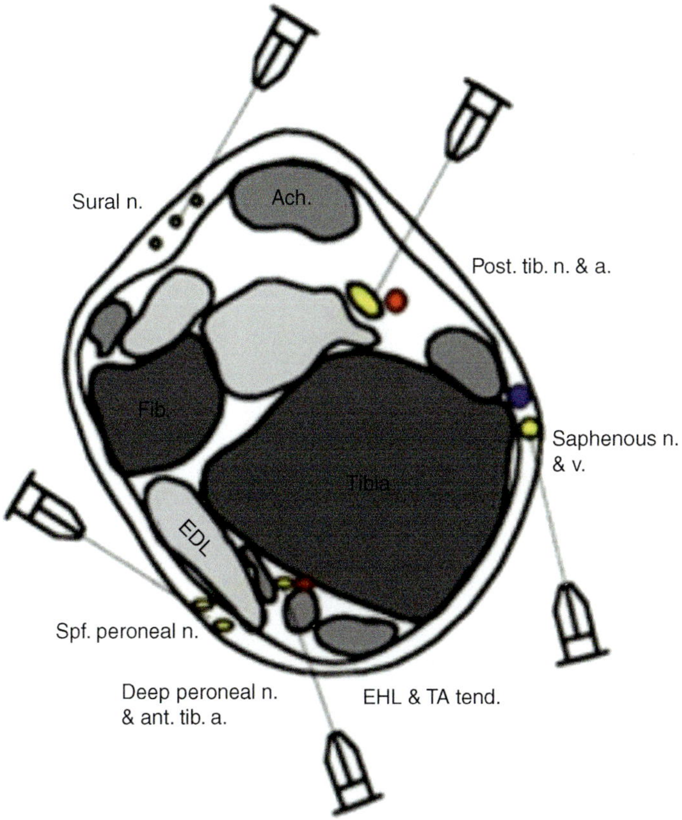

Figure 2.17 Cross-sectional view of five insertion points for ankle block. (Reprinted from Conrad III ES, Delonnay PB, Halaszynski TM. Regional anesthesia for foot and ankle aurgery. In: Scuderi GR, Tria AJ, editors. Minimally invasive surgery in orthopedics. Switzerland: Springer International Publishing; 2015. p. 1–9. With permission from Springer Nature)

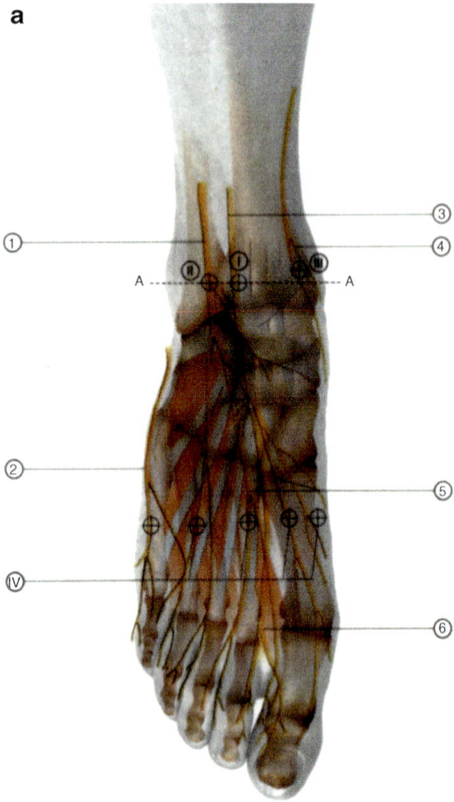

FIGURE 2.18 Ankle block anatomy and insertion points: (**a**) anterior block (I. injection site for deep peroneal nerve block; II. injection site for superficial peroneal nerve block; III. injection site for saphenous nerve block; IV. injection site for metatarsal nerve block; A---A line. Line along which infiltration is carried out; (1) superficial peroneal nerve; (2) sural nerve; (3) deep peroneal nerve; (4) saphenous nerve; (5) medial and lateral terminal branches of peroneal nerve; (6) dorsal digital nerves); (**b**) posterior block (I. injection site for tibial nerve block; II. injection site for sural nerve block; A---A line. Line along which infiltration is carried out; (1) tibial nerve alongside posterior tibial artery; (2) medial malleolus; (3) flexor retinaculum; (4) sural nerve; (5) lateral malleolus). (**a**, **b**: Reprinted from Raj P, Nolte H, Stanton-Hicks M. Anterior ankle and metatarsal block. In: Illustrated manual of regional anesthesia. Berlin/Heidelberg: Springer; 1988. p. 217–24. With permission from Springer Nature)

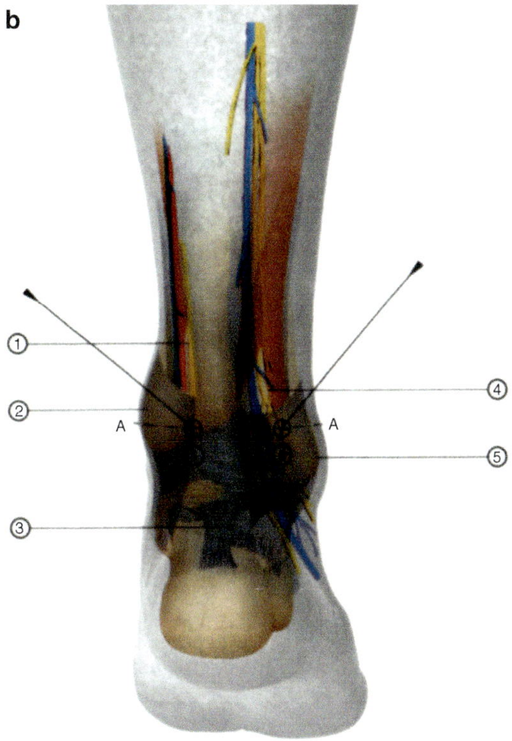

FIGURE 2.18 (continued)

Technique:

- ***Positioning:***
  - Stabilize ankle/foot in neutral position.
  - Identify nerve course between extensor hallucis longus (EHL) and tibialis anterior (TA) tendons at malleoli level. ***Ankle dorsiflexion can help identify TA tendon, while great toe extension can help identify EHL****
  - Insert needle until extensor retinaculum is penetrated; inject ~5 cc superficial to the periosteum, lateral to EHL tendon. Withdraw slightly, and fan 30° medial and lateral to maximize block.

    Aspirate prior to injection to confirm anterior tibial/dorsalis pedis artery, immediately medial, has not been penetrated* (See Fig. 2.22)

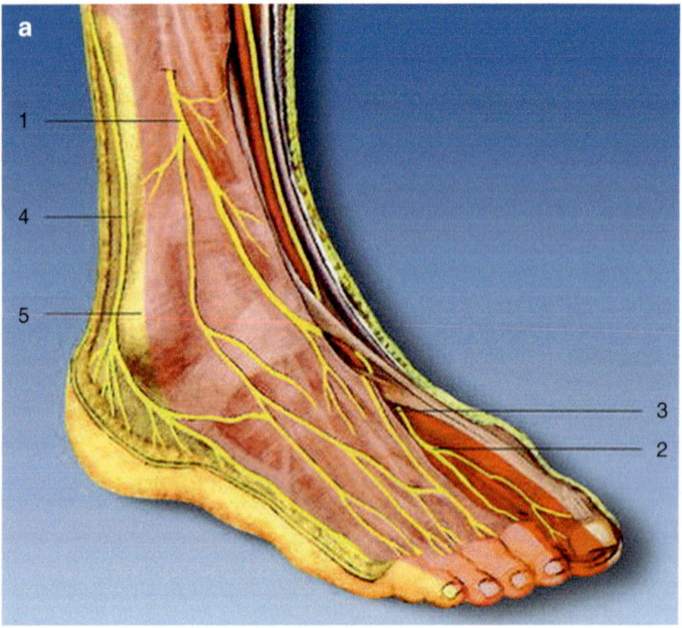

FIGURE 2.19 Ankle block areas of innervation: (**a**) lateral view (1) superficial peroneal nerve, (2) deep peroneal nerve, (3) dorsalis pedis artery, (4) sural nerve, (5) sural nerve distribution); (**b**) dorsal view (1) superficial peroneal nerve, (2) deep peroneal nerve, (3) saphenous nerve, (4) sural nerve, (5) sural nerve distribution). (**a**, **b**: Reprinted from Peng PWH. Peripheral nerve block in the ankle joint region. In: Regional nerve blocks in anesthesia and pain therapy. Cham: Springer; 2015. p. 863–74. With permission from Springer Nature)

C. ***Saphenous nerve:***

- Provides anesthesia to medial aspect of ankle (See Fig. 2.23).

Technique:

- ***Positioning:***
  - Foot in neutral position.
  - Inject ~5 cc anesthetic ~1.5 cm superior and anterior to medial malleolus (just medial to tibialis anterior tendon).

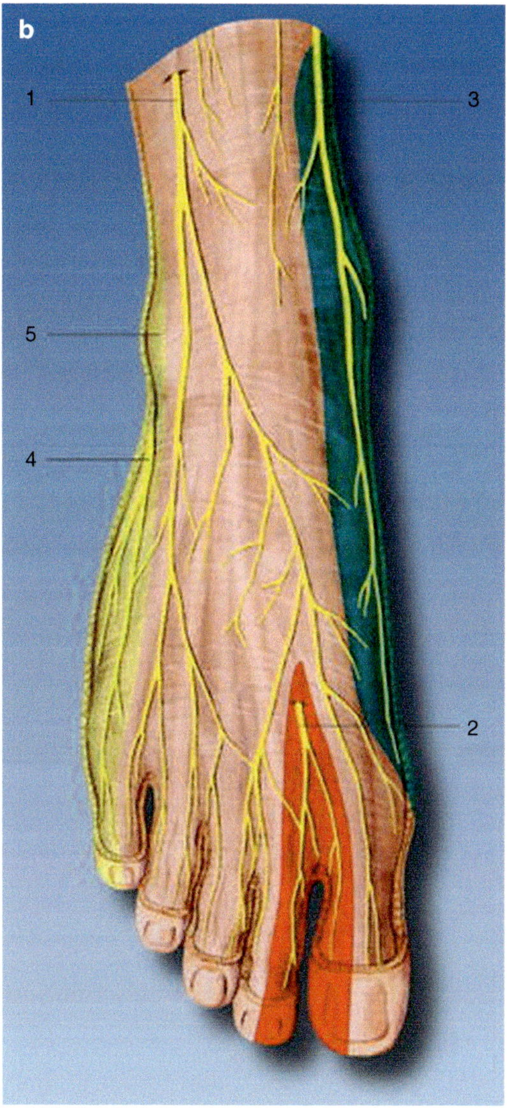

FIGURE 2.19 (continued)

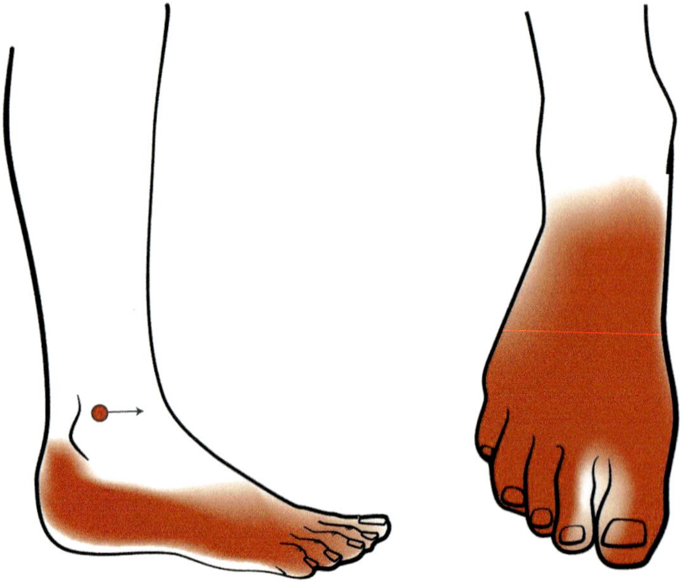

FIGURE 2.20 Superficial peroneal nerve block. (Image reprinted with permission from Medscape Drugs & Diseases (http://emedicine.medscape.com/), Ankle Block, 2017, available at: https://emedicine.medscape.com/article/1999563-overview)

– Allows for penetration of sulcus between tibialis anterior tendon and anterior bony tibial ridge; needle trajectory should be directed toward the lateral malleolus (See Fig. 2.24).

Posterior Block

A. ***Tibial nerve:***

- Provides anesthesia to plantar aspect of foot through the medial and lateral plantar nerves.
  - ***Medial plantar nerve:*** provides cutaneous innervation to medial sole and medial 3.5 toes (including nail beds).
  - ***Lateral plantar nerve:*** provides cutaneous innervation to lateral sole and lateral 1.5 toes (See Fig. 2.25).

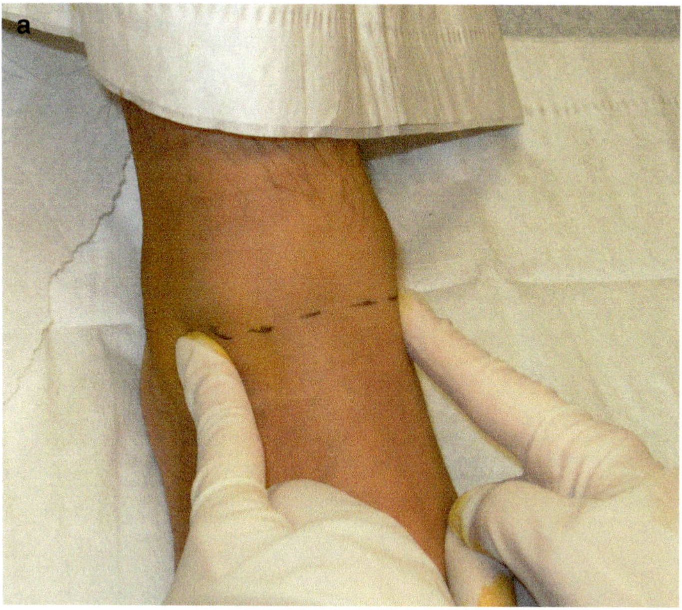

FIGURE 2.21 (**a**, **b**) Superficial peroneal nerve block technique. (**a**, **b**: Images reprinted with permission from Medscape Drugs & Diseases (http://emedicine.medscape.com/), 2016, available at: http://emedicine.medscape.com/article/83218-overview)

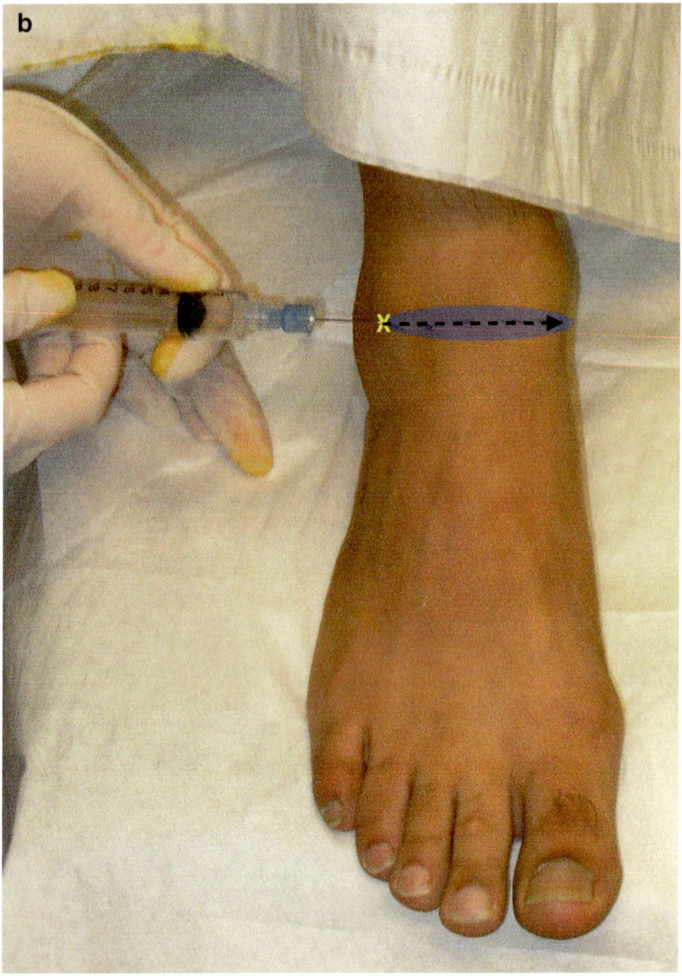

FIGURE 2.21 (continued)

Technique:

- ***Positioning:***
  - Patient supine versus prone, with ankle in slight dorsiflexion.
  - Locate nerve just proximal and posterior to medial malleolus *(posterior to posterior tibial artery).*

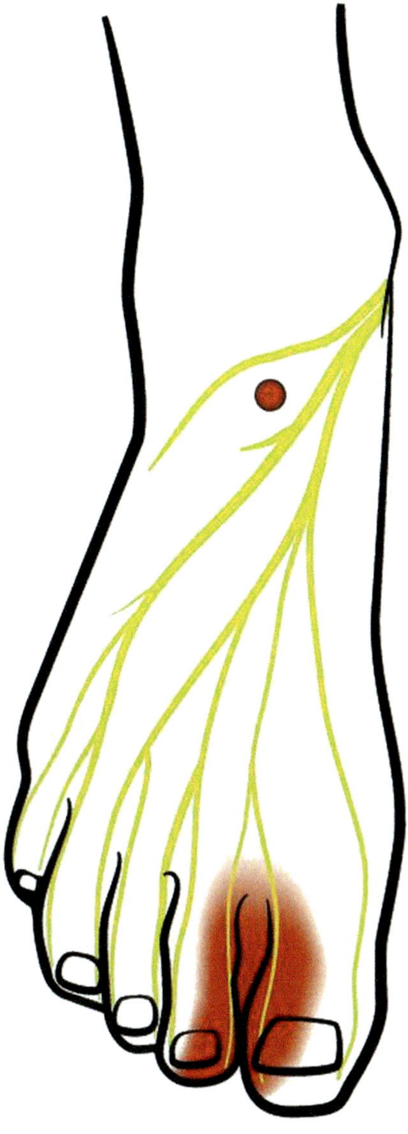

FIGURE 2.22 Deep peroneal nerve block. (Image reprinted with permission from Medscape Drugs & Diseases (http://emedicine.medscape.com/), Ankle Block, 2017, available at: https://emedicine.medscape.com/article/1999563-overview)

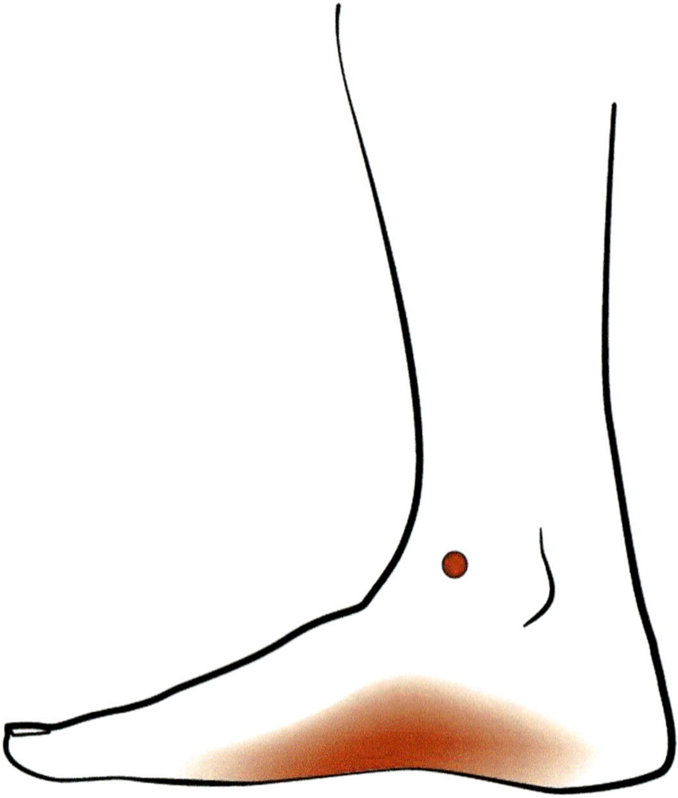

FIGURE 2.23 Saphenous nerve block. (Image reprinted with permission from Medscape Drugs & Diseases (http://emedicine.medscape.com/), Ankle Block, 2017, available at: https://emedicine.medscape.com/article/1999563-overview)

– Place skin wheal, and then penetrate flexor retinaculum. Inject ~5 cc anesthetic +/– adjust needle trajectory, aiming 30° medially and laterally, injecting ~2 cc on each side to ensure adequate analgesia.
  If cannot palpate pulse, inject ~ 1 cm superior to medial malleolus, just anterior to Achilles tendon
  (See Fig. 2.26)

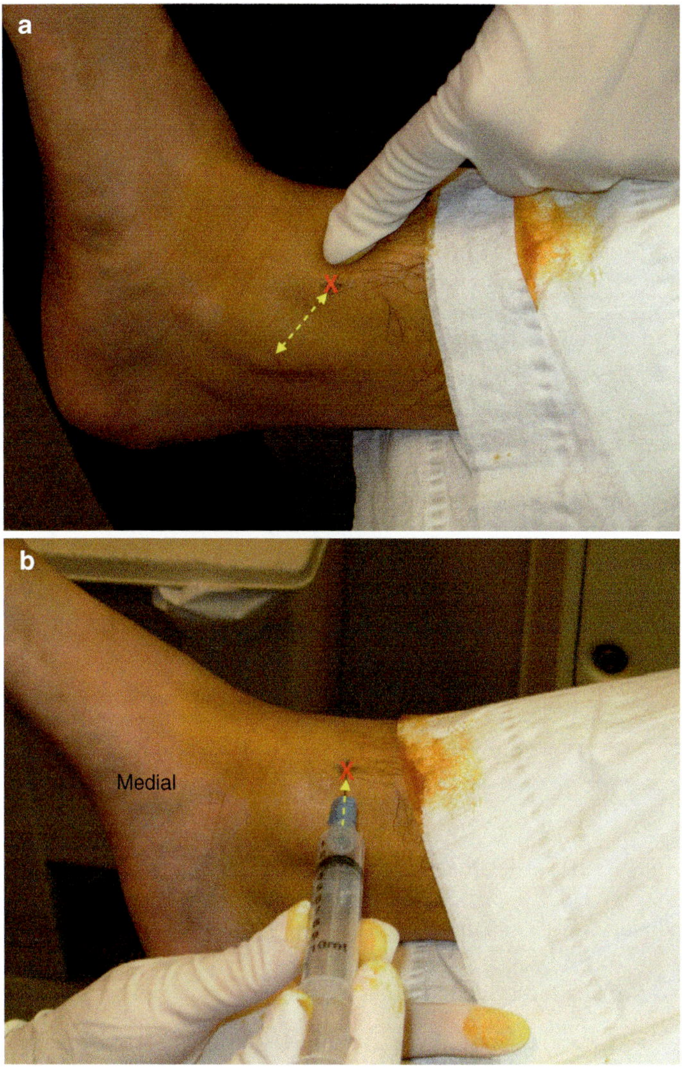

FIGURE 2.24 (**a**, **b**) Saphenous nerve block technique: anesthetization site between tibialis anterior tendon and anterior bony tibial ridge. (**a**, **b**: Images reprinted with permission from Medscape Drugs & Diseases (http://emedicine.medscape.com/), 2016, available at: http://emedicine.medscape.com/article/83237-overview)

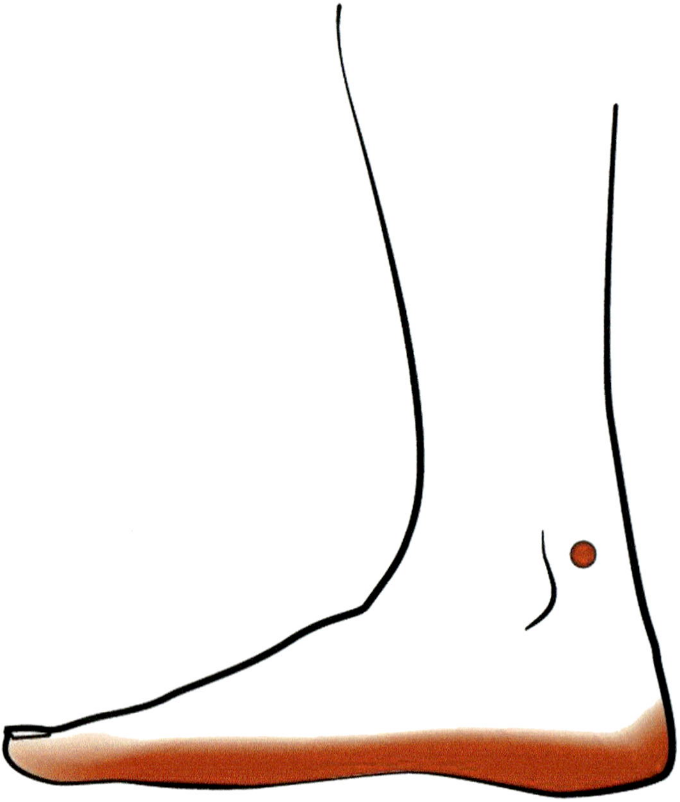

Figure 2.25 Tibial nerve block. (Image reprinted with permission from Medscape Drugs & Diseases (http://emedicine.medscape.com/), Ankle Block, 2017, available at: https://emedicine.medscape.com/article/1999563-overview)

B. ***Sural nerve:***

- Provides anesthesia to posterolateral calf and dorsolateral aspect of heel/sole of foot (See Fig. 2.27).

Technique:

- ***Positioning:***
  - Patient supine with foot in neutral, slight internal rotation, or prone with ankle in slight dorsiflexion.

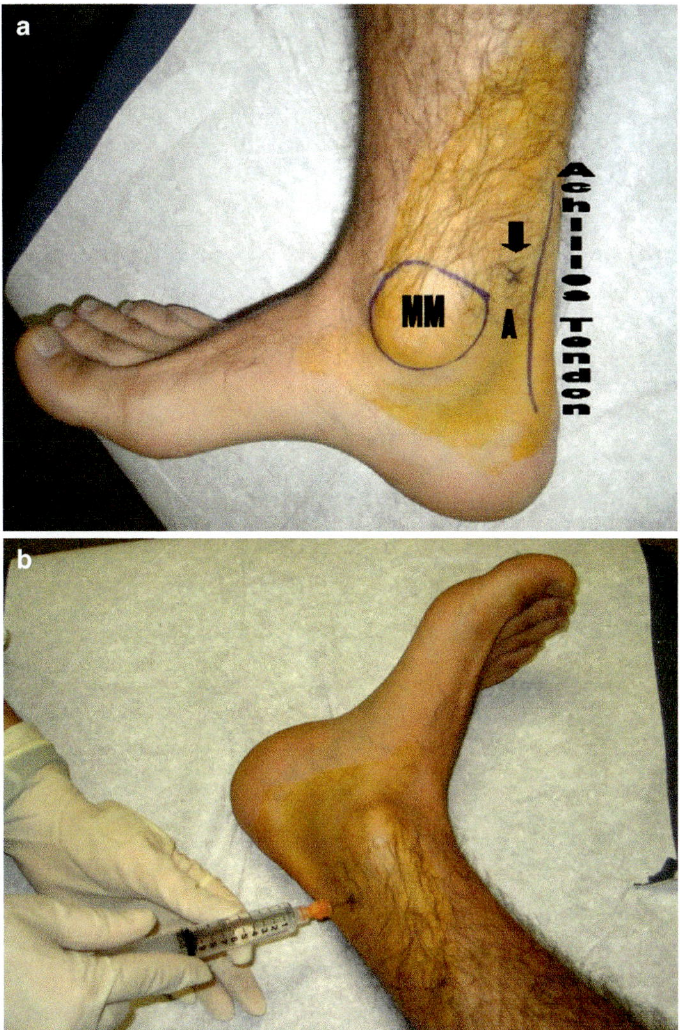

FIGURE 2.26 (**a**, **b**) Tibial nerve block technique. (**a**, **b**: Images reprinted with permission from Heather Tassone, DO, Jacobi and Montefiore Medical Centers, and Matthew A Silver, MD, Kaiser Permanente, San Diego Medical Center, published by Medscape Drugs & Diseases (http://emedicine.medscape.com/), 2017, available at: http://emedicine.medscape.com/article/83135-overview)

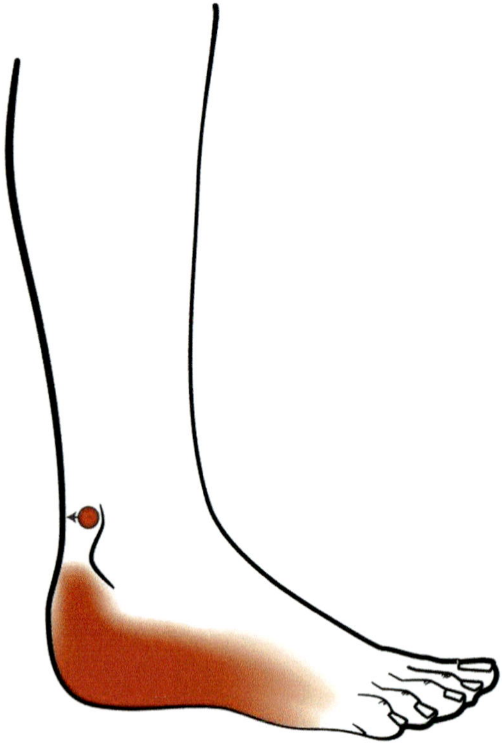

FIGURE 2.27 Sural nerve block. (Image reprinted with permission from Medscape Drugs & Diseases (http://emedicine.medscape.com/), Ankle Block, 2017, available at: https://emedicine.medscape.com/article/1999563-overview)

- Inject ~5 cc anesthetic in subcutaneous space at superolateral border lateral malleolus in fan-shaped pattern.
  Avoid direct injection into Achilles tendon because of risk of atrophy/rupture (See Fig. 2.28)

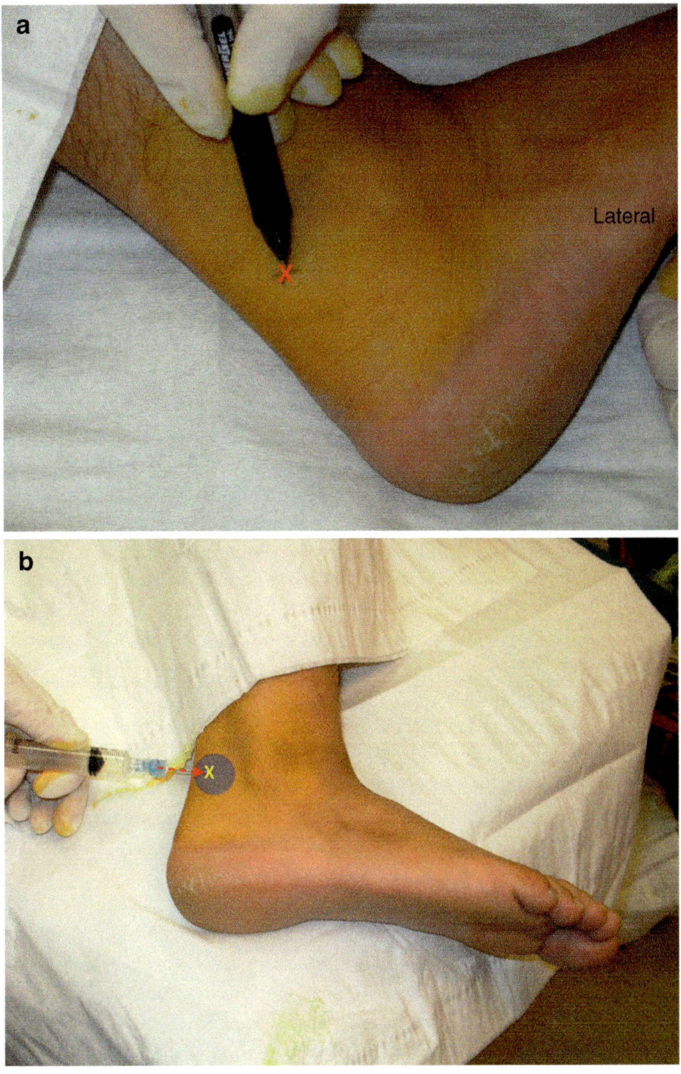

FIGURE 2.28 (**a**, **b**) Sural nerve block technique. (**a**, **b**: Images reprinted with permission from Medscape Drugs & Diseases (http://emedicine.medscape.com/), 2016, available at: http://emedicine.medscape.com/article/83199-overview)

Suggested Reading

1. Chiu DTW. Transthecal digital block: flexor tendon sheath used for anesthetic infusion. J Hand Surg. 1990;15:471–3.
2. Crystal CS, Blankenship RB. Local anesthetics and peripheral nerve blocks in the emergency department. Emerg Med Clin North Am. 2005;23(2):477–502.
3. Denkler K. A comprehensive review of epinephrine in the finger: to do or not to do. Plast Reconstr Surg. 2001;108(1):114–24.
4. Dillion DC, Gibbs MA. Chapter 40. Local and regional anesthesia. In: Tintinalli JE, Stapczynski JS, Cline DM, Ma OJ, Cydulka RK, Meckler GD, editors. Tintinalli's emergency medicine: a comprehensive study guide. 7th ed. New York: McGraw-Hill; 2011.
5. Flarity-Reed K. Methods of digital block. J Emerg Nurs. 2002;28:351.
6. Gmyrek R. (2018). Local and Regional Anesthesia: Overview, Indications, Contraindications. [online] Emedicine.medscape.com. Available at: https://emedicine.medscape.com/article/1831870-overview [Accessed 6 Oct. 2017].
7. Hill RG Jr, Patterson JW, Parker JC, Bauer J, Wright E, Heller MB. Comparison of transthecal digital block and traditional digital block for anesthesia of the finger. Ann Emerg Med. 1995;25(5):604–7.
8. Kay J, Delmonte RJ, Greenberg PM. Ankle block. In:Textbook of regional anesthesia. New York: McGraw-Hill; 2007. p. 546–553/39.
9. Kelly JJ, Spektor M. Nerve blocks of the thorax and extremities. In: Roberts JR, Hedges JR, editors. Clinical procedures in emergency medicine. 4th ed. Philadelphia: WB Saunders Company; 2004. p. 584–9.
10. Lawrence SJ, Botte MJ. The deep peroneal nerve in the foot and ankle: an anatomic study. Foot Ankle Int. 1995;16(11):724–8.
11. McGee D. Local and topical anesthesia. In: Roberts JR, Hedges JR, editors. Clinical procedures in emergency medicine. 4th ed. Philadelphia: WB Saunders; 2004. p. 541–5.
12. Myerson MS, Ruland CM, Allon SM. Regional anesthesia for foot and ankle surgery. Foot Ankle. 1992;13(5):282–8.
13. The New York School of Regional anesthesia. Wrist Block. Available at http://www.nysora.com.
14. Organ GE Jr, Mikhail MS, Murray MJ. Chapter 17. Peripheral nerve blocks. In: Morgan Jr GE, Mikhail MS, Murray MJ, editors. Clinical anesthesiology. 4th ed. New York: McGraw-Hill; 2006.

15. Overbaugh RH. Peripheral nerve blocks of the upper extremity. In: Waldman SD, editor. Pain management. 2nd ed. Philadelphia: Saunders Elsevier; 2007. Chap 146. p. 1233.
16. Reichman EF, Tolson DR. Regional nerve blocks (regional anesthesia). In: Reichman EF, Simon RR, editors. Emergency medicine procedures. New York: McGraw-Hill; 2004. p. 965–81.
17. Schabort D, Boon JM, Becker PJ, Meiring JH. Easily identifiable bony landmarks as an aid in targeted regional ankle blockade. Clin Anat. 2005;18(7):518–26.
18. Salam G. Regional anesthesia for office procedures: part II. Extremity and inguinal area surgeries. Am Fam Phys. 2004;69(4):896–900.
19. Sarhadi NS, Shaw-Dunn J. Transthecal digital nerve block. An anatomical appraisal. J Hand Surg (Br). 1998;23:490.
20. Tintinalli JE, Stapczynski JS, Ma OJ, Cline DM, Cydulka R, Meckler G, editors. Tintinalli's emergency medicine. 7th ed. New York: McGraw-Hill; 2011. Figures 40-2, 40-3, 40-6, 40-7, 40-12: http://www.accessmedicine.com.
21. Volfson D. (2018). Digital Nerve Block: Background, Indications, Contraindications. [online] Emedicine.medscape.com. Available at: https://emedicine.medscape.com/article/80887-overview [Accessed 6 Oct. 2017].

Chapter 3
Acute Compartment Syndrome

Daniel Purcell, Bryan A. Terry, and Brian R. Sharp

Definition

- Limb and life-threatening condition that involves compression of nerves, blood vessels, and muscle tissue within an enclosed space (compartment).
- Rigid surrounding/encircling connective tissue resists expansion, leading to heightened interstitial pressures, thereby reducing arterial inflow and venous outflow.
- Subsequent lack of tissue oxygenation/reduced tissue metabolite removal results in ischemia, with potential for local tissue death/muscle necrosis and associated deleterious systemic effects (e.g., hyperkalemia/dysrhythmia, rhabdomyolysis/acute renal failure) (See Fig. 3.1).

D. Purcell (✉)
Emergency Department, New York University Langone Medical Center Brooklyn, New York, NY, USA
e-mail: daniel.purcell@nyumc.org

B. A. Terry
The Brooklyn Hospital Center, Brooklyn, NY, USA

B. R. Sharp
BerbeeWalsh Department of Emergency Medicine, University of Wisconsin School of Medicine and Public Health, Madison, WI, USA

D. Purcell et al. (eds.), *Emergency Orthopedics Handbook*,
https://doi.org/10.1007/978-3-030-00707-2_3

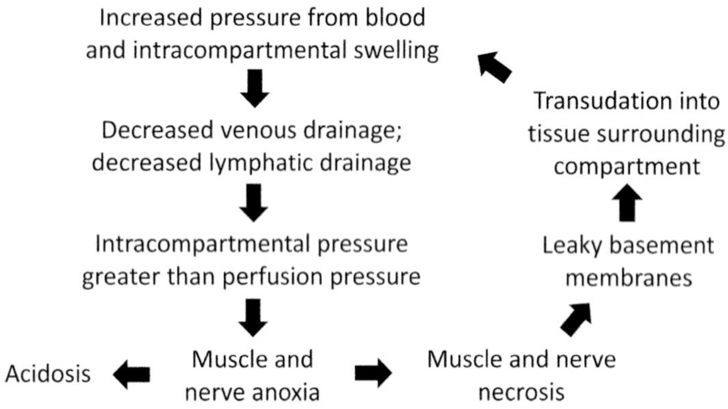

FIGURE 3.1 Compartment syndrome pathogenesis

- Most commonly involves the lower extremity ***(anterior compartment lower leg most often involved; deep posterior compartment lower leg most frequently missed)***.
- **SURGICAL EMERGENCY!!!**

History

- Most commonly seen following long bone fractures **(can also occur following "open" fractures)**.
- Other potential causes:
  - Blunt or penetrating soft tissue trauma without fracture (e.g., gunshot wounds)
  - Prolonged limb compression/burns/crush injuries
  - Poor casting/splinting technique, with constricting wraps/tight dressings in acute injury period
  - Invasive surgical procedures that cause soft tissue swelling
  - Tight closure of deep fascial wounds
  - Ischemic reperfusion following injury
  - Vigorous IO infusion/rehydration
  - Attempts at cannulating vessels in patients on systemic anticoagulants and/or patients treated with thrombolytic drugs

- Remember to always assess and document baseline neuromotor and vascular status, presence of coagulopathy, and systemic infiltrative/congenital disease processes.

Findings

- **CLINICAL DIAGNOSIS!!!**
- The six Ps:
  - ***Pain out of proportion*** to the injury: most reliable clinical feature, especially when muscle within an affected compartment is placed under *passive stretch* (e.g., great toe extension with anterior lower leg compartment syndrome).
  - ***Pallor***: cyanotic color change.
  - ***Pulselessness: rarely occurs, and if present, very late finding!***
    - Pressures that cause compartment syndrome are often well below arterial pressures supplying affected compartments.
    - Generally only occurs if a relevant artery is contained within an affected compartment (e.g., deep compartment lower leg and posterior tibial artery).
  - ***Paresis/paralysis***: poor limb movement and/or function.
  - ***Paresthesias***: "pins and needles"/burning/tingling; sensory nerves typically affected earlier than motor nerves (decreased 2-point discrimination is usually the earliest sensory component finding).
  - ***Poikilothermia***: decreased ability to regulate temperature of the affected extremity.
- If injury mechanism predisposes to development of compartment syndrome (e.g., transverse tibia/fibula fracture), strictly document pain medication administration and refrain from implementing PCA (increasing demand of narcotics may be only clue to insidiously evolving diagnosis).

Diagnostics

- Very useful if the patient cannot provide reliable feedback (e.g., altered/unconscious/intoxicated patients).
- Otherwise, if clinically suspected, treat accordingly with early surgical consultation.
  Time management critical—if compartment syndrome clinically suspected, fasciotomy is the only definitive treatment*
- Measuring compartment pressures:
  - Supplies:
    1. Commercially available intra-compartmental pressure monitoring system (e.g., Stryker).
    2. Arterial line.
    3. Mercury manometer system.

  Needle insertion: ***Know the anatomy—avoid neurovascular structures****

    1. Measure compartment of interest with extremity elevated to heart level.
    2. Always use sterile technique.
    3. Measure as close to fracture site as possible to avoid underestimation of pressure ***(testing within 5 cm of fracture site generally yields "peak" pressure).***
    4. Skin entry site should be infiltrated with local anesthetic.
       Do not inject anesthetic into fascia/muscle as can falsely elevate compartment pressure*
    5. Make sure instrument has been calibrated prior to pressure reading.
    6. Enter needle perpendicular to the skin.
    7. Resting compartment pressure measurement interpretation (*approximate values*):

  - 0–12 mm Hg = normal.
  - >20 mm Hg = can impair vascular inflow/outflow.
  - >30 mm Hg = potential indication for fasciotomy.
  - Commonly used decision guideline: comparison of individual compartment pressure to systemic diastolic

blood pressure (ΔP); if individual compartment measurement is within 30 mmHg of diastolic pressure, another indication for emergent fasciotomy ***(+/– within 20 mm Hg of diastolic pressure if patient profoundly hypotensive).***

Lower Leg Compartment Anatomy (See Fig. 3.2)

Treatment:

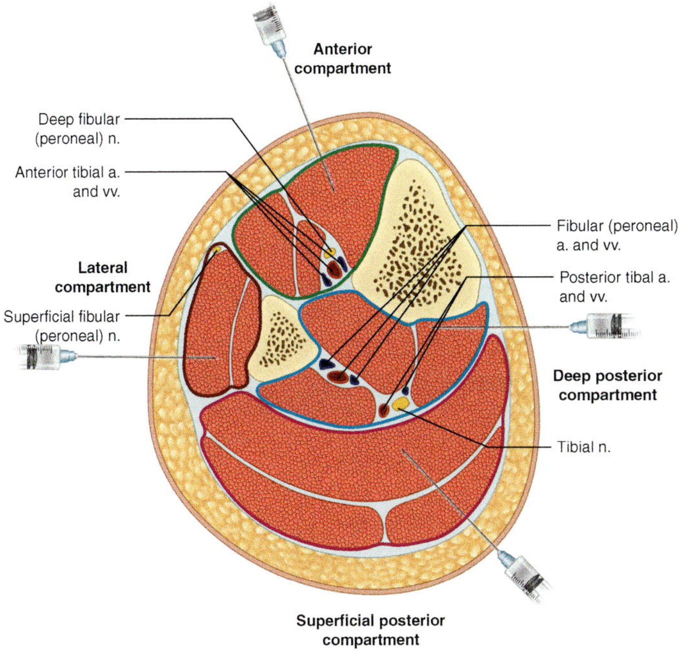

FIGURE 3.2 Compartments of the lower leg: anterior (insert needle to depth ~1–3 cm), superficial posterior compartment (insert to depth ~2–4 cm), deep posterior compartment (insert to depth ~ 2–4 cm), lateral (insert to depth ~ 1–1.5 cm)

- ***Interim*** (<6 hr from injury/onset of symptoms): if diagnosis is unclear, can observe until clinical picture declares itself, ***but get consultants on board early.***
  - Remove all constricting bandages and immobilization devices while maintaining stabilization of injury.
  - Do not elevate extremity above level of heart (impairs tissue perfusion, reducing the arterial-venous pressure gradient).
  - Strictly document analgesia requirements.
  - Perform serial neurovascular examinations at frequent intervals.
- ***Definitive:*** fasciotomy—goal is to perform within 6 hr; if delayed, irreversible nerve and muscle damage can occur leading to decreased/absent limb function ***(+/− need for amputation).***

Suggested Reading

1. Arato E, Kurthy M, Sinay L, et al. Pathology and diagnostic options of lower limb compartment syndrome. Clin Hemorheol Microcirc. 2009;41(1):1–8.
2. Defraigne JO, et al. Local and systemic consequences of severe ischemia and reperfusion of the skeletal muscle. Physiopathology and prevention. Acta Chir Belg. 1998;98(4):176.
3. Elliot KG, et al. Diagnosing acute compartment syndrome. J Bone Joint Surg Br. 2003;85(5):625.
4. Frankel N, Villarin L. Compartment syndrome evaluation. In: Roberts JR, Hedges J, editors. Clinical procedures in emergency medicine. 4th ed. Philadelphia: Saunders Elsevier; 2004. p. 1058–71.
5. Haller P. Compartment syndrome. In: Tintinalli's emergency medicine. 6th ed. New York: McGraw-Hill; 2004. p. 1746–9.
6. Hammerberg EM, et al. The reliability of measurement of tissue pressure in compartment syndrome. J Orthop Trauma. 2012;26(1):24–31; discussion 32.
7. Kostler W, et al. Acute compartment syndrome of the limb. Injury. 2005;36(8):992.

8. Mar GJ, Barrington MJ, McGuirk BR. Acute compartment syndrome of the lower limb and the effect of postoperative analgesia on diagnosis. Br J Anaesth. 2009;102(1):3–11.
9. Matsen FA 3rd, Winquist RA, Krugmire RB Jr. Diagnosis and management of compartmental syndromes. J Bone Joint Surg Am. 1980;62(2):286–91.
10. McQueen MM, Chrisstie J, Court-Brown CM. Acute compartment syndrome in tibial diaphyseal fractures. J Bone Joint Surg Br. 1996;78-B:95.
11. McQueen MM, Court-Brown CM. Compartment monitoring in tibial fractures. The pressure threshold for decompression. J Bone Joint Surg Br. 1996;78(1):99–104.
12. Olson SA, et al. Acute compartment syndrome in lower extremity musculoskeletal trauma. J Am Acad Orthop Surg. 2005;13(7):436.
13. Prasam ML, et al. Acute compartment syndrome of the upper extremity. J Am Acad Orthop Surg. 2011;19:49–58.
14. Rizvi S, et al. Responding promptly to acute compartment syndrome. Emerg Med. 2008;40:12.
15. Shadgan B, Pereira G, Menon M, et al. Risk factors for acute compartment syndrome of the leg associated with tibial diaphyseal fractures in adults. J Orthop Traumatol. 2015;16:185–92.

Chapter 4
Joint Arthrocentesis

Daniel Purcell, Bryan A. Terry, and Brian R. Sharp

Indications

- ***Diagnostic:***
  - Diagnosis of non-traumatic injuries by joint synovial fluid analysis (e.g., septic arthritis, crystal arthropathy).
  - Evaluate for intra-articular penetrating injuries—instill saline +/– methylene blue for investigation.
- ***Therapeutic:***
  - Drain traumatic effusions/hemarthroses that stretch joint capsule to increase joint mobility and provide pain relief via instillation of:

D. Purcell (✉)
Emergency Department, New York University Langone Medical Center Brooklyn, New York, NY, USA
e-mail: daniel.purcell@nyumc.org

B. A. Terry
The Brooklyn Hospital Center, Brooklyn, NY, USA

B. R. Sharp
BerbeeWalsh Department of Emergency Medicine, University of Wisconsin School of Medicine and Public Health, Madison, WI, USA

D. Purcell et al. (eds.), *Emergency Orthopedics Handbook*,
https://doi.org/10.1007/978-3-030-00707-2_4

  - Analgesia (e.g., evaluating continuity of knee/elbow extensor mechanism)
  - Anti-inflammatory medications (e.g., corticosteroids for osteoarthritis/rheumatoid arthritis)
  - Joint preservation products (e.g., injection of hyaluronic acid derivatives)

Relative contraindications (no absolute contraindications)

- Needle point of entry with overlying cellulitis/inflammation (risk of seeding joint).
- Coagulopathy: necessity of joint fluid for analysis and/or pain relief versus creation/worsening of iatrogenic hemarthrosis.
- Prosthetic joints: ***always consult orthopedics prior to performing procedure!***
  - May not want to perform at present time (observation and conservative management often preferred, at least initially).
  - May want own team member to perform (considered more difficult secondary to scar tissue formation/altered anatomic relationships).
  - May want to perform more definitive procedure (formal I&D with/without removal of implant) in OR based upon current history and established treatment protocol.

Technique

General Considerations

- Obtain informed consent.
- Patient comfort imperative; familiar positioning and appropriate analgesia should be implemented to enhance potential for success.
- Aseptic technique (e.g., Betadine/Chloraprep) should surround region to create a sterile field.
- Local anesthetic should be injected over determined aspiration site (e.g., Lidocaine); do not inject deeper than sub-

cutaneous tissue because it can potentially interfere with joint fluid analysis.

- Aspirate/inject with 18–22 gauge needle of appropriate length (based upon joint of interest and patient body habitus).
- Know the anatomy to avoid penetration of neurovascular/ soft tissue structures (e.g., tendons).
- If correctly placed, needle insertion should not encounter resistance; if resistance is encountered, withdraw and redirect.

1. ***KNEE***

   - ***Anatomic landmarks:*** quadriceps/patellar tendon, patella, and tibial plateau (joint line).

   A. ***Suprapatellar approach:***

      - Knee slightly flexed (~15–20°).
      - Insert 18-gauge needle ~1 cm proximal to supero-medial/superolateral border of the patella.
      - Needle then directed toward intercondylar notch of femur (See Fig. 4.1).

   B. ***Parapatellar approach:***

      - Knee slightly flexed (~15–20°).
      - Insert 18-gauge needle at midpoint of lateral/ medial border of patella.
      - Needle then directed perpendicular to long axis of leg, toward intercondylar notch of femur.

   C. ***Infrapatellar approach:***

      - Knee in ~90° flexion (patient upright, knee bent over edge of stretcher-allows gravity to assist in opening joint cavity).
      - Insert 18-gauge needle ~0.5 cm below inferior border of patella, at level of joint line, just medial/ lateral to patellar tendon.
      - Needle then directed perpendicular to long axis of leg, toward intercondylar notch of femur (See Fig. 4.2).

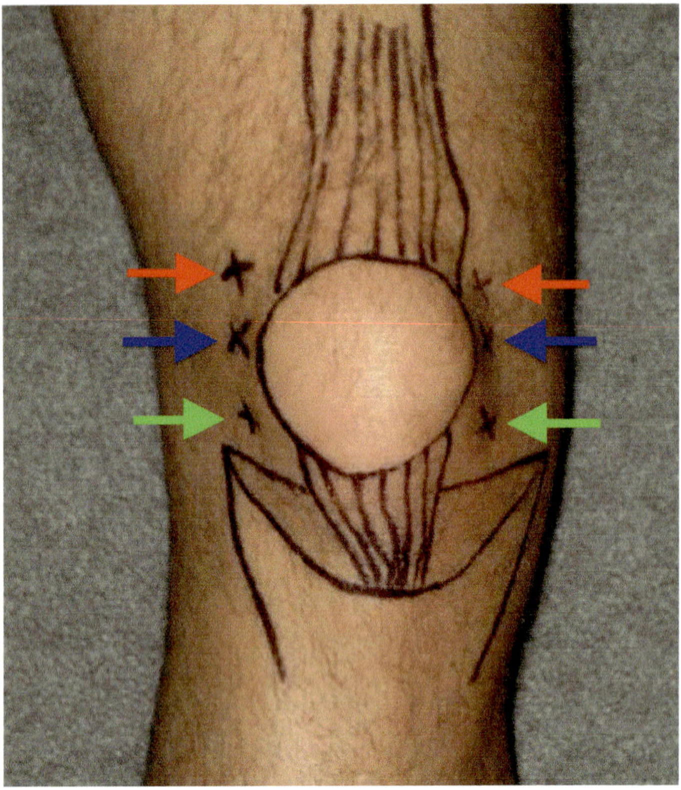

FIGURE 4.1 Anatomical landmarks for knee arthrocentesis: Red arrows demonstrate Suprapatellar approach, Blue arrows Parapatellar approach and Green arrows Infrapatellar approach. (Image reprinted with permission from Gil Z. Shlamovitz, MD, FACEP, Keck School of Medicine of the University of Southern California, published by Medscape Drugs & Diseases. (http://emedicine.medscape.com/), 2016, available at: http://emedicine.medscape.com/article/79956-overview OR http://emedicine.medscape.com/article/79994-overview)

Pearls:

- If utilizing either suprapatellar or parapatellar approaches, place small "bump" (rolled up towel) under posterior knee (popliteal space) to maintain slight flexion; allows for relaxation of quadriceps muscles (easier joint penetration).

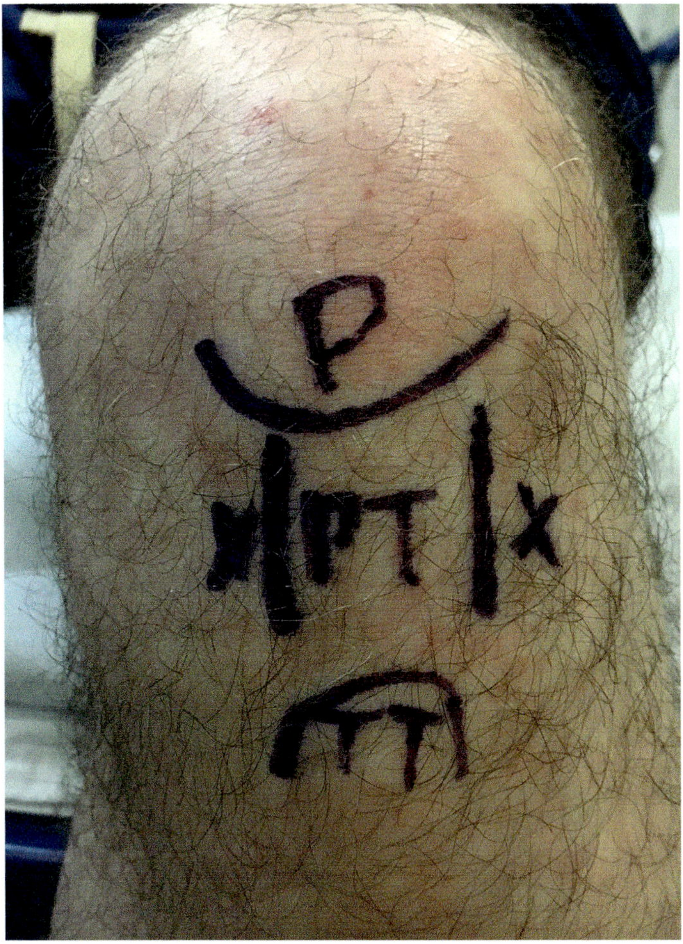

FIGURE 4.2 Infrapatellar approach: note the patellar tendon (PT), tibial tuberosity (TT), and joint access points (X)

- Knee effusion is common manifestation of Lyme disease. In young patient with monoarticular involvement +/– systemic symptoms, especially outdoorsmen, do not forget to measure Lyme titers. Also consider gonococcal arthritis in the appropriate clinical scenario.

2. ***SHOULDER***

- ***Anatomic landmarks:*** Coracoid process of scapula (anteromedially), proximal humerus/acromion (laterally), and spine of scapula (posteriorly).

  A. ***Anterior Approach:***

  - Patient seated upright with humerus adducted and internally rotated (hand on abdomen).
  - Locate coracoid process and insert 18–20-gauge needle just inferolateral, in groove between coracoid process and humeral head.
  - Needle then directed slightly superiorly, laterally, and posteriorly toward glenoid rim.
  - A sudden loss of resistance will be noted once glenohumeral joint correctly entered.

    *****Take care to avoid entering nearby neurovascular bundle***** (See Fig. 4.3)

  B. ***Lateral approach:***

  - Patient seated upright with arm at side.
  - Insert 18–20-gauge needle just inferior to lateral surface of acromion and above greater tuberosity of humerus.
  - Needle then directed medially and slightly posterior.

  C. ***Posterior approach:***

  - Patient seated upright with palm of affected arm on anterior surface of opposite shoulder.
  - Locate posterior border of acromion process (where spine of scapula turns anterior to become acromion) and place non-dominant thumb here, with tip of non-dominant index finger on coracoid process.
  - Insert 18–20-gauge needle ~1–2 cm below thumb, parallel to floor, and advance toward index finger (See Fig. 4.4).

Pearls:

- Diabetic patient presenting with symptoms consistent with septic shoulder: think *syrinx*.
- Patient with infected shoulder replacement: propionibacterium acnes is most commonly isolated bacterium.

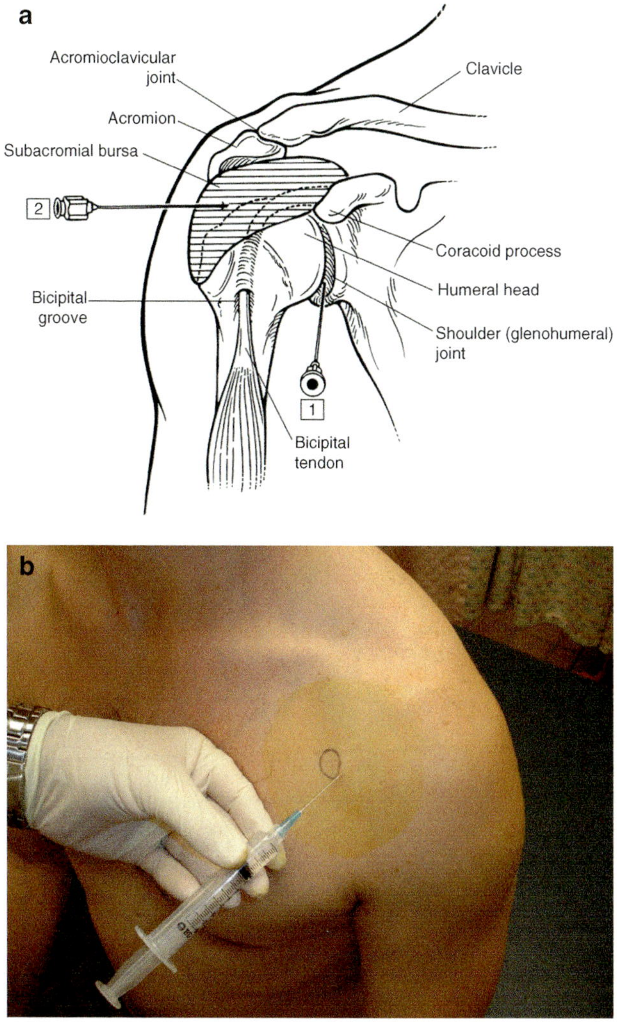

FIGURE 4.3 Shoulder arthrocentesis: (**a**) anatomical landmarks for anterior (1) lateral (2) approaches. (**b**) Anterior approach. (**a**: Image reprinted with permission from RheumaNow, (http://www.rheumaknowledgy.com/), available at: http://www.rheumaknowledgy.com/shoulder-glenohumeral-arthrocentesis/. **b**: Image reprinted with permission from Medscape Drugs & Diseases (http://emedicine.medscape.com/), 2017, available at: http://emedicine.medscape.com/article/80013-overview)

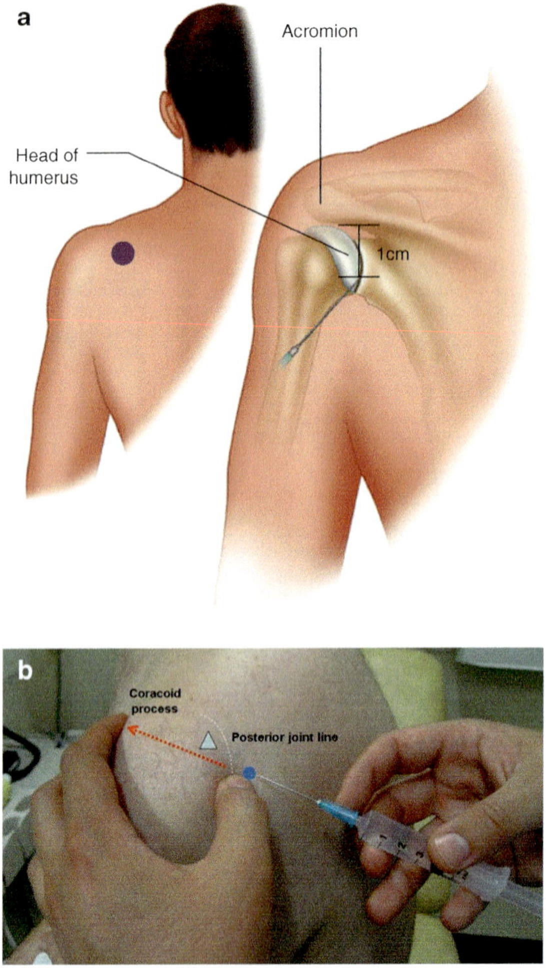

FIGURE 4.4 Shoulder arthrocentesis posterior approach: (**a**) anatomic landmarks (**b**) posterior approach initiated just inferior to posterior border of acromion. (**a**: Reprinted from Kothakota B, Waseem M. Intra-articular injection. In: Ganti L, editor. Atlas of emergency medicine procedures. New York: Springer Verlag; 2016. p. 623–9. With permission from Springer Verlag. **b**: Reprinted from Zayat AS, Wakefield RJ. Arthrocentesis in the elderly. In: Nakasato Y, Yung RL, editors. Geriatric rheumatology. New York: Springer Verlag; 2011. p. 113–24. With permission from Springer Verlag)

3. ***ANKLE***

- ***Anatomic landmarks:*** medial/lateral malleolus, tibial plafond/talus (joint line), EHL tendon (identify via resistance to great toe extension), TA tendon (identify via resistance to ankle dorsiflexion), EDL tendon (identify by extending lesser toes against resistance) (See Fig. 4.5).

A. ***Medial approach:***

- Patient positioned supine or upright on examination table.
- Insert 18–22-gauge needle perpendicular to long axis of tibia, anterolateral to medial malleolus, and slightly medial to TA tendon and/or EHL tendon (*TA tendon landmark preferred*).
- Needle should be inserted ~2–3 cm to reach joint space.

B. ***Lateral approach:***

- Patient positioned supine or upright on examination table.
- Insert 18–22-gauge needle perpendicular to long axis of fibula, midway between base of lateral malleolus and lateral border of EDL tendon.
- Needle should be inserted ~1–2 cm to reach joint space (See Fig. 4.6).

Pearls:

- If using EHL tendon as injection landmark, *dorsalis pedis artery* and *deep peroneal nerve* course immediately lateral.
- Slight plantar flexion of foot may assist in enlarging effective joint space.
- Avoid injuring underlying cartilage (avascular tissue) by implementing proper insertion placement based upon surface landmarks and associated proper advancement technique.

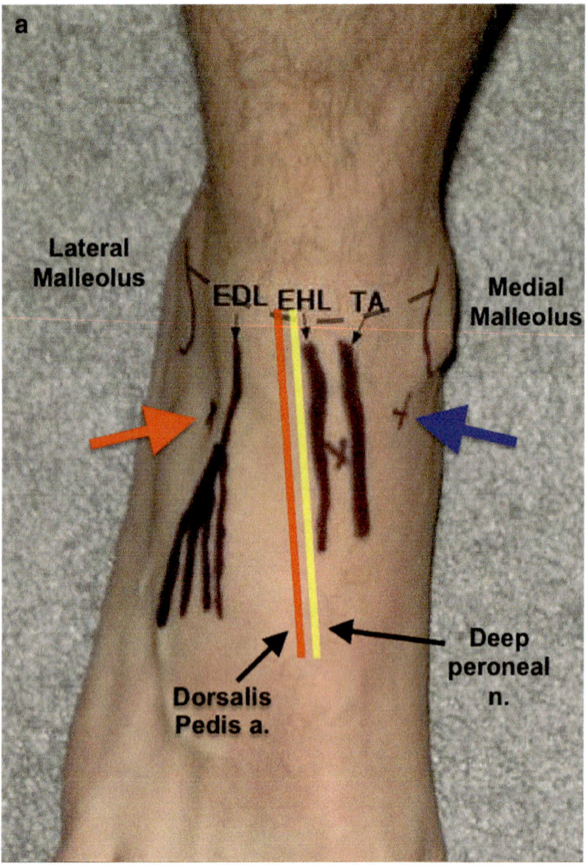

FIGURE 4.5 Anatomic landmarks for ankle arthrocentesis: (**a**) blue arrow demonstrates medial approach and red arrow, lateral approach. Note the neurovascular structures: EDL (extensor digitorum longus), EHL (extensor hallucis longus), and TA (tibialis anterior tendon). (**b**) Needle entry for lateral and medial approaches. (**a**: Image reprinted with permission from Gil Z. Shlamovitz, MD, FACEP, Keck School of Medicine of the University of Southern California, published by Medscape Drugs & Diseases (http://emedicine.medscape.com/), 2016, available. at: http://emedicine.medscape.com/article/79956-overview OR http://emedicine.medscape.com/article/79994-overview. **b**: Image reprinted with permission from RheumaNow, (http://www.rheumaknowledgy.com/), available at: http://www.rheumaknowledgy.com/ankle-arthrocentesis/)

b

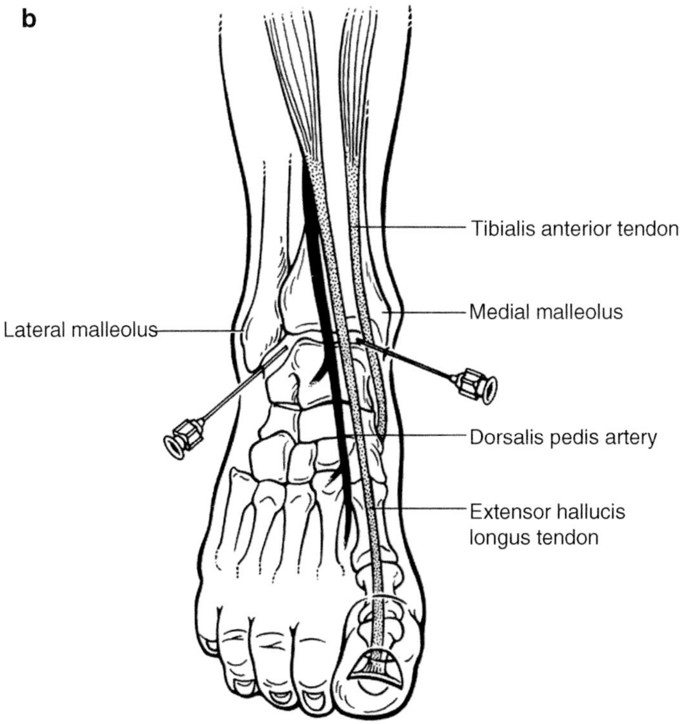

FIGURE 4.5 (continued)

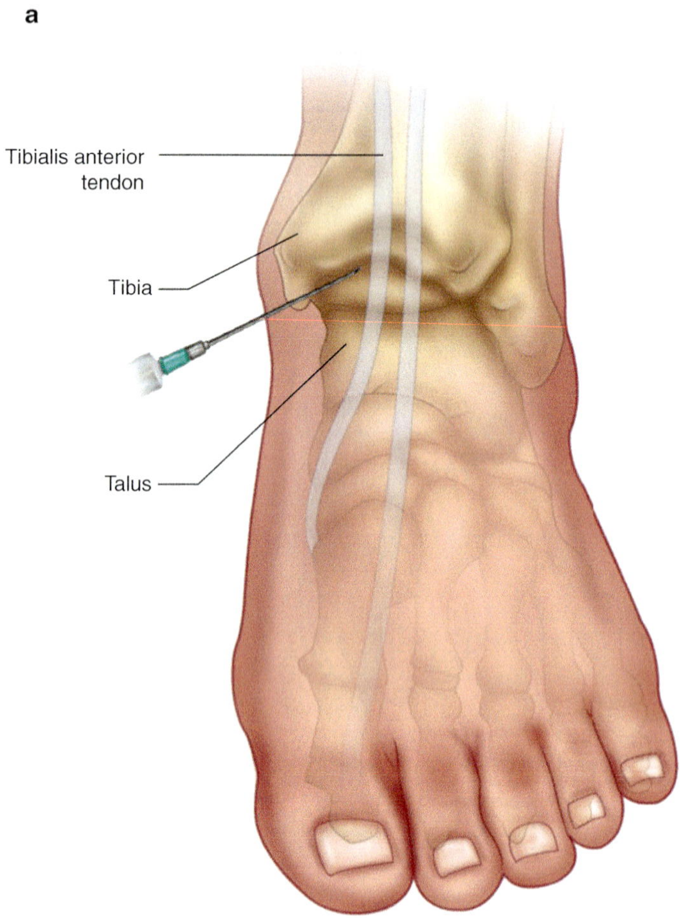

FIGURE 4.6 Ankle arthrocentesis: (**a**) medial approach and (**b**) lateral approach (red circle denotes needle entry point). (**a**: Reprinted from Kothakota B, Waseem M. Intra-articular Injection. In: Ganti L, editor. Atlas of emergency medicine procedures. New York: Springer Verlag; 2016. p. 623–9. With permission from Springer Verlag. **b**: Reprinted from da Silva JAP, Woolf AD. Regional syndromes the foot and ankle. In: da Silva JAP, Woolf AD, editors. Rheumatology in practice. London: Springer Verlag; 2010. p. 141–9. With permission from Springer Verlag)

b

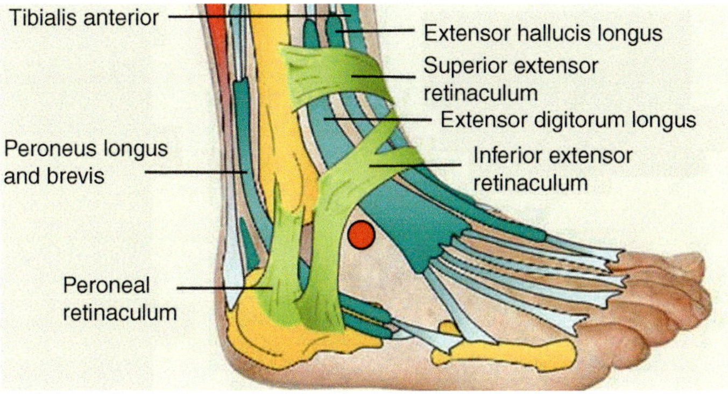

FIGURE 4.6 (continued)

4. ***ELBOW***

- ***Anatomic landmarks:*** Radial head, tip of olecranon process, and lateral epicondyle of humerus (***structures form a triangle***).
- ***Lateral approach:***
  - Patient supine or upright with arm supported, elbow flexed 45–90°, and forearm pronated—palm down (***pronation of hand moves radial nerve/PIN out of intended aspiration path and widens synovial cavity***).
  - Identify depression located proximal to radial head, distal to lateral epicondyle, and anterior to tip of olecranon process.
  - Insert 18–22-gauge needle perpendicular to the skin into depression and advance to depth up to ~2 cm (See Fig. 4.7).

Pearls:

- Presence of posterior fat pad on imaging should raise suspicion for "occult" fracture.
- Surface landmarks are easier to elucidate if the arm is initially extended to locate area of depression and then flexed/pronated.

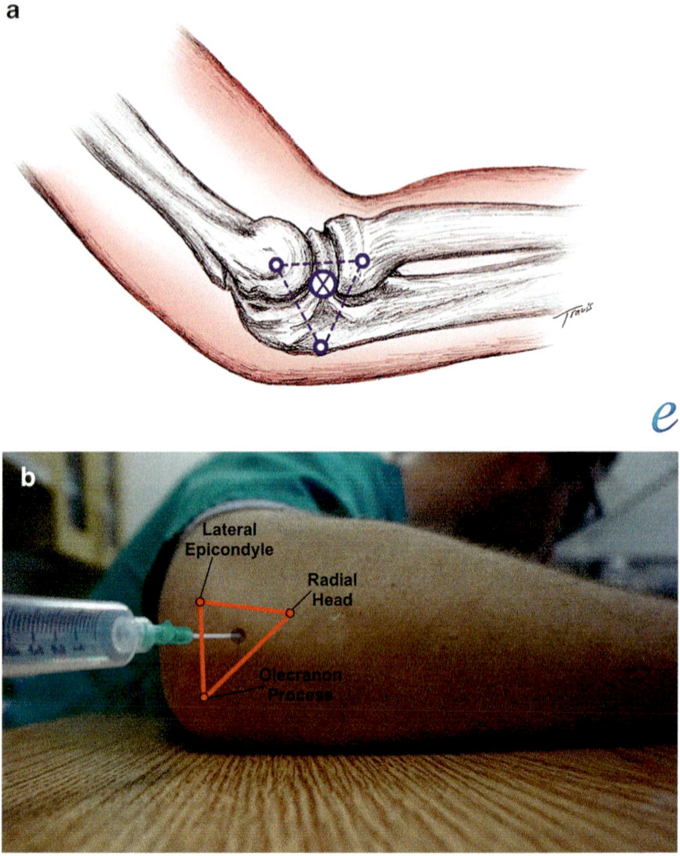

Figure 4.7 Elbow arthrocentesis: (**a**) anatomic landmarks and (**b**) needle entry into triangle. (**a**: Image reprinted with permission from Medscape Drugs & Diseases (http://emedicine.medscape.com/), 2016, available at: http://emedicine.medscape.com/article/79975-overview)

- Do not confuse olecranon bursitis with elbow joint effusion; olecranon bursitis is located posteriorly over olecranon process.
- Do not attempt *medial approach* based upon proximity of ulnar nerve and superior ulnar collateral artery.

5. ***WRIST***

- ***Anatomic landmarks:*** Distal radius/ulna, Lister's tubercle (bony prominence on dorsal aspect of distal radius), EPL tendon (courses just radial to Lister's tubercle).
- ***Dorsal approach:***
  - Patient supine or upright with 20–50° of wrist flexion and slight ulnar deviation (examiner non-dominant hand should apply continuous gentle ulnar traction to increase effective joint space).
  - Insert 20–22-gauge needle immediately distal to Lister's tubercle, just ulnar to EPL tendon.
  - Needle should pass freely through extra-articular tissue, +/– a "pop" upon reaching wrist joint (See Fig. 4.8).

Pearls:

- Can have patient extend thumb against resistance to better identify EPL tendon.
- Do not contact and/or inject into tendon proper; can potentiate tendon rupture (e.g., corticosteroid injection) (See Fig. 4.9).

Complications:

- "Dry tap": potential causes are incorrect needle placement, absent/minimal effusion, and/or mechanical obstruction.
- Hemarthrosis is generally self-limiting versus coagulopathic patients who may require further evaluation/monitoring (e.g., hematology consultation).
- Aseptic technique and meticulous needle placement/advancement can dramatically reduce risk of introducing infection.
- Allergic reactions can occur secondary to hypersensitivity to local anesthesia.
- Articular cartilage injury can occur following improper needle placement/advancement, or unnecessary needle movement within the joint space; cartilage is avascular,

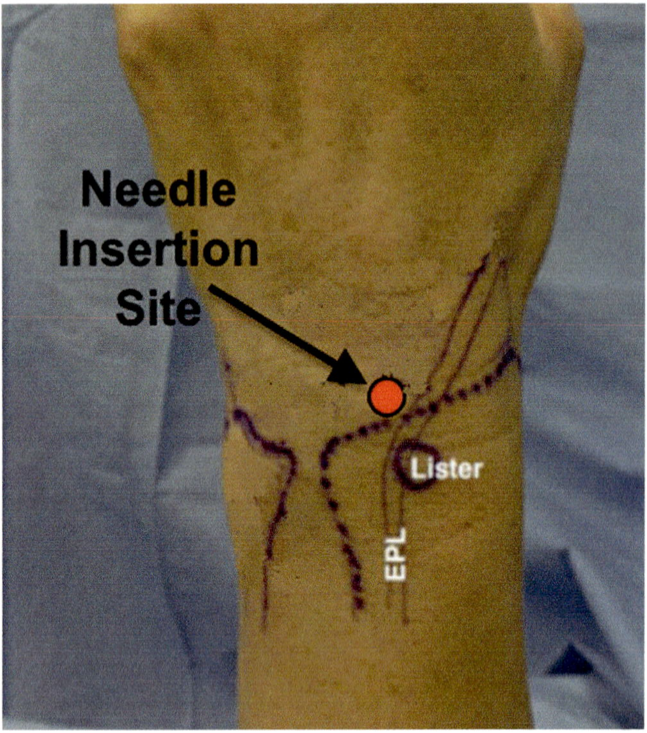

FIGURE 4.8 Wrist arthrocentesis: Anatomic landmarks, red circle denotes needle entry point; EPL (extensor pollicis longus). (Reprinted from Badur N, Luchetti R, Atzei A. Arthroscopic wrist anatomy and setup. In: Geissler WB, editor. Wrist and elbow arthroscopy. New York: Springer Verlag; 2015. p. 1–28. With permission from Springer Verlag)

thus iatrogenic injuries do not overwhelmingly heal, and may lead to focal degenerative changes and/or become a nidus for future infection.

Pearls:

- Joint infection can occur by (a) hematogenous spread—most common scenario (b) spread from a contiguous source of infection (c) direct implantation (d) postoperative contamination (e) trauma.
- Joint fluid analysis examination: cell count (RBC, WBC, differential), crystals, protein, glucose, gram stain/culture,

Diagnosis	Appearance	WBCs/mm^3	PMNs (%)	Glucose: % blood level	Crystals under polarized Light	Culture
Normal	Clear	<200	<25	95–100	None	Negative
Septic arthritis	Purulent/turbid; bloody, white	5000–>50,000	>90	<50	None	Positive (usually)
Acute gout	Turbid	200–50,000	>75	80–100	Monosodium urate crystals (needle shaped, negatively birefringent, parallel = yellow, perpendicular = blue)	Negative
Pseudogout	Turbid	2000–50,000	>75	80–100	Pseudogout = calcium pyrophosphate crystals (rhomboid, positively birefringent, perpendicular = yellow, parallel = blue)	Negative
Rheumatoid arthritis	Turbid	2000–50,000	50–75	~75	None	Negative

FIGURE 4.9 Arthrocentesis fluid analysis

and associated specialized studies (e.g., rheumatoid factor).

- Different parameters exist for analysis of possible prosthetic joint infection: in immediate/subacute postoperative period, hematologic values as low as ***1100 WBC and 64% PMNs may suggest joint infection.***
- Traumatic effusions may be grossly bloody (contain large amount of RBCs). This is a diagnostic clue for intra-articular fracture and/or soft tissue structural disruption. Synovial fluid can be evaluated for fat globules released from marrow cavity of fractured bone, confirming presence of intra-articular pathology despite negative radiographic findings.
- Recommended appropriate volume of saline injection (+/– methylene blue) to detect intra-articular penetration: knee, 100–200 mL; elbow, 20–30 mL; ankle, 20–30 mL; wrist, 5 mL; and shoulder, 40–60 mL.

Suggested Reading

1. Ahmed I, et al. Safety of arthrocentesis and joint injection in patients receiving anticoagulation at therapeutic levels. Am J Med. 2012;125(3):265–9.
2. Bauer T, et al. Diagnosis of periprosthetic joint infection. JBJS. 2006;88:869–82.
3. Bork S, et al. Elbow arthrocentesis. Medscape.com.

4. Burton J. Acute disorders of the joints and bursae. In: Tintinalli's emergency medicine. 6th ed. New York: McGraw-Hill; 2004. p. 1795–800.
5. Cardone DA, Tallia AF. Diagnostic and therapeutic injection of the elbow region. Am Fam Phys. 2002;66:2097–100.
6. Cardone DA, Tallia AF. Diagnostic and therapeutic injection of the hip and knee region. Am Fam Phys. 2003;67:2147–52.
7. Krause R, et al. Wrist arthrocentesis. Medscape.com.
8. Parillo S, Fisher J. Arthrocentesis. In: Roberts JR, Hedges J, editors. Clinical procedures in emergency medicine. 4th ed. Philadelphia: Saunders Elsevier; 2004. p. 1042–57.
9. Reichman E, et al. Joint arthrocentesis. Emerg Med Proc. 2003;65:559–84.
10. Siva C, Velazquez C, Mody A, Brasington R. Diagnosing acute monoarthritis in adults: a practical approach for the family physician. Am Fam Phys. 2003;68(1):83–90.
11. Sclamovitz G, et al. Knee arthrocentesis technique. Medscape.com.
12. Tallia AF, et al. Diagnostic and therapeutic injection of the ankle and foot. Am Fam Phys. 2003;68(7):1356–63.
13. Tallia AF, Cardone DA. Diagnostic and therapeutic injection of the shoulder region. Am Fam Phys. 2003;67:1271–8.
14. Tallia AF, Cardone DA. Diagnostic and therapeutic injection of the wrist and hand region. Am Fam Phys. 2003;67:745–50.
15. Wise C. Arthrocentesis and injection of joints and soft tissue. In: Kelley's textbook of rheumatology. 8th ed. Philadelphia: Saunders Elsevier; 2009.
16. Woodward TW, Best TM. The painful shoulder: part II. Acute and chronic disorders. Am Fam Phys. 2000;61:3291–300.
17. Zink B, Raukar N. Bone and joint infections. In: Rosen's emergency medicine. 7th ed. Philadelphia: Saunders Elsevier; 2010. p. 1830–5.
18. Zuber TJ. Knee joint aspiration and injection. Am Fam Phys. 2002;66(8):1497–500, 1503–4, 1507.

Chapter 5
Dislocation(s)/Reduction(s)

Daniel Purcell, Bryan A. Terry, and Brandon R. Allen

General Considerations

- Assessment of the patient with a dislocation necessitates examination for other serious injuries based upon a high-energy mechanism ***(especially hip, knee, and posterior sternoclavicular dislocations)***.
- All dislocations (+/− fracture) require a detailed, documented neurovascular examination before consideration of reduction *and* following manipulation.
- No rigid, generally accepted practice guidelines exist regarding use of pharmacologic adjuncts in management; however, generous use of analgesia +/− sedation is

D. Purcell (✉)
Emergency Department, New York University Langone Medical Center Brooklyn, New York, NY, USA
e-mail: daniel.purcell@nyumc.org

B. A. Terry
The Brooklyn Hospital Center, Brooklyn, NY, USA

B. R. Allen
Department of Emergency Medicine, University of Florida Health, University of Florida, Gainesville, FL, USA

D. Purcell et al. (eds.), *Emergency Orthopedics Handbook*,
https://doi.org/10.1007/978-3-030-00707-2_5

recommended, remembering each patient presentation is unique and should be approached accordingly.

- Understanding injury mechanism is imperative, as application of an opposite force is generally required for successful reduction.
- Proper positioning, essential equipment, and a meticulous plan of action are necessary to optimize potential outcome.
- Always obtain post-reduction imaging to assess appropriateness of reduction, position of immobilization, and integrity of immobilization method (splint/cast).
- Do not delay reduction in limbs with obvious neurovascular impairment; only patients with evidence of maintained perfusion should undergo pre-reduction radiographs.
- After each reduction attempt, assess neurovascular status to ensure no sensory/motor compromise has developed and peripheral perfusion has been maintained.
- Osseous fragments/soft tissue structures can become interposed/entrapped making closed reduction in certain circumstances ***impossible***; repeated forceful attempts will only cause additional injury (iatrogenic fractures/soft tissue disruption with potential for ***transforming a closed fracture into an "open" fracture***).
- If attempting repeat reduction, understand why the initial attempt was unsuccessful; implement a different strategy/physical maneuver versus consider consulting orthopedic service for further management.
- Always evaluate skin integrity/potential of open fractures.

ANKLE

- Ankle joint mortise is inherently stable; dislocation requires a high-energy mechanism.
- Ligamentous structures are often stronger than osseous architecture, thus associated fractures are commonplace.
- Ligamentous disruption and soft tissue injury vary according to type and direction of dislocation.

- ***Dislocation is described according to position of the talus in relation to the tibia.***
- Most common direction of dislocation is posterior (talus moves posterior to the distal tibia); ankle plantar flexion (smaller surface area of posterior talus) creates diminished ankle mortise stability in contrast to the dorsiflexed position (See Fig. 5.1).
- Inversion injuries generally lead to posteromedial displacement of talus relative to the tibia, with associated tears of the ATFL and CTFL ligaments.
- Eversion injuries generally produce lateral dislocations, with talo-tibial ligament and medial joint capsule rupture.
- Anesthesia: local/regional block of the ankle joint versus conscious sedation.

Posterior ankle dislocation reduction technique:

1. Patient supine versus upright on stretcher (depends upon patient tolerance/provider preference); hip and knee flexed **(relaxes gastrocnemius muscle)** with foot in plantar flexion **(recreates original injury mechanism)**.
2. If assistant available, provide extremity stabilization with proximal, posterior traction on the lower leg.
3. Place one hand behind heel and one hand on dorsal foot; apply downward and anterior traction.
4. May hear "clunk" upon reduction, with return of essential perfusion.
5. Immobilize in 90° of ankle flexion **(neutral position)** with posterior short leg **(limits flexion/extension)** and associated "U" stirrup splint **(limits rotation)** (See Fig. 5.2).

Pearls:

- Evaluation of injury must sufficiently demonstrate ankle versus subtalar dislocation. Subtalar dislocations can have similar presentation, yet are reduced quite differently, leading to heightened patient morbidity.

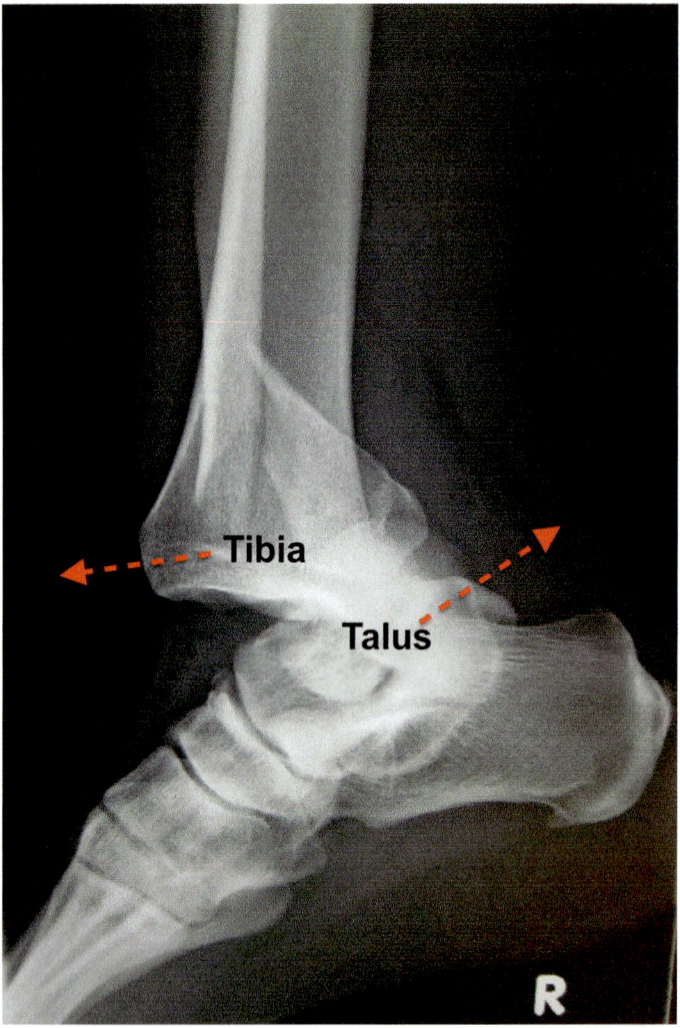

FIGURE 5.1 Posterior ankle (tibiotalar joint) dislocation. (Reprinted from James Heilman, MD: https://commons.wikimedia.org/wiki/File:Ankledislocation.JPG. With permission from Creative Commons Attribution: https://creativecommons.org/licenses/by-sa/3.0/deed.en)

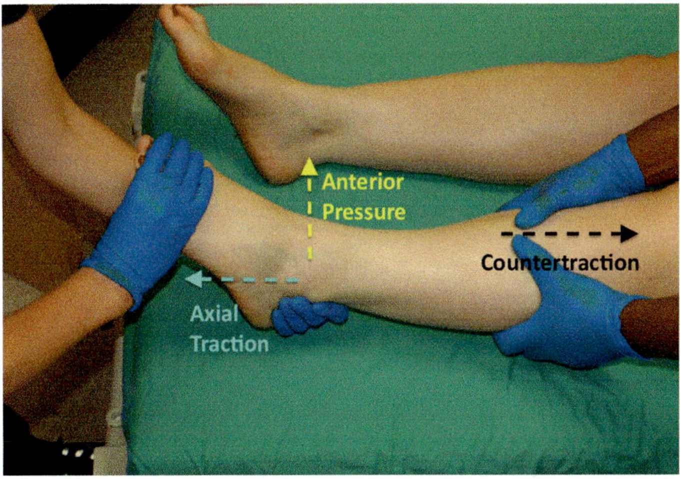

FIGURE 5.2 Posterior ankle dislocation reduction method. (Reprinted from John K, Kile J, Aghera A. Ankle dislocation reduction. In: Ganti L, editor. Atlas of emergency medicine procedures. New York: Springer; 2016. p. 615–8. With permission from Springer Nature)

- Keep knee flexed to aid in reduction; eliminate effect of gastrocnemius muscle that crosses both knee and ankle joints.
- ***Vascular compromise/"tented" skin is susceptible to ischemic necrosis/pending "open" fracture: reduce promptly and delay radiographic studies until after gross reduction/peripheral perfusion is restored.***
- **Subtalar dislocation: direction of dislocation delineated with respect to the position of the foot/calcaneus** (See Fig. 5.3).
  - Medial dislocations are more common, yet lateral dislocations are more likely to present with "open" injuries.
  - Foot will be locked in supination with medial dislocations versus pronation with lateral dislocations.

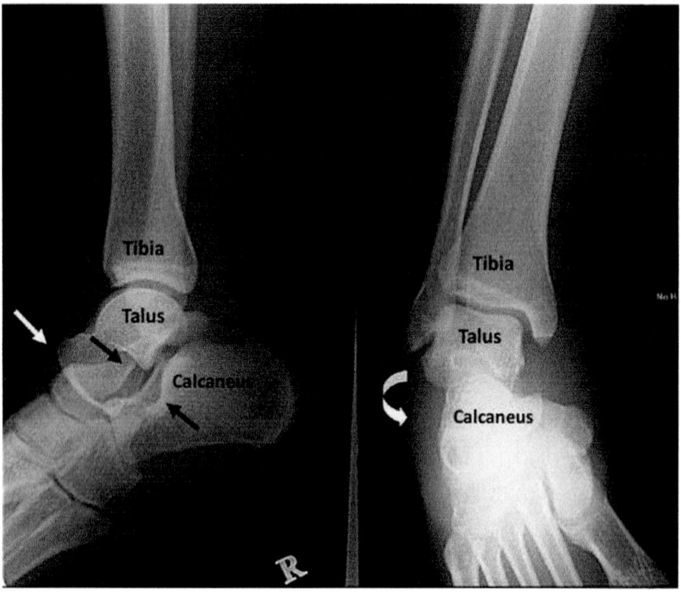

FIGURE 5.3 Medial subtalar ankle dislocation: (Left) Imaging of right ankle shows loss of talonavicular alignment (white arrow) and widening of the talocalcaneal joint (black arrows). (Right) Midfoot is medially displaced in relation to the ankle (curved arrow). (Reprinted from Pua U. Subtalar dislocation: rare and often forgotten. Int J Emerg Med. 2009;2(1):51–2. With permission from Springer Nature)

- Talar head will be superior to the navicular on lateral imaging in medial dislocations and co-linear/inferior with lateral injuries.
- Reduction maneuvers involve knee flexion, ankle plantarflexion, distraction and hindfoot inversion/eversion depending on the direction of dislocation.
- Medial dislocation reduction can be hindered by lateral soft tissue structures including the peroneal tendons and extensor digitorum brevis, while lateral dislocation reduction can be complicated by interposed medial structures, including the posterior tibial and flexor digitorum/hallucis tendons.

KNEE

- ***Orthopedic emergency - requires immediate reduction.***
- Dislocation uncommon due to strong ligamentous support (anterior/posterior cruciate and medial/lateral collateral ligaments).
- Direction of dislocation is described with respect to the position of the tibia in relation to the femur (See Fig. 5.4).
- Requires at least three of the four major knee ligaments to be disrupted.
- ***Most important aspect of clinical assessment: perfusion status of distal extremity (10–30% have associated vascular injury which may be limb threatening).***
- Injury to popliteal artery is commonplace secondary to tethering both proximally and distally (proximally as it

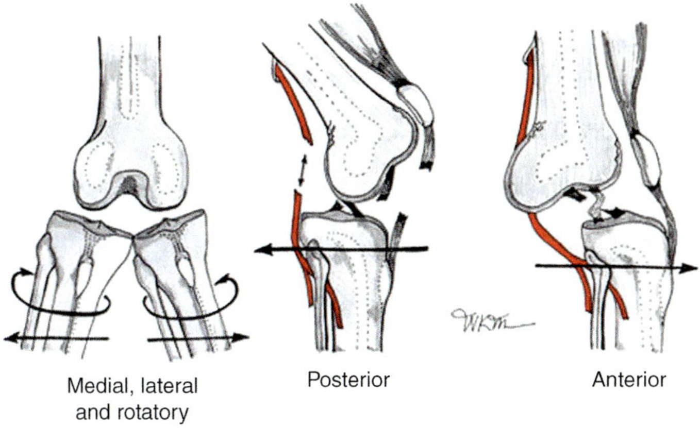

FIGURE 5.4 Knee dislocation: Direction delineated by position of the tibia. (Image reprinted with permission from Diku Mandavia, MD, FACEP, FRCPC, Cedars-Sinai Medical Center and Los Angeles County-USC Medical Center, published by Medscape Drugs & Diseases (http://emedicine.medscape.com/), 2017, available at: http://emedicine.medscape.com/article/823589-overview)

emerges from the adductor hiatus and distally at the tendinous arch of the soleus muscle).

- Anterior dislocations can exert traction effects on the popliteal artery resulting in intimal tears, while posterior dislocations generally result in complete tears.
- ***Can have normal pulses with popliteal artery injury***, thus check ankle-brachial index (ABI) to assess distal perfusion (<0.9 requires vascular consult +/– an arteriogram).
- Dorsalis pedis pulse: palpated on dorsum of foot immediately lateral to the EHL tendon, just distal to the most prominent aspect of the navicular bone.
- Posterior tibial pulse: palpated at level of the ankle joint, midway posterior to the medial malleolus, and anterior to the Achilles tendon (Pimenta's point).

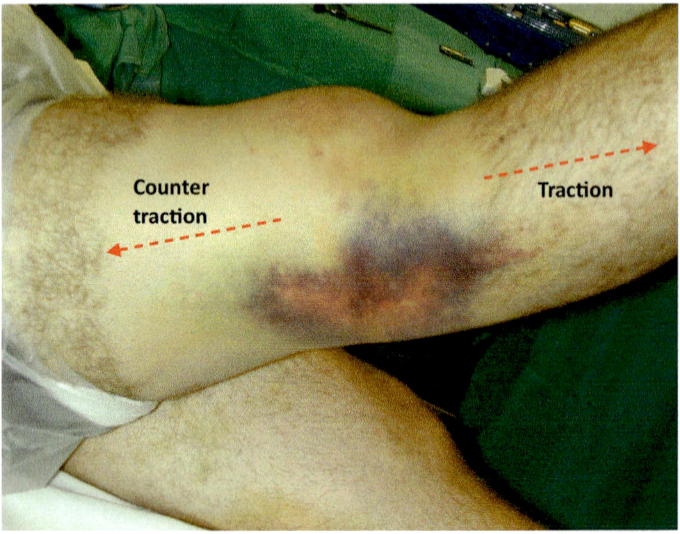

FIGURE 5.5 Global reduction mechanism for knee dislocation. (Image reprinted with permission from Brett D Owens, MD, Keller Army Hospital and Uniformed Services University of the Health Sciences, published by Medscape Drugs & Diseases (http://emedicine.medscape.com/), 2016, available at: http://emedicine.medscape.com/article/1250829-overview)

Anterior dislocation reduction technique:

1. Assistant provides gentle longitudinal traction.
2. One hand lifts femur anteriorly, while one guides tibia posteriorly.
3. Place in posterior splint in ~20° of flexion or knee immobilizer (KI) (See Fig. 5.6).

Posterior dislocation reduction technique:

1. Assistant provides gentle longitudinal traction.
2. One hand directs the femur posteriorly, while one lifts the tibia anteriorly.
3. Place in posterior splint in ~20° of flexion versus KI (See Fig. 5.7).

Pearls:

- Be sure to correct for any rotational component that may be present.
- Beware of "spontaneous" reduction (50% of knee dislocations spontaneously reduce prior to initial evaluation); requires a high index of suspicion based upon injury mechanism and clinical presentation.
- Exam clues: knee pain, hemarthrosis with posterior knee/calf hemorrhage and/or ecchymosis, and diffuse ligamentous laxity/instability.
- Reduction assessment: ***lateral X-ray is key; must be anatomic or will require supplemental rigid fixation.***
- "Hard signs" of arterial injury can be delayed 24–48 hrs with popliteal artery disruption; thus evaluation of ABI is a better assessment of distal perfusion.
- ***All knee dislocations require hospital admission for serial monitoring:***
  - ABI >0.9 requires observation for serial perfusion assessment, while ABI <0.9 requires vascular surgery assessment +/– arteriogram/revascularization.

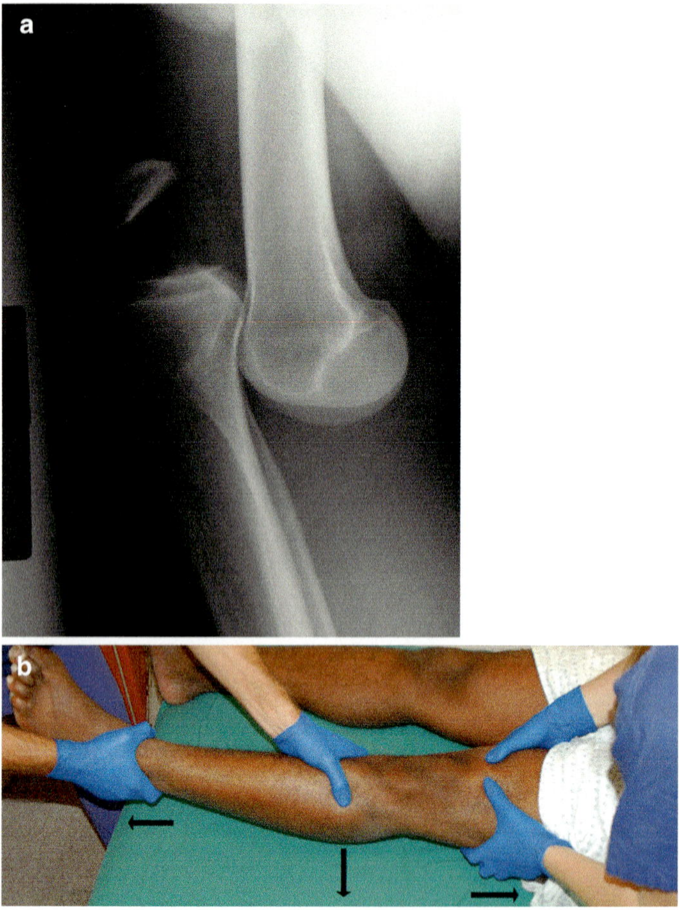

FIGURE 5.6 Anterior knee dislocation: (**a**) lateral X-ray, (**b**) reduction technique. (**a**: Image reprinted with permission from Brett D Owens, MD, F Edward Hebert School of Medicine, Uniformed Services University of Health Sciences, Keller Army Hospital, and Texas Tech University Health Sciences Center, Paul L Foster School of Medicine, published by Medscape Drugs & Diseases (http://emedicine.medscape.com/), 2017, available at: http://emedicine.medscape.com/article/1250829-overview. **b**: Reprinted from John K, Kile J, Aghera A. Knee dislocation reduction. In: Ganti L, editor. Atlas of emergency medicine procedures. New York: Springer; 2016. p. 607–13. With permission from Springer Science + Business Media)

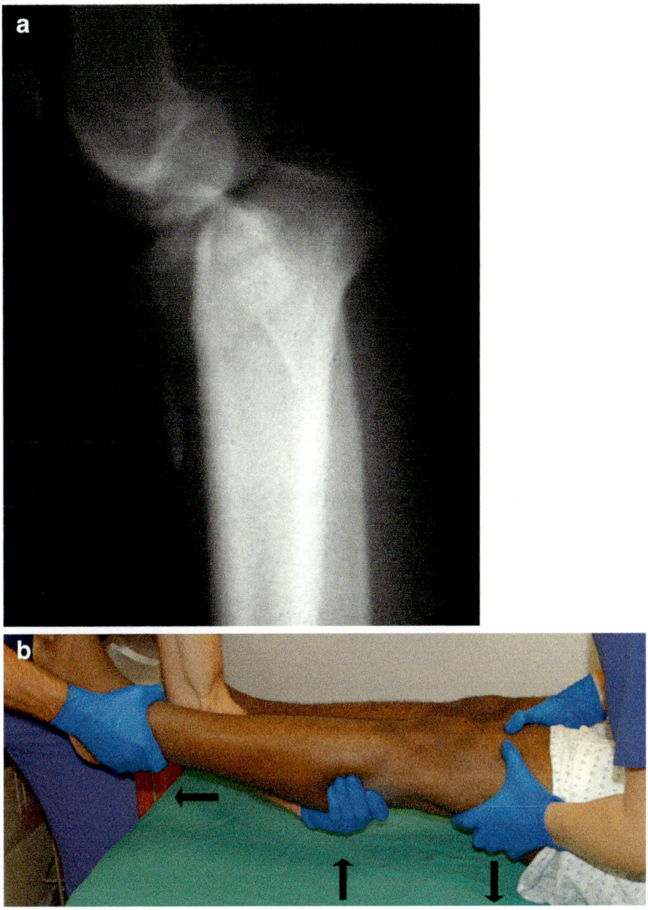

FIGURE 5.7 Posterior knee dislocation (**a**): lateral X-ray, (**b**) reduction technique. (**a**: Image reprinted with permission from Diku Mandavia, MD, FACEP, FRCPC, Cedars-Sinai Medical Center and Los Angeles County-USC Medical Center, published by Medscape Drugs & Diseases (http://emedicine.medscape.com/), 2017, available at: http://emedicine.medscape.com/article/823589-overview. **b**: Reprinted from John K, Kile J, Aghera A. Knee dislocation reduction. In: Ganti L, editor. Atlas of emergency medicine procedures. New York: Springer; 2016. p. 607–13. With permission from Springer Science + Business Media)

- Revascularization, if necessary, should be performed within 8 hrs of injury, +/– external fixation, and/or lower extremity fasciotomy to prevent reperfusion damage and optimize long-term outcomes.
- Nerve injury is less common, but peroneal nerve damage is a highly recognized complication (25–35% of patients); manifests with decreased sensation at first dorsal web space and impaired ankle dorsiflexion (50% of neurological deficits are permanent).
- Posterolateral dislocations may be irreducible secondary to medial femoral condyle "buttonholing" through medial joint capsule (manifests as "dimple sign" at medial joint line).
- Posterior knee dislocations are common in dashboard injuries (axial loading of flexed knee); occurs in combination with PCL/PLC injuries, posterior hip dislocations, and/or acetabular injuries (posterior wall most common).
- Be wary of dislocation following total knee arthroplasty (less common than following total hip replacement). ***If distal perfusion impaired, treat as native dislocation emergency***; otherwise contact orthopedics for treatment directives.

PATELLA

- Most common direction of dislocation: lateral
- Typically caused by direct blow or sudden twisting, +/– rotation of lower extremity; causes forced internal/external rotation of femur on firmly planted tibia with knee in flexion. Can also occur with forced contraction of the quadriceps with the knee in flexion
- Patient presentation: inability to extend an obviously deformed knee; with spontaneous reduction, can have similar presentation to those that have experienced isolated/combined ligamentous and/or meniscal injuries (See Fig. 5.8)

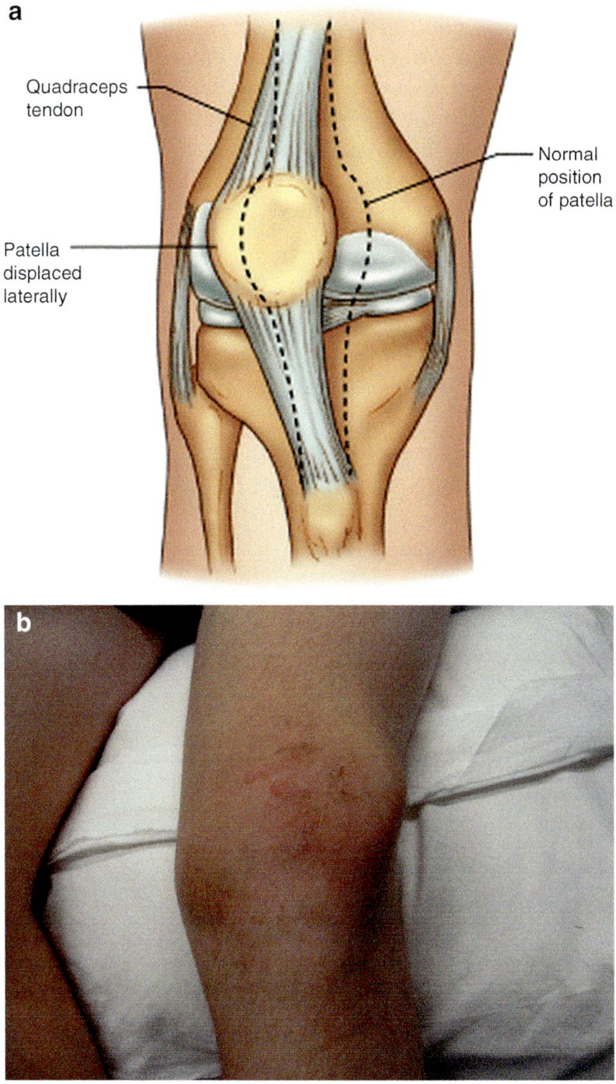

FIGURE 5.8 Lateral patella dislocation: (**a**) Schematic demonstrating abnormal patella movement (**b**) Note lateral position of patella. (**a**: © 2017 Reed Group, Ltd. Reproduced from MDGuidelines® with permission from Reed Group. All rights reserved. **b**: Used with permission from: http://lifeinthefastlane.com/patella-dislocation/)

Lateral dislocation reduction technique:

- Patient placed in supine versus upright position, with affected leg placed over edge of stretcher.
- Extension of lower leg in combination with gentle medial pressure, lifting lateral patellar edge over femoral condyle, generally allows for patella relocation (See Fig. 5.9).

Pearls:

- ***Patella dislocations are extremely different than knee dislocations*, with the latter being life/limb threatening!**
- Obtain axial imaging of knee joint to assess patella congruence, +/– patella tilt, and adequacy of the trochlear groove.
- Significant tenderness near medial retinaculum may suggest torn tendinous structure; MPFL (medial patellofemoral ligament) is major medial soft-tissue restraint against lateral patella dislocation.

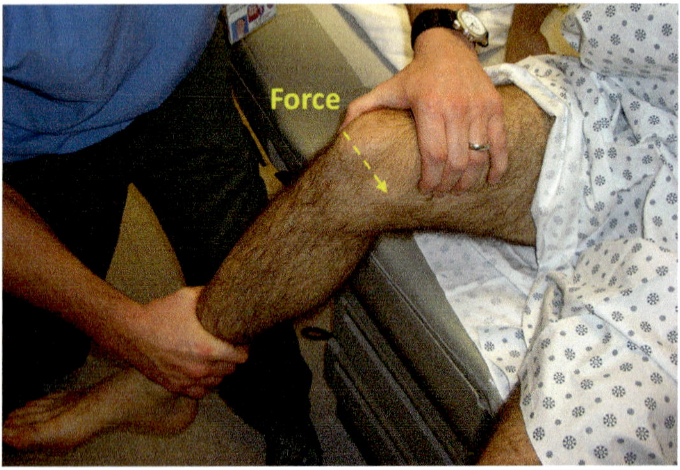

Figure 5.9 Lateral patella dislocation reduction technique. (Image reprinted with permission from Medscape Drugs & Diseases (http://emedicine.medscape.com/), 2016, available at: http://emedicine.medscape.com/article/109263-overview)

- Post-reduction: place in static knee immobilizer, obtain x-ray (assess patella height/location, presence of fractures, etc.) and provide orthopedic follow-up for re-evaluation.
- If unsure of post-reduction assessment (e.g., patella height), image contralateral knee for comparison.
- Immediate goals are to reduce inflammation, relieve pain, and refrain from activities that place excessive load(s) across the patellofemoral joint (e.g., kneeling, squatting, etc.).
- *PRICE principles:* protection of injured joint, relative rest, ice, compression, and elevation.
- Aggressive physical therapy should be implemented as appropriate to heighten quadriceps tone/strength, particularly the VMO (vastus medial obliquus) muscle.

HIP

- *****Native hip dislocation = Orthopedic emergency requires immediate reduction.*****
- Native hip dislocations require inherently massive forces based upon intrinsic stability of hip joint. Timely reduction, assessment of stability, and detection of associated injuries are paramount to achieving an enduring functional result.
- ***Any patient with a native hip dislocation must be evaluated for femoral neck fracture prior to manipulation***. Missing this associated injury may dramatically alter treatment, heighten risk of avascular necrosis (AVN), and cause associated life-altering consequences.
- Up to 50% of patients sustain concomitant fractures at time of dislocation ***(most common: posterior wall acetabular fractures)***.
- ***Majority of dislocations are posterior*** (~90%) and occur secondary to axial loading of flexed/adducted hip, leading to a ***shortened, adducted and internally rotated extremity*** (consider along with knee dislocations, PCL/PLC injuries, and acetabular injuries in dashboard injury mechanism).
- Sciatic nerve palsy is present in ~10–15% of cases, with the peroneal division (e.g., ankle dorsiflexion) preferentially affected.

- ***Anterior dislocations*** assume an abducted and externally rotated position, with the degree of hip flexion at the time of injury determining whether the dislocation is also inferior/superior (See Fig. 5.10).

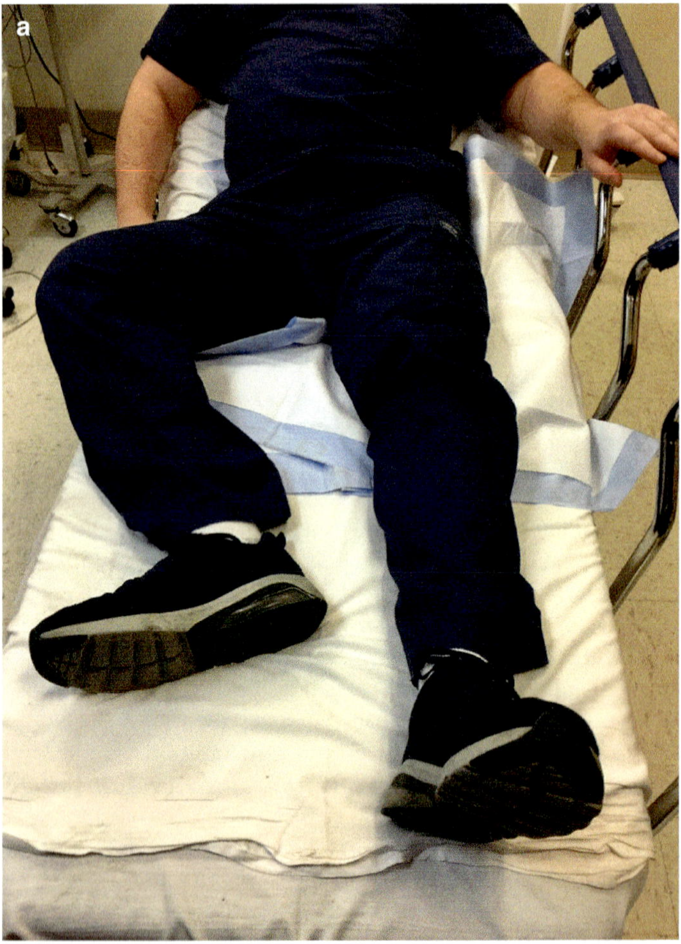

FIGURE 5.10 Anterior hip dislocation: (**a**) leg abducted and externally rotated, (**b**) AP X-ray, (**c**) lateral X-ray. (**b**, **c**: Reprinted from Kim J, Bishop C, Lycans D, Day JB. Hip dislocations. In: Eltorai A, Eberson C, Daniels A, editors. Orthopedic surgery clerkship. Cham: Springer; 2017. p. 267–71. With permission from Springer Nature)

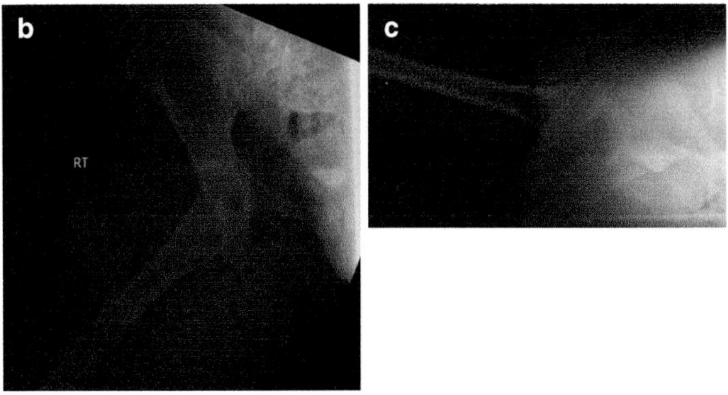

FIGURE 5.10 (continued)

Posterior hip dislocation reduction techniques:

A. Allis maneuver (*Reverse Stimson*):

1. Patient placed supine on stretcher, with hip and knee flexed to 90°.
2. Assistant secures patient pelvis to stretcher to provide stabilization against distraction.
3. While standing above the patient, initially apply an inferior force to disengage the femoral head from behind the acetabulum, and then apply upward traction to proximal/posterior calf +/− gentle internal/external rotation.
4. Successful reduction usually signified via an audible and/or palpable clunk, with return of appreciable leg length (See Fig. 5.11).

B. Captain Morgan:

1. Patient placed supine, hip and knee flexed to ~90°; patient pelvis stabilized as above.
2. Physician places one foot on stretcher, flexing knee of affected leg, and allowing patient calf to rest on examiner's knee.
3. Stabilize lower extremity of patient, while exerting upward force by performing calf raise (plantar-flexing your ankle) +/− external/internal rotation of lower leg to effect reduction (See Fig. 5.12).

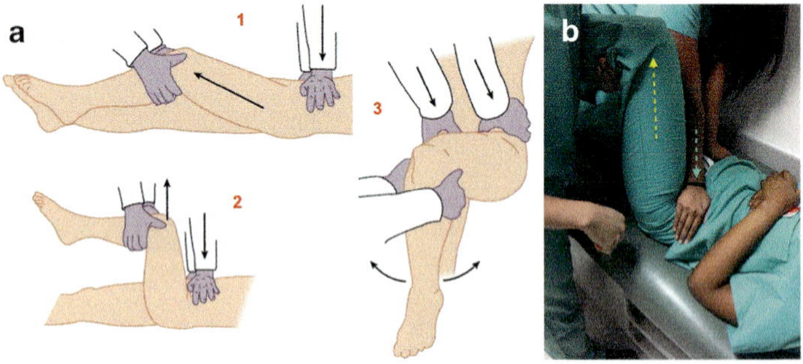

FIGURE 5.11 Allis maneuver: (**a**) (1) note the initial force to disengage the femoral head from behind the acetabulum, (2) traction and countertraction, (3) gentle internal/external rotation (**b**) 90° flexion of the hip with continued traction away from the pelvis. (**a**: Reprinted from: https://wikem.org/wiki/File:Hip_Reduction.jpg#filelinks. With permission from Creative Commons Attribution: https://creativecommons.org/licenses/by-sa/4.0/)

C. Whistler technique:

1. Unaffected leg slightly flexed, with affected hip flexed to ~90° (assistant stabilizes patient pelvis).
2. Examiner places his/her forearm in popliteal fossa under affected leg and grasps knee of the unaffected leg.
3. Free hand then secures control of the distal tibial region of the affected leg.
4. While pulling inferior traction on the lower leg of the affected extremity, this effectively flexes the knee, pulling traction along the proximal femur; internal/external rotation of the lower leg can also facilitate reduction (See Fig. 5.13).

Pearls:

- Classic injury presentations can be dramatically altered with accompanying pathology. High level of suspicion must exist in patients unable to provide a history of injury events.
- AP pelvis view: femoral head will appear smaller on affected side versus uninjured side in posterior dislocations, and will appear larger in anterior dislocations.

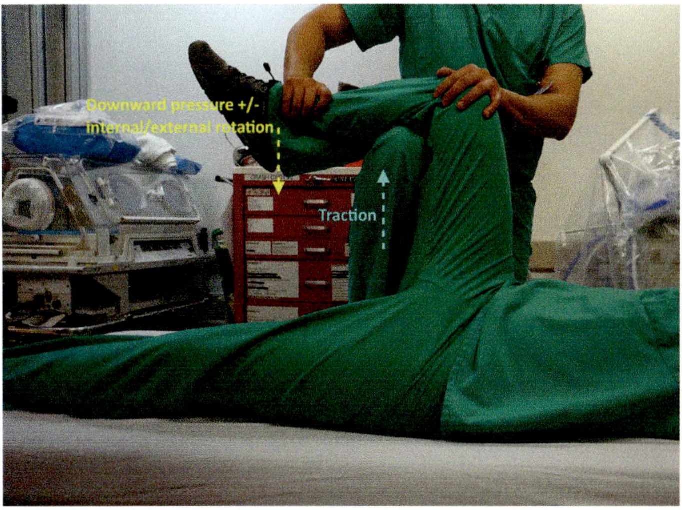

FIGURE 5.12 Captain Morgan technique: allows application of three traction forces across the femur (pelvic stabilization required prior to initiation)

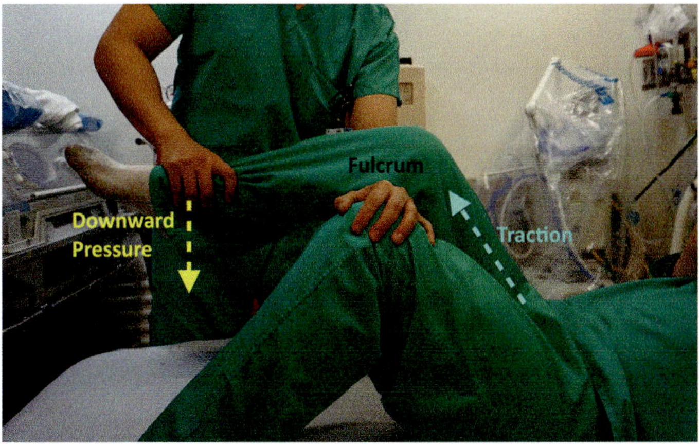

FIGURE 5.13 Whistler technique: Examiner forearm serves as fulcrum, while the affected lower leg comprises the lever (pelvic stabilization required prior to initiation)

- AVN is commonly associated with hip dislocations because the medial femoral circumflex artery (dominant blood supply to femoral head) can be stretched and/or occluded. Overall rate of AVN following hip dislocations is 15%, but increases to 20% with associated femoral head fractures.
- ***Appropriate sedation is an often overlooked component; patient/muscle relaxation will facilitate reduction.***
- Sciatic nerve palsy is another common complication: 10–15% of adult traumatic hip dislocations are accompanied by sciatic nerve palsy; 60–70% of cases will partially or entirely resolve; documentation of sciatic nerve function should be performed ***before and after*** any attempts at reduction.
- Appropriate consent, including risks of sedation, fracture, loss/diminished sciatic nerve function and potential of unsuccessful result necessitating need for "open" reduction, must be obtained.
- Once reduced, hip joint stability and maintenance of concentric reduction must be assessed via active hip flexion, post-reduction radiographs +/– CT scan.
- If the hip joint is irreducible, there may be an anatomic block to reduction (requiring surgery), or the joint may be too unstable with respect to associated injuries (e.g., large posterior wall acetabular fracture).
- If repeat hip dislocation occurs upon dynamic testing (70–90° of flexion, neutral rotation, with posterior-directed force), the joint may require temporary traction pin placement to maintain congruency. However, this modality must be considered with respect to patient age (generally contraindicated in pediatric patients and is questionable in elderly osteoporotic patients), as well as in those with associated injuries (open wounds, ipsilateral extremity fractures, etc.).
- Posterior dislocation management: if determined stable, static knee immobilizer protects against excessive flexion, adduction, and internal rotation. If no fracture is present, protected weight-bearing with associated activity precautions may be implemented until orthopedic re-evaluation.

Anterior hip dislocation reduction technique:

– The patient is placed supine on the stretcher, and an assistant applies downward pressure on the femoral head.

- Longitudinal traction is applied in line with the femur.
- The hip is then hyperextended and internally rotated to allow for reduction.
- **Prosthetic hip dislocation:** major causes include patients assuming positions that exceed stability of prosthesis, soft tissue imbalance, and/or component malposition.

ELBOW

- In adults, the elbow is the second most frequently dislocated major joint following the shoulder; it is the most commonly dislocated joint in children.

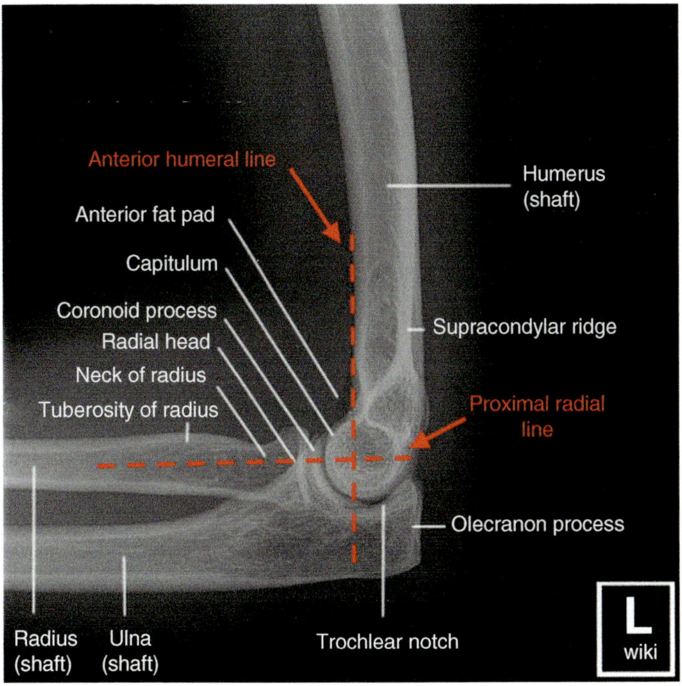

FIGURE 5.14 Normal lateral elbow X-ray. (Used with permission from: http://www.wikiradiography.net/page/Lateral+Scapula+Radiography)

- Direction of dislocation is determined by position of the ulna in relation to the distal humerus: ***>90% dislocations are posterior*** (See Fig. 5.15).
- Coronoid process of the ulna disengages from the trochlea of the humerus; mechanism typically involves a fall onto an outstretched hand (FOOSH) with the elbow in extension.
- Simple posterior dislocations (without fracture) generally require correction of medial/lateral displacement, longitudinal traction, and flexion for successful reduction.

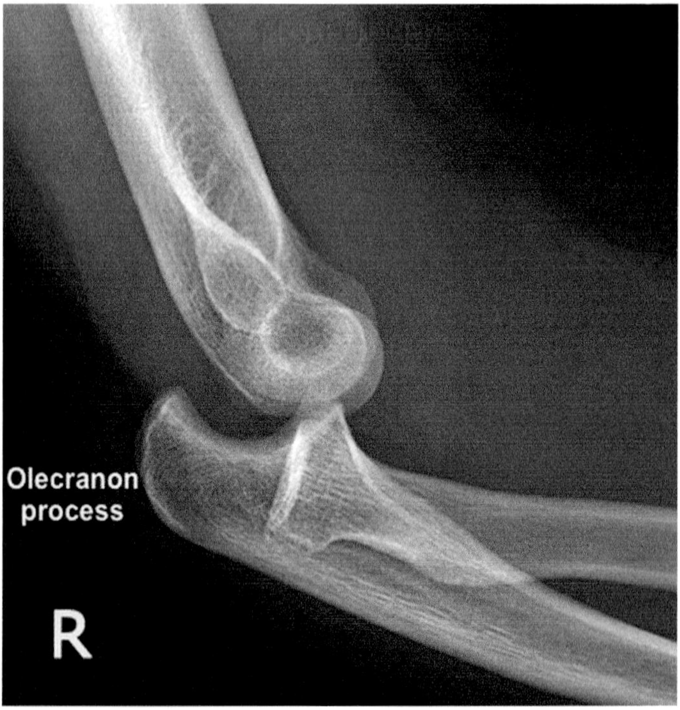

FIGURE 5.15 Posterior elbow dislocation. (Used with permission from: http://www.wikiradiography.net/page/Elbow+Dislocations)

Posterior elbow reduction techniques:

A. ***Parvin method:***

1. Patient is placed in prone position with humerus resting on stretcher and forearm hanging in perpendicular fashion (humerus should be supported, with padding just proximal to the elbow joint).
2. Apply 5–10 lbs of weight to wrist and/or gently pull down at wrist while guiding olecranon into place (See Fig. 5.16).

B. ***Flexion-traction method:***

****Supine positioning may be better for obese patients or those with potential for respiratory compromise.****

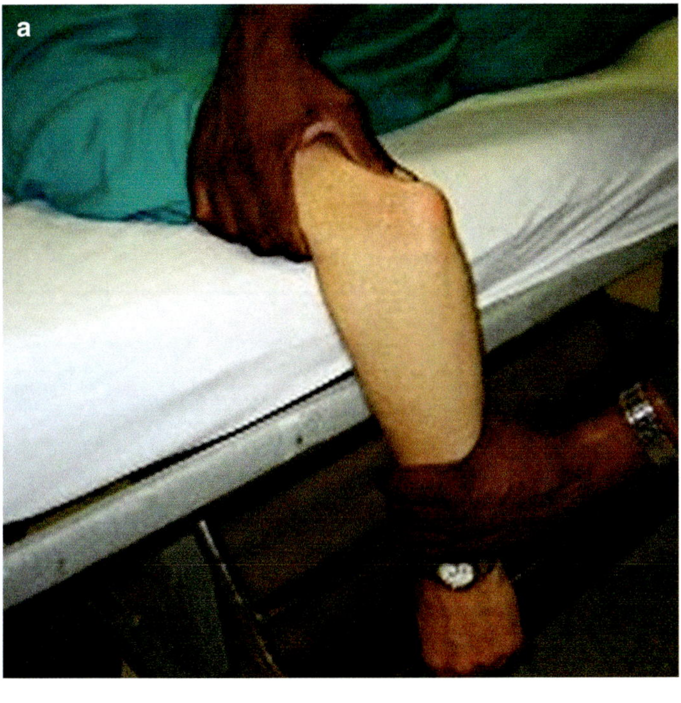

FIGURE 5.16 Elbow reduction techniques: (**a**) Parvin method alone; (**b**) with assistant. (**a**, **b**: Image reprinted with permission from Medscape Drugs & Diseases (http://emedicine.medscape.com/), 2016, available at: http://emedicine.medscape.com/article/109168-overview)

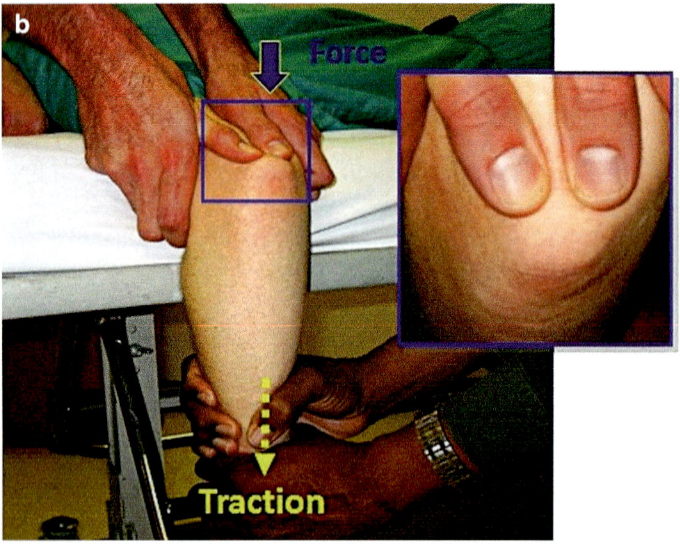

FIGURE 5.16 (continued)

1. Patient is placed in supine/upright position while assistant stabilizes humerus with forearm in supination.
2. Examiner then grasps the wrist and applies slow, steady in-line traction with wrist supinated, simultaneously correcting medial/lateral displacement.

Be sure to maintain the elbow in a slightly flexed position to avoid engaging the triceps mechanism.

3. Reduction is signified by audible/palpable clunk as the olecranon once again engages the humeral articular surface (See Fig. 5.17).

Pearls:

- Examine ipsilateral upper extremity for associated injuries (neurovascular deficits, shoulder/wrist fractures, disruption of distal radioulnar joint (DRUJ), etc.).
- ***Radial pulse* can be present even with *brachial artery injury*** secondary to effects of collateral circulation.

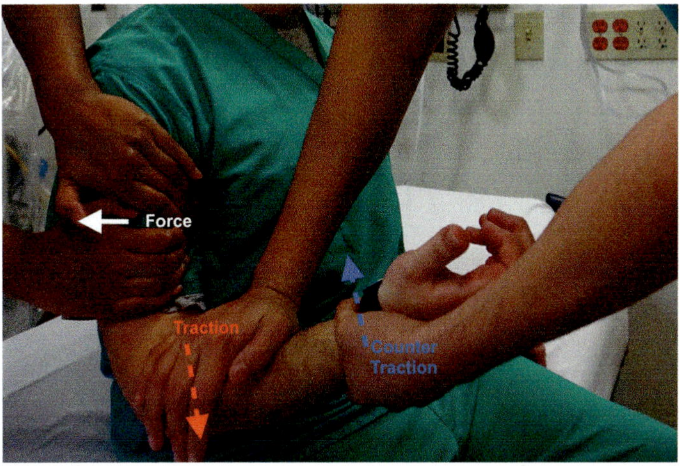

FIGURE 5.17 Flexion-traction method: Note traction and counter-traction

- Ulnar nerve is the most commonly injured neurologic structure. Always test its motor function (finger abduction/adduction) and sensory function (ulnar side dorsal hand) ***before and after*** reduction.
- Assure appropriate analgesia +/– sedation before reduction attempt to optimize potential outcome.
- Ulnar collateral ligament (UCL): anterior bundle is the primary valgus (medial) stabilizer of the elbow joint.
- Once reduction achieved, elbow joint should immediately be placed through gentle ROM to ensure reduction is stable and no mechanical block to movement exists.
- Elbow usually stable in >90° flexion, however, is clinically more relevant if stable at 30° flexion with respect to potential need for surgical intervention and long-term outcomes. If unstable at 30° flexion, maximally pronate forearm to heighten stress on the UCL, which generally prohibits posterolateral subluxation ***(immobilize in pronation)***.
- Post-reduction immobilization requires a posterior long-arm splint with an accompanying sling for comfort.

- Always obtain post-reduction radiographs to assess elbow joint congruency +/− presence of associated fractures.
- **Potential complications:**
  - Loss of elbow motion (commonly experience decreased elbow extension with prolonged immobilization); orthopedic re-evaluation should take place within 1 week, whereby gentle ROM usually initiated to diminish this potential (assuming no significant instability exists).
  - Valgus instability.
  - Neurovascular injury.
  - Heterotopic ossification.

- **Terrible triad injury:** elbow dislocation, radial head/neck, and coronoid process fractures.
- Anterior dislocations **(RARE)**: more commonly associated with severe injuries (consider early orthopedic consultation); reduction involves in-line traction with a posterior-directed force placed on the proximal forearm; as above, an assistant should provide countertraction with respect to stabilization of the humerus.

RADIAL HEAD

- Dislocation occurs most frequently in combination with other injuries (e.g., elbow dislocations, Monteggia fractures, etc.); ***isolated radial head dislocations are rare***.
- Patient typically holds the elbow flexed at 90°, resists elbow ROM (including pronation and supination), and is tender to palpation over radial head region.

Reduction techniques:

A. Supination/flexion maneuver:

1. Patient seated upright, comfortable, with elbow flexed to 90°.

2. The examiner grasps affected side wrist with one hand and elbow with the other hand; thumb should be placed over radial head.
3. Forearm should be supinated first and then flexed in one continuous motion until reduction achieved (See Fig. 5.18).

B. Hyper-pronation maneuver:

1. Patient positioned as above.
2. Same positioning by examiner, but forearm instead hyper-pronated and then flexed to effect reduction.

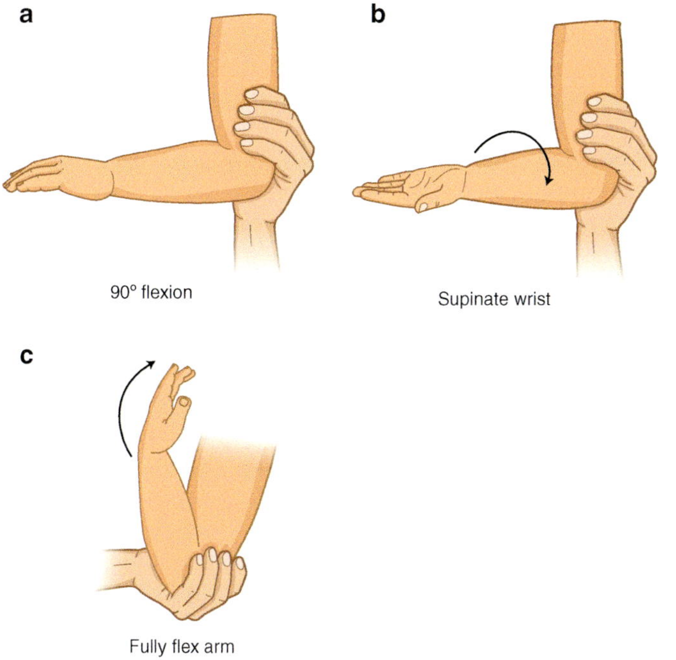

FIGURE 5.18 (**a**–**c**) Flexion/supination maneuver. (Images reprinted with permission from Medscape Drugs & Diseases (http://emedicine.medscape.com/), 2017, available at: http://emedicine.medscape.com/article/104158-overview)

Pearls:

- Most injuries occur in pronated position, thus immobilization should occur in posterior long arm versus sugar tong splint, with forearm in supinated position at ~90° elbow flexion.
- Posterior interosseous nerve (PIN) is most commonly injured neurovascular structure; damage results in weakness of finger and/or thumb extension; post-reduction neurapraxia is often a temporary problem, generally resolving spontaneously.
- ***Nursemaid's elbow:*** pediatric isolated radial head dislocation: classic mechanism involves longitudinal traction on arm with wrist in pronation (e.g., child lifted up by wrist). Pathologic lesion is interposition/tear of the annular ligament attachment to the radial neck periosteum that becomes entrapped between the radial head and capitellum.
  ****Reduction methods are identical to those described for adult radial head dislocations.****

  - Typical patient presents in no distress, with arm held slightly flexed and pronated at side. Radiographs generally not needed with minimally tender radial head region, regardless of history. Reduction generally performed without pre-medication, with full, unrestricted arm use generally evident within 15–30 min; no immobilization/post-reduction radiographs are necessary. *****Many encounters will not elicit audible/palpable click despite successful reduction.*****
  - Because other pathology may rarely mimic this condition (e.g., occult fractures, osteomyelitis, joint infection, tumors, etc.), full, unrestricted, and painless use of the arm should be evident by 24 hrs after reduction, or further evaluation should be initiated.

Radial head dislocations are easily missed on radiographs, thus requiring high index of suspicion (See Fig. 5.19).

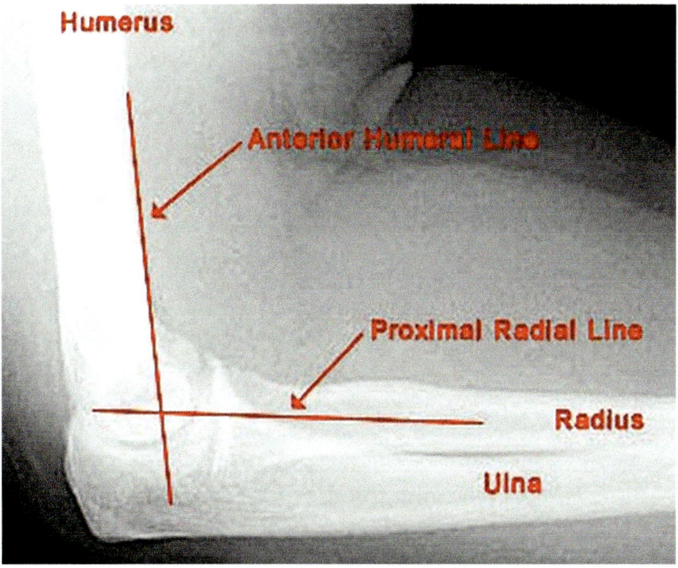

FIGURE 5.19 Normal elbow radiograph: Anterior humeral line should intersect the middle third of the capitulum, and the radial line should engage its center. (Reprinted from: http://skeletaltrauma.wikispaces.com/Elbow. With permission from Creative Commons Attribution: https://creativecommons.org/licenses/by-sa/3.0/)

SHOULDER

Anterior dislocations:

- Most common direction of dislocation (>90% of presentations).
- Typically presents with "squared-off" shoulder (humeral head located inferomedially relative to normal anatomic position).
- Patients with anterior dislocation generally hold injured extremity slightly abducted, in external rotation *(adduction/IR are limited).*
- Routine imaging includes anteroposterior (AP) and axillary lateral views. ("Scapular Y" view is often substituted for the

latter). ***Key image is* the axillary view**; if cannot be obtained (consider Velpeau view), CT scan recommended to ensure "true orthogonal" imaging (false negative results possible when employing "Scapular Y" view).

- AP view: anteriorly dislocated humeral head lies in subcoracoid/subglenoid position.
- **Axillary view:** humeral head falls anterior to glenoid *(identify coracoid process, an anterior structure, to assess A-P orientation).*
- **"Scapular Y" view** is taken with beam directed parallel to scapular body; Y formed by scapular body, spine, and coracoid process; glenoid falls in center of Y. With an anterior dislocation, humeral head will appear medial/anterior to Y formation (See Fig. 5.20).
- Anterior dislocations can be associated with:
  - **Hill-Sachs lesion**: compression fracture of posterolateral humeral head
  - **Bankart lesion/fracture**: detachment of anteroinferior aspect of glenoid rim +/− fracture (Bony Bankart); occurs following humeral head forcefully contacting glenoid rim during dislocation process
  - Greater tuberosity fractures with concomitant rotator cuff tears and/or avulsions (See Fig. 5.21)

Posterior dislocations:

- Associated with seizures, electrical injuries, and/or voluntary dislocations.
- Mechanism of injury is a combination of flexion, adduction, and IR.
- Usually results from forceful contraction of internal rotator musculature (subscapularis, latissimus dorsi, pectoralis major), which is significantly more forceful than external rotator grouping.

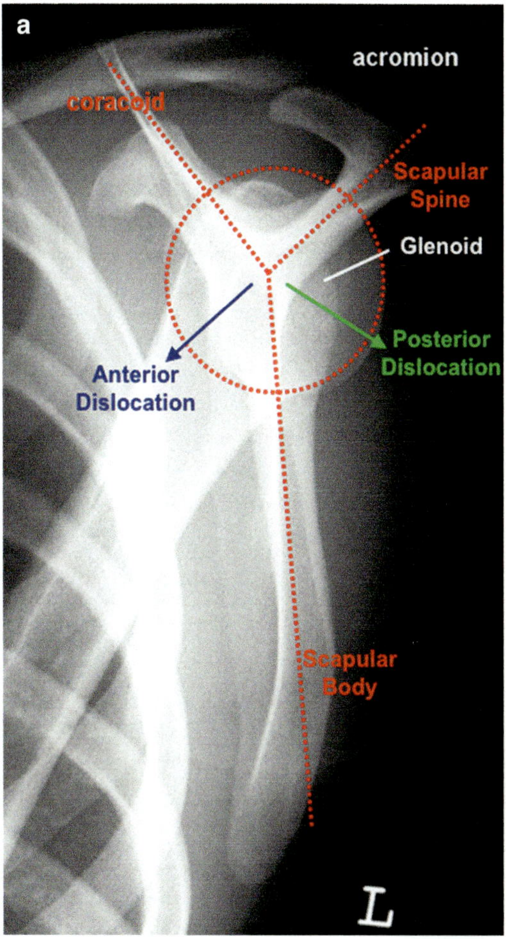

FIGURE 5.20 Scapular "Y" view: (**a**) normal, (**b**) anteroinferior shoulder dislocation. (**a**: Used with permission from: http://www.wikiradiography.net/page/Lateral+Scapula+Radiography. **b**: Image reprinted with permission from Medscape Drugs & Diseases (http://emedicine.medscape.com/), Shoulder Dislocation Imaging, 2017, available at: http://emedicine.medscape.com/article/395520-overview)

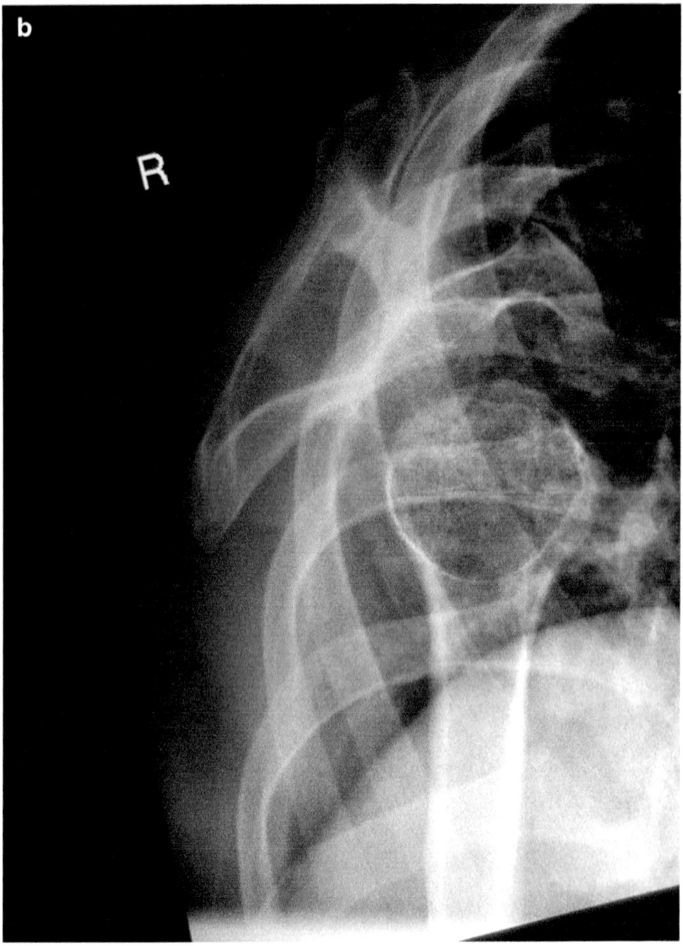

FIGURE 5.20 (continued)

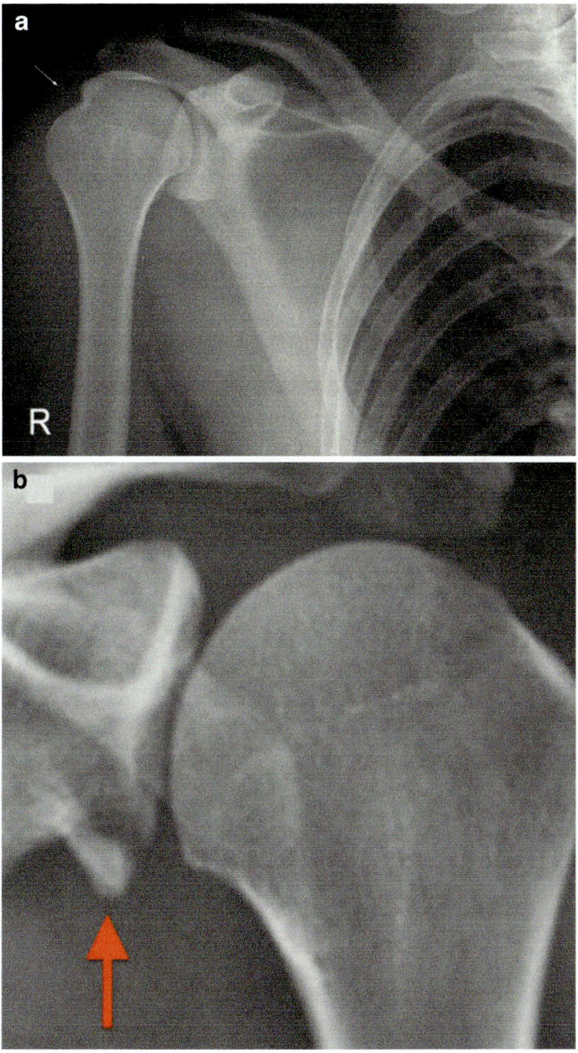

FIGURE 5.21 Shoulder X-ray: (**a**) Hill-Sachs lesion. (**b**) Bony Bankart lesion. (**a**: Used with permission from: http://www.wikiradiography.net/page/Hill-Sachs+and+Bankart+Lesions. **b**: Reprinted from Jaeger M, Izadpanah K, Südkamp NP. Posttraumatic shoulder instability. In: Oestern HJ, Trentz O, Uranues S, editors. Bone and joint injuries. European manual of medicine. Berlin/Heidelberg: Springer-Verlag; 2014. p. 13–23. With permission from Springer Nature)

- Patient will generally hold affected extremity in adduction/internal rotation and likely not be able to fully/actively externally rotate arm at 90° of elbow flexion.
- ***Extension of elbow with forearm in supination can obscure meaningful loss of external rotation***; failure to diagnose and treat a posterior dislocation can lead to recurrent dislocation/instability, AVN of humeral head, accelerated degenerative disease, limited active ROM, and chronic pain (See Figs. 5.22 and 5.23).

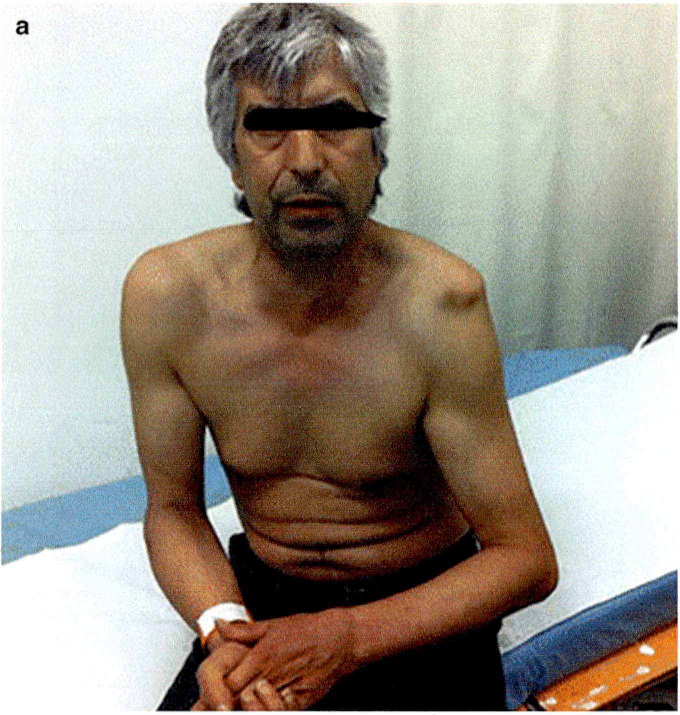

FIGURE 5.22 External appearance shoulder dislocation: (**a**) Anterior dislocation; (**b**) Posterior dislocation **Note prominence of coracoid process anteriorly**. (**a**: Reprinted from Gomes N, Sevivas N, Randelli P, Safran M. Shoulder instability. In: Espregueira-Mendes J, et al., editors. Injuries and health problems in football. Berlin/Heidelberg: Springer; 2017. p. 335–52. With permission from Springer Nature. **b**: Courtesy of Martin Krause)

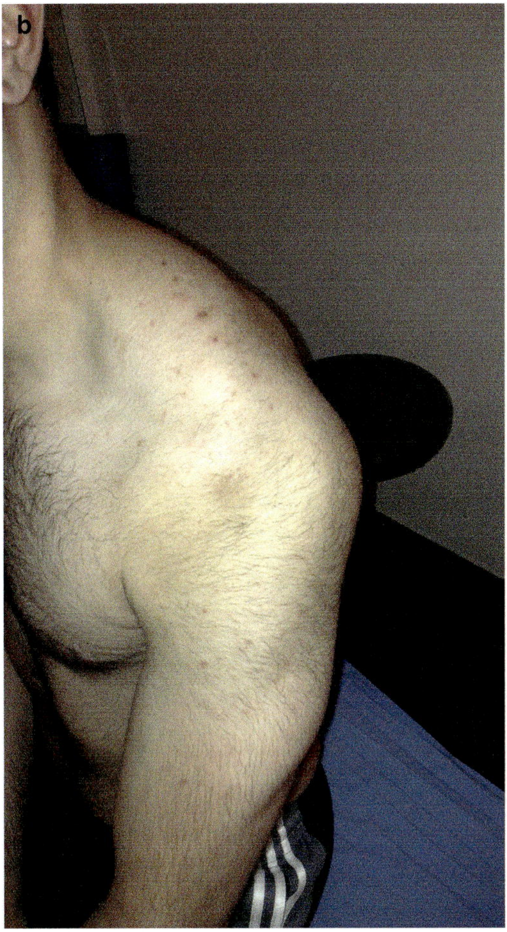

FIGURE 5.22 (continued)

Imaging clues to posterior dislocation:

- AP imaging: internally rotated humeral head may appear symmetric in shape of "light bulb" (depending upon amount of rotation) versus normal club-shaped appearance created by native greater tuberosity.

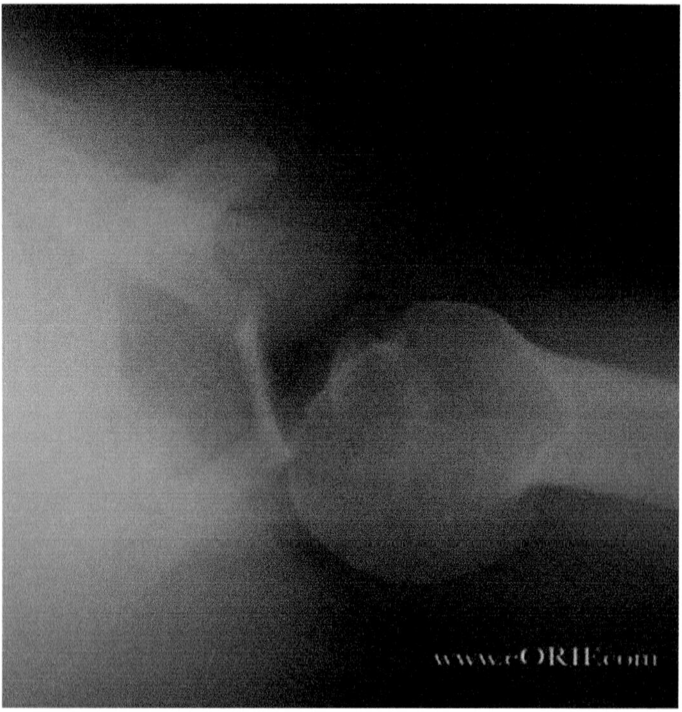

Figure 5.23 Posterior dislocation axillary view. (Reprinted from http://eorif.com/shoulder-dislocation-images. With permission from eORIF, LLC)

- Axillary view: demonstrates humeral head posterior to glenoid.
- Scapular Y view: displays humeral head lateral to glenoid and beneath acromion.

Analgesia techniques:

- Options
  - PO, IV analgesia
  - Intra-articular injection +/– PO, IV analgesia
  - Conscious sedation

Intra-articular injection:

- Under sterile conditions, insert 18–20 gauge spinal needle ~2 cm inferior and ~2 cm medial to palpated superolateral edge of acromion into glenohumeral joint.
- Alternative technique (lateral): insert similar gauge needle ~1 cm inferolateral to palpated acromial edge, direct medially and caudally into glenohumeral joint.
- Following aspiration (hemarthrosis confirms in joint), inject ~10–20 mL of 1% lidocaine +/– bupivacaine (See Fig. 5.24).

Anterior dislocation reduction methods: (*not all inclusive*):

- ***Traction/countertraction***
- ***Milch***
- ***Scapular manipulation***
- ***External rotation***

A. ***Traction/countertraction technique:***

(a) Equipment: sheet or wide strap.
(b) Position: patient supine on stretcher, bed elevated to height of operator comfort for assurance of smooth, enduring muscle force application.
(c) Technique:

- Place sheet/strap over patient's upper chest, under back/axilla of affected shoulder; confirm both ends are of equal length and open to unaffected side.
- Standing on unaffected side, assistant should take firm hold of each end of sheet or securely tie sheet around his or her waist.
- Assistant will slowly begin to lean back to initiate continuous countertraction, implementing their body weight.
- While maintaining affected arm at 90° of elbow flexion, with both hands securely around forearm, examiner will then also apply continuous traction

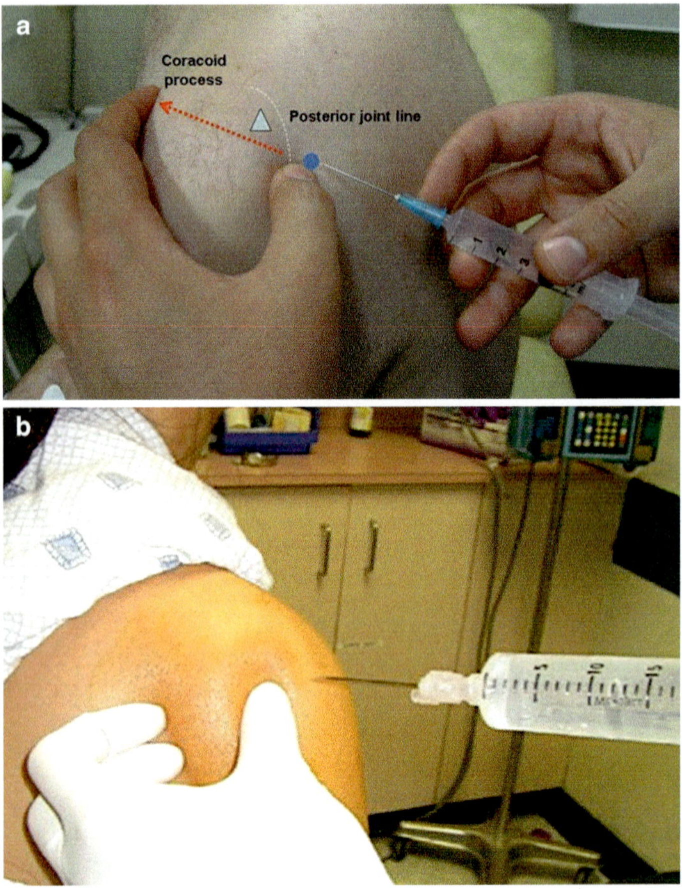

Figure 5.24 Intra-articular injection of glenohumeral joint: (**a**) posterior, (**b**) lateral. (**a**: Reprinted from Zayat AS, Wakefield RJ. Arthrocentesis in the elderly. In: Nakasato Y, Yung RL, editors. Geriatric rheumatology. New York: Springer Verlag; 2011. p. 113–24. With permission from Springer Verlag. **b**: Image reprinted with permission from Medscape Drugs & Diseases (http://emedicine.medscape.com/), 2016, available at: http://emedicine.medscape.com/article/109130-overview)

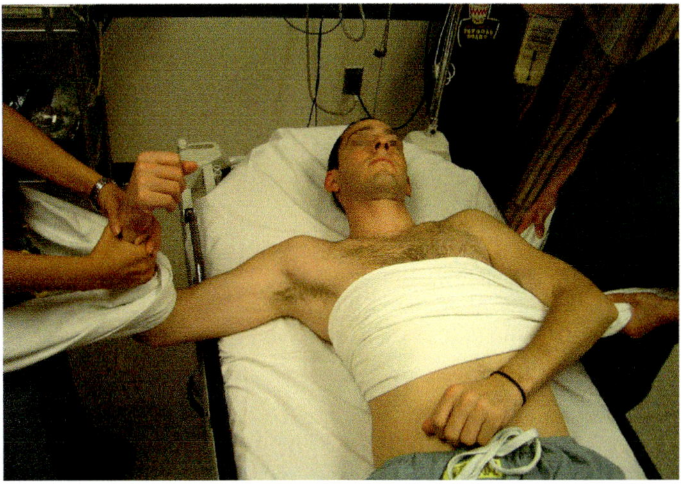

FIGURE 5.25 Traction/countertraction technique. (Image reprinted with permission from Medscape Drugs & Diseases (http://emedicine.medscape.com/), 2016, available at: http://emedicine.medscape.com/article/109130-overview)

along axis of dislocation in opposite direction by leaning backward.

- Continue this constant, gentle traction until patient musculature fatigues and reduction is attained *(slight IR/ER may help foster reduction)* (See Fig. 5.25).

(d) Advantages: familiar to most clinicians, high rate of success, and useful in patients with heightened apprehension and/or severe muscle spasm/pain.

(e) Disadvantages: procedural sedation may be required, requires more than one operator, and prolonged force/endurance is often necessary.

B. Milch technique:

(a) Equipment: none
(b) Position: supine with affected shoulder near edge of the stretcher.
(c) Technique:

- Place patient arm in full abduction, and apply constant longitudinal traction with gentle external rotation.
- Thumb of other hand can be used to assist in relocating humeral head, with gradual adduction of extended arm while still in traction (See Fig. 5.26).

(d) Advantages: well tolerated, can usually be done without sedation, and does not require assistant.
(e) Disadvantages: may be difficult in anxious and uncooperative patients.

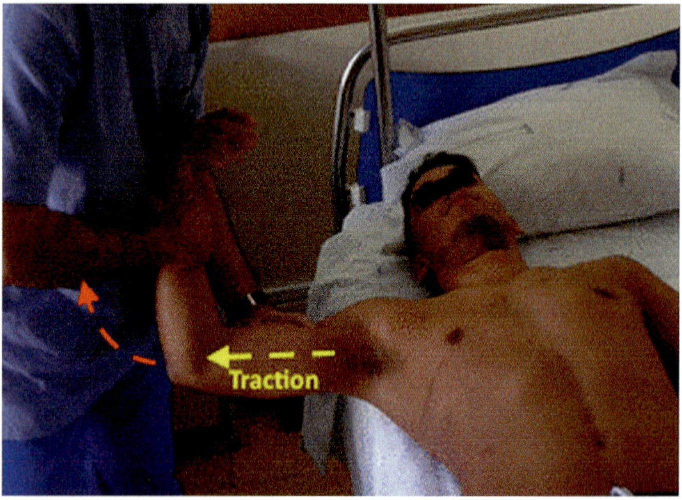

FIGURE 5.26 Milch technique. (Reprinted from Gomes N, Sevivas N, Randelli P, Safran M. Shoulder instability. In: Espregueira-Mendes J, et al., editors. Injuries and health problems in football. Berlin/Heidelberg: Springer; 2017. p. 335–52. With permission from Springer Nature)

C. Scapular manipulation technique:

(a) Equipment: none.
(b) Position: seated or prone with patient back exposed.
(c) Technique:

1. Place affected arm in 90° forward flexion; can have an assistant apply steady forward traction parallel to floor, with countertraction implemented using other arm, which is extended, resting on patient clavicle.
2. Stabilize scapula by placing palm of one hand on lateral shoulder with thumb securely on superolateral border of scapula.
3. Place other palm over inferior tip of scapula, with that thumb on the inferolateral border.
4. Use both hands to rotate inferior tip of the scapula medially and the superior aspect of the scapula laterally (See Fig. 5.27).

(d) Advantages: well tolerated and minimal force require to achieve reduction.
(e) Disadvantages: distinct borders of scapula may be difficult to locate in obese patients, and assistance may be required for patient stabilization/implementation of maneuver.

D. External rotation method:

(a) Equipment: none.
(b) Position: supine.
(c) Technique:

- Adduct affected arm tightly to side of patient.
- Grasp wrist securely, flex elbow to 90°, and apply an associated ER force without traction.
- Continue to methodically externally rotate the forearm until reduction is achieved. Generally takes place between 70° and 110° of ER, but occasionally occurs instead during IR, upon returning patient arm to the starting position (See Fig. 5.28).

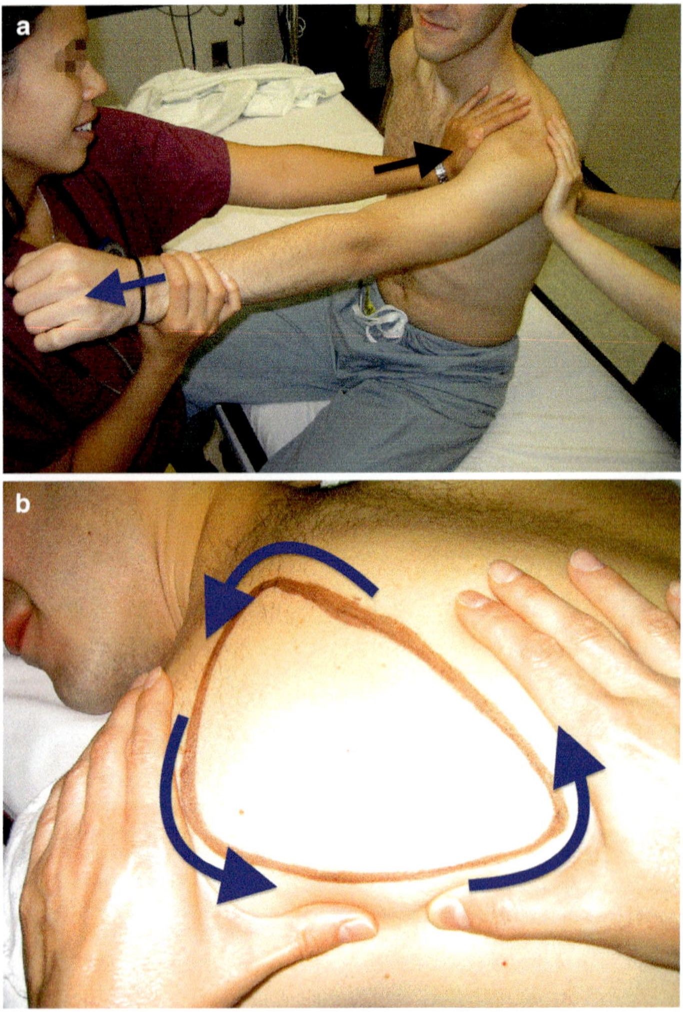

FIGURE 5.27 Scapular manipulation technique: (**a**) seated position, traction and countertraction, (**b**) scapular manipulation, rotate inferior tip medially. (**a**, **b**: Image reprinted with permission from Medscape Drugs & Diseases (http://emedicine.medscape.com/), 2016, available at: http://emedicine.medscape.com/article/109130-overview)

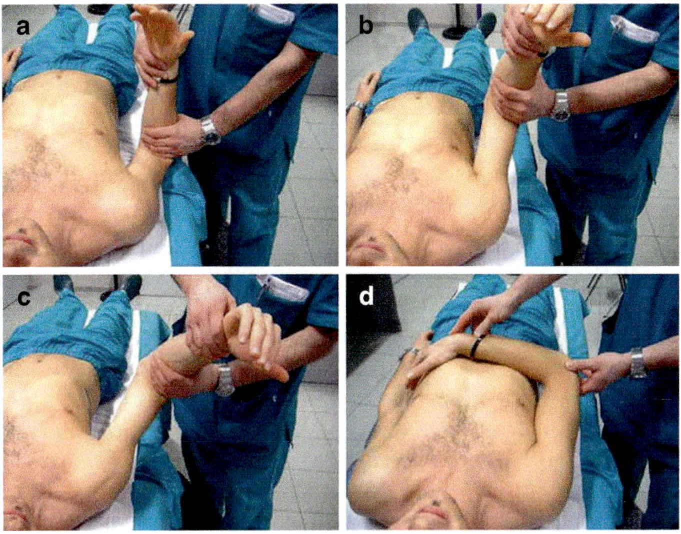

Figure 5.28 External rotation technique: (**a**) place forearm ~90° flexion; (**b**) arm adduction with 20° forward flexion; (**c**) externally rotate shoulder until forearm in coronal plane; (**d**) internally rotate arm into adducted position. (Reprinted from Marinelli M, de Palma L. The external rotation method for reduction of acute anterior shoulder dislocations. J Orthopaed Traumatol. 2009;10(1):17–20. With permission from Springer Nature)

(d) Advantages: well tolerated, sedation generally not necessary, can be performed without assistant, and minimal force generally required to exact reduction.
(e) Disadvantages: requires patient cooperation.

Pearls:

- When choosing a reduction technique, be mindful of available equipment, ancillary staff, and time requirements.
- Consider intra-articular injection analgesia in patients with narcotic issues or contraindications to conscious sedation.

- Elderly and pediatric patients require special attention when applying traction with leverage techniques because they can easily suffer iatrogenic skin friction and/or sloughing injuries.
- Perform/document neurovascular examination and assess for the presence of any fractures/dislocations ***before and after*** any attempts at manipulation/reduction.
- Shoulder should be immobilized in sling in position of comfort and discharged with orthopedic *follow-up within 1 week* for re-evaluation (splinting in ER has not proven to reduce future risk of dislocation and is impractical in many cases).
- Risk for future dislocations is most closely associated with age at time of first dislocation ***(age at time of dislocation inversely related to rate of potential recurrence)***.
- ***Axillary nerve:*** most commonly injured nerve in anterior shoulder dislocations; evaluate sensation of superolateral arm and motor function by palpating for deltoid contraction as patient attempts to abduct the humerus.
- Rotator cuff tears after anterior dislocations are uncommon in younger patients, but occur in >50% of patients over age 40.
- Axillary artery injury upon reduction attempt is rare—more common in older patients with chronic dislocations; generally occurs in patients >50 years of age secondary to joint capsule adhesions and/or atherosclerosis with loss of vessel elasticity. Clues to diagnosis: increasing upper extremity pain, diminished pulse, and/or development of large hematoma. Treatment involves emergent reduction followed by immediate axillary angiography.
- Venous (axillary vein) injury can also occur; usually presents as pain/swelling in affected extremity secondary to venous thrombosis. As above, requires immediate vascular evaluation (+/− systemic anti-coagulation, local fibrinolysis, and/or surgical intervention).

Posterior dislocations:

(a) Can be seen in football offensive linemen, as arm forward flexed to 90° while engaging in blocking technique; inherent shoulder stability is overcome by larger posteriorly directed force transmitted by engaging defensive player.

(b) Can be reduced by traction/counter-traction method, with minor adjustments to application of in-line traction, and gentle lifting of humeral head (+/– lateral traction to unlock humeral head from behind glenoid).

(c) If dislocated >3 weeks (common in elderly, debilitated/demented patients) or there is an anterior humeral articular injury (reverse Hill-Sachs lesion) that involves >20% of the articular surface, closed reduction is generally contraindicated.

STERNOCLAVICULAR JOINT (SCJ)

- Only 50% of medial end of clavicle articulates with the manubrium; thus the SCJ has little inherent stability; largely depends upon ligamentous attachments for structural support:
  - Posterior capsular ligament: provides anterior-posterior stability
  - Anterior SC ligament: primary restraint to superior displacement of medial clavicle

- Anterior dislocations are more common versus posterior dislocations, but ***posterior dislocations are much more concerning (brachial plexus/major vascular structures lie immediately behind medial clavicle)***.
- Posterior SCJ dislocations have an estimated 25% complication rate (pneumothorax, superior vena cava laceration, subclavian artery/vein occlusion, and/or tracheal disruption).
- Injury mechanism:
  - ***Anterior dislocation:*** generally results from an indirect mechanism (e.g., direct blow to anterior shoulder, rotating scapula posteriorly, while simultaneously transmitting an anterior stress to SCJ).

  - ***Posterior dislocation:*** traumatic force drives the shoulder forward or via a direct posterior impact to sternal/medial clavicular surface.

Presentation:

1. ***Anterior dislocation:***

   - Palpable deformity that increases with arm abduction and/or elevation

2. ***Posterior dislocation:***

   - Dyspnea, dysphagia, tachypnea, stridor worse when supine.
   - Clavicle appears shortened/thrust forward, with decreased arm ROM and/or paresthesias (head turn to affected side may help relieve discomfort).

Reduction techniques:

1. ***Anterior dislocation:***

   - ***Acute:***
     - Place patient supine
     - Arm placed at edge of the stretcher
     - Abduct/extend arm while applying axial traction and posterior directed pressure over medial aspect of clavicle

   *****Reduction not always stable, but more about cosmesis than long-term discomfort/diminished function.*****

   - ***Chronic (>3 weeks)***
     - ***Irreducible, unstable:*** accept deformity (most preferable) with sling for comfort.
     - Surgical repair.

2. ***Posterior dislocation:***

*****Generally performed in OR with cardiothoracic surgeon/orthopedic teams present. However, if patient develops aerodigestive/neurovascular symptoms, reduction must be attempted urgently in the emergency room +/− CT/Ortho surgery present if available.*****

- ***Acute:***
  - Place patient supine, with roll/bump between scapulae, and arm at edge of stretcher.
  - Have assistant abduct/extend arm, while applying axial traction and manipulate medial end of clavicle with towel clip or fingers.
  - Reduction stable: sling and swathe for 3 weeks, elbow exercises at 3 weeks, with return to sports at ~3 months.

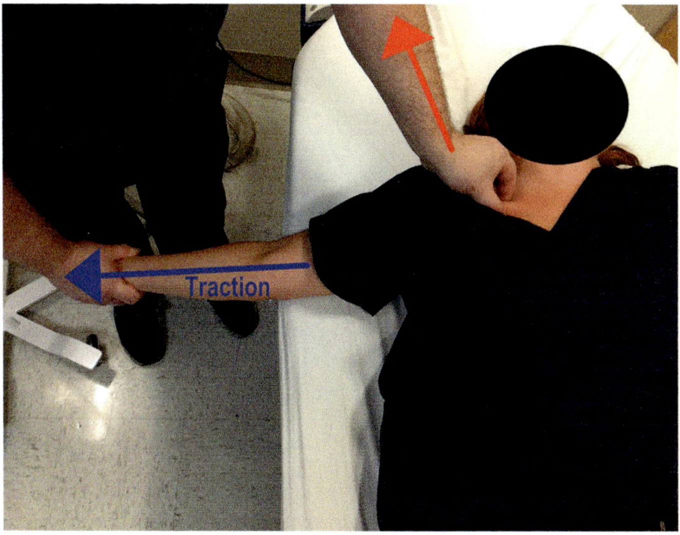

FIGURE 5.29 Posterior SCJ dislocation technique: initiate downward/posterior traction of the arm, while simultaneously pulling the medial aspect of the clavicle anteriorly

- ***Chronic (>3 weeks):***
  - ***Asymptomatic:*** non-operative management, accept deformity, provide sling for comfort; return to unrestricted activity at ~3 months.

Pearls:

- ***Posterior dislocations***: closely monitor vital signs, ***especially respiratory status and adequacy of circulation*** (venous congestion of head, neck, or affected arm can be present).
- ***Serendipity view:*** may allow for better visualization/ detection of a SCJ injury; obtained as AP image with a 40° cephalic tilt; imaging beam should be centered on manubrium (See Fig. 5.30)

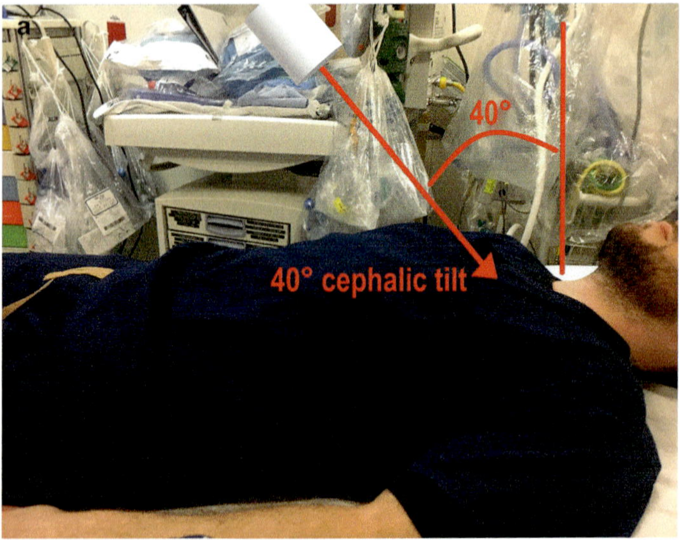

FIGURE 5.30 Serendipity view: (**a**) image technique (**b**) Image appearance: Anterior dislocation-medial clavicle lies above inter-clavicular line; Posterior dislocation lies below inter-clavicular line. (**b**: Reprinted from Pace AM, Neumann L. Sternoclavicular joint and medial clavicle injuries. In: Bentley G, editor. European surgical orthopaedics and traumatology. Berlin/Heidelberg: Springer; 2014. p. 977–91. With permission from Springer Nature)

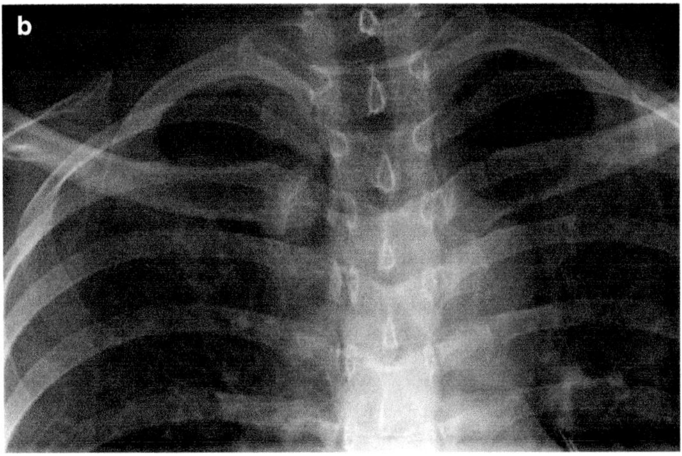

FIGURE 5.30 (continued)

- *Atraumatic subluxation:* often occurs with overhead arm elevation in younger, hyper-lax patients; majority are not painful and usually reduce with lowering of arm: treatment involves reassurance and local symptomatic measures (e.g., ice and sling immobilization).
- CT imaging may be better able to distinguish medial clavicle injuries versus true SCJ dislocations, as well as detect concomitant injuries not readily apparent on plain imaging.
- Medial clavicle physis is last growth plate to ossify at ~20–30 years of age, thus many SC joint dislocations are actually medial physeal fractures/injuries.

Suggested Reading

1. Hendey GW. Bone chillin' orthopedic reductions and regional block. Course lecture presented at: American College of Emergency Physicians 2009 Scientific Assembly, October 5, 2009; Boston MA.
2. Ufberg J, McNamara R. Management of common dislocations. In: Roberts JR, Hedges JR, editors. Clinical procedures

in emergency medicine. 4th ed. Philadelphia: WB Saunders Company; 2004. p. 984–6.
3. Hollis JD, Daley B, et al. 10-year review of knee dislocations: is arteriography always necessary? J Trauma. 2005;59(3):672–5.
4. Hendey GW, Avila A. The captain morgan technique for the reduction of the dislocated hip. Ann Emerg Med. 2011;58(6):536–40.
5. Walden PD, Hamer JR. Whistler technique used to reduce traumatic hip dislocation of the hip in the emergency department setting. J Emerg Med. 1999;17(3):441–4.
6. McDonald J, Whitelaw C, Goldsmith LJ. Radial head subluxation: comparing two methods of reduction. Acad Emerg Med. 1999;6(7):715–8.
7. Baykal B, Sener S, Turkan H. Scapular manipulation technique for reduction of traumatic anterior shoulder dislocations: experiences of an academic emergency department. Emerg Med J. 2005;22:336–8.
8. Cunningham N. Techniques for reduction of anteroinferior shoulder dislocation. Em Med Aust. 2005;17:463–71.
9. Malanga G, et al. Patellar injury and dislocation. Emedicine/Medscape.com. Kelleher B, et al. Knee dislocation in emergency medicine. EmedicineMedscape.com.
10. Keany JE. Ankle dislocation in emergency medicine. Background, pathophysiology, epidemiology. https://emedicine.medscape.com/article/823087-overview. Published April 28, 2016. Accessed 16 Mar 2018.
11. Elstrom JA, Virkus WW, Pankovich A. Handbook of fractures. 3rd ed. New York: McGraw Hill Professional; 2006. p. 362–9.
12. Cornwall R, Radomisli TE. Nerve injury in traumatic dislocation of the hip. Clin Orthop Relat Res. 2000;377:84–91.
13. Yang EC, Cornwall R. Initial treatment of traumatic hip dislocations in the adult. Clin Orthop Relat Res. 2000;377:24–31.
14. Schuberth JM. Diagnosis of ankle injuries: the essentials. J Foot Ankle Surg. 1994;33(2):214.
15. Davenport M. Reduction of posterior hip dislocation. Background, indications, contraindications. https://emedicine.medscape.com/article/109225-overview. Published February 26, 2018. Accessed 16 Mar 2018.
16. Arendt EA, Fithian DC, Cohen E. Current concepts of lateral patella dislocation. Clin Sports Med. 2002;21(3):499–519.
17. Cash JD, Hughston JC. Treatment of acute patellar dislocation. Am J Sports Med. 1988;16(3):244–9.

18. Chapman MW, editor. Chapman's orthopaedic surgery, vol. 2. 3rd ed. Baltimore: Lippincott Williams & Wilkins; 1993.
19. Purcell D. Musculoskeletal medicine for medical students. Orthop One [ePub]. 2011.
20. Foulk D, et al. Hip dislocation: evaluation and management. J Am Acad Orthop Surg. 2010;18:199–2.
21. Good L, et al. The dislocated knee. JAAOS. 1995;3:284–29.
22. Lent GS. Reduction of radial head dislocation. Background, Indications, Contraindications. https://emedicine.medscape.com/article/80051-overview. Published August 2, 2017. Accessed 16 Mar 2018.
23. Perron AD, et al. Orthopedic pitfalls in the ED: galeazzi and monteggia fracture-dislocation. Am J Emerg Med. 2001;19(3):225–8.
24. Weatherford B. Sternoclavicular dislocation. Sternoclavicular dislocation – trauma – orthobullets. https://www.orthobullets.com/trauma/1009/sternoclavicular-dislocation. Published 2012. Accessed Mar 2017.
25. Mallia AK. Reduction of shoulder dislocation. Background, indications, contraindications. https://emedicine.medscape.com/article/109130-overview. Published August 9, 2017. Accessed 16 Mar 2018.
26. Ceroni D, et al. Radiographic evaluation of anterior dislocation of the shoulder. Acta Radiol. 2000;41:658–61.
27. Wen DY. Current concepts in the treatment of anterior shoulder dislocations. Am J Emerg Med. 1999;17:401–7.
28. Riebel GD, et al. Anterior shoulder dislocation: a review of reduction techniques. Am J Emerg Med. 1991;9:180–8.
29. McNamara RM. Reduction of anterior shoulder dislocations by scapular manipulation. Ann Emerg Med. 1993;22:1140–4.
30. Wolfson AB, Hendey GW. Harwood-Nuss clinical practice of emergency medicine. 5th ed. Philadelphia: Wolters Kluwer; 2010.
31. Davenport M. Reduction of ankle dislocation. Background, indications, contraindications. https://emedicine.medscape.com/article/109244-overview. Published February 26, 2018. Accessed 16 Mar 2018.

Chapter 6
Immobilization

Sneha A. Chinai, Laura Walker, Matthew R. Rebesco, Bryan A. Terry, and Daniel Purcell

Indications

A. Suspected/confirmed fracture(s) and/or dislocation(s) (+/− reduction)
B. Sprain(s)/strain(s)
C. Inflammatory disorders: tenosynovitis, arthritic flare (RA), gout, etc.
D. Contusions, abrasions, and/or lacerations that extend to or involve joint surface

---

S. A. Chinai
Department of Emergency Medicine, University of Massachusetts Medical School, Worcester, MA, USA

L. Walker
Department of Emergency Medicine, Mayo Clinic, Rochester, MN, USA

M. R. Rebesco (✉)
Department of Emergency Medicine, UMass Memorial Medical Center, Worcester, MA, USA
e-mail: matthew.rebesco@umassmemorial.org

B. A. Terry
The Brooklyn Hospital Center, Brooklyn, NY, USA

D. Purcell
Emergency Department, New York University Langone Medical Center Brooklyn, New York, NY, USA

D. Purcell et al. (eds.), *Emergency Orthopedics Handbook*,
https://doi.org/10.1007/978-3-030-00707-2_6

E. Puncture wounds/human, animal bites (hands/feet)
F. Infection/burns

Immobilization protects injury, diminishes pain, maintains bony alignment, promotes healing, and compensates for surrounding muscular deficits/weakness.

Initial approach to casting/splinting requires a thorough assessment of the skin/soft tissues, neurovascular status, and bony structures to accurately diagnose and thoroughly evaluate injury.

Splinting

- Non-circumferential immobilization is the generally preferred method of acute immobilization secondary to persistent post-injury swelling
- Can be static (prevent motion) or dynamic (functional) to assist with controlled motion
- Can use plaster, fiberglass materials, or other prefabricated devices (See Fig. 6.1)

A. ***Plaster*** (See Figs. 6.2, 6.3, 6.4, and 6.5)

Advantages

- Allows for post-injury swelling during acute inflammatory phase (increased pliability)
- Decreased pressure-related complications (skin breakdown, compartment syndrome) versus *casting*
- Easily removed for injury inspection

Disadvantages

- Potential for easy removal (non-compliant patients)
- Poor resistance to water, low strength-weight ratio, heavier (thicker) vs. *fiberglass*
- Not considered definitive treatment for unstable injuries (e.g., increased motion at injury site versus *casting*)

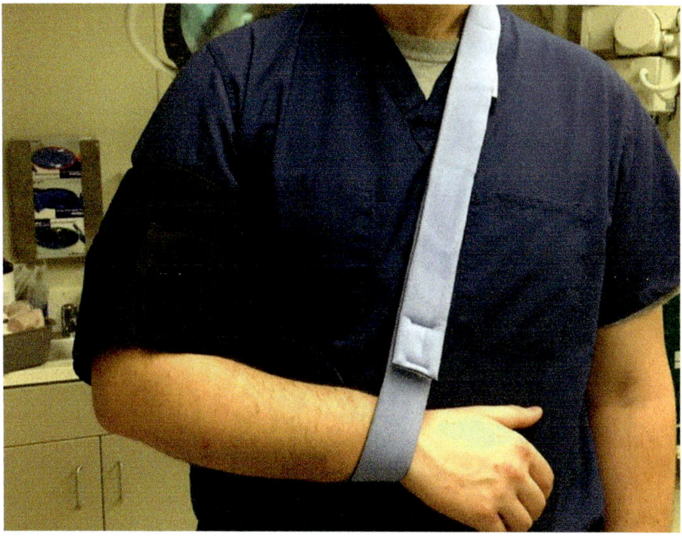

FIGURE 6.1 "Functional brace" – used to assist with controlled range of motion during healing

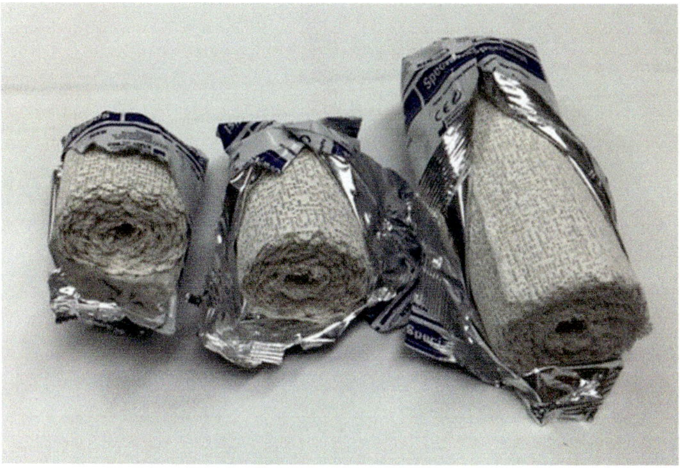

FIGURE 6.2 "Plaster material" – can be used for splinting/casting

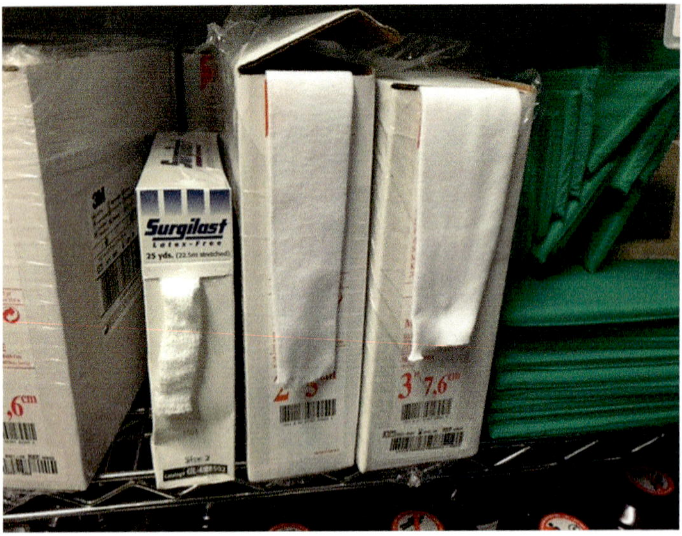

FIGURE 6.3 "Stockinette" – proper size will depend on the site of immobilization and the size of the patient's extremity

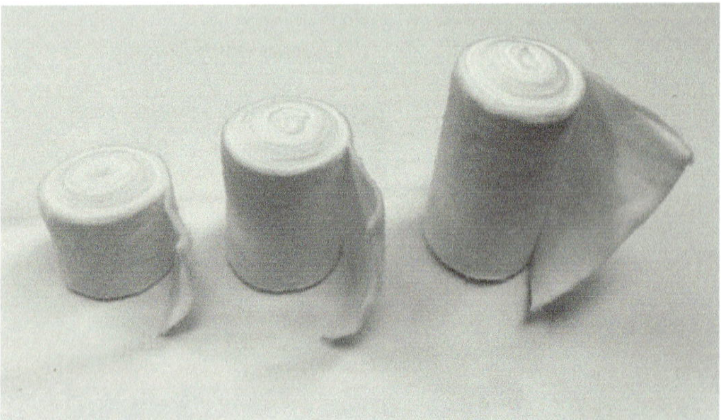

FIGURE 6.4 "Webril" – proper size will depend on the site of immobilization and the size of the patient's extremity

B. ***Prefabricated Fiberglass Splints*** *(e.g., ORTHO-GLASS, 3M)* (See Fig. 6.6)

Advantages

- Fast application (easily cut/molded to injured extremity)
- Lightweight, yet strong material (high stiffness)
- Less material required versus *plaster* (unclear if cost effective)
- Less thermal energy generated during curing process, wicks moisture away from skin

Disadvantages

- More difficult to mold and maintain desired position of immobilization versus *plaster*
- Expensive (unclear if cost-effective)
- Not available in all settings

C. ***Plaster Splint Technique***

Perform/document neurovascular exam prior to immobilization.

Arrange comfortable/appropriate position for patient/provider before application.

Place extremity in "position of function" before and after padding/splint application to avoid areas of excess wrinkling/pressure.

1. Estimate length of stockinette/padding/plaster splint material:

   (a) Stockinette (if implemented) should extend ~5–10 cm beyond indicated immobilization.
   (b) Consider additional ~1–2 cm plaster length to allow for "shrinkage" during wetting, molding, and drying.

- Upper extremity injuries require 3–4 inch width stockinette, lower extremity 4–6 inch width.
- Upper extremity injuries require ~8–10 layers of plaster, lower extremity ~10–12 layers.

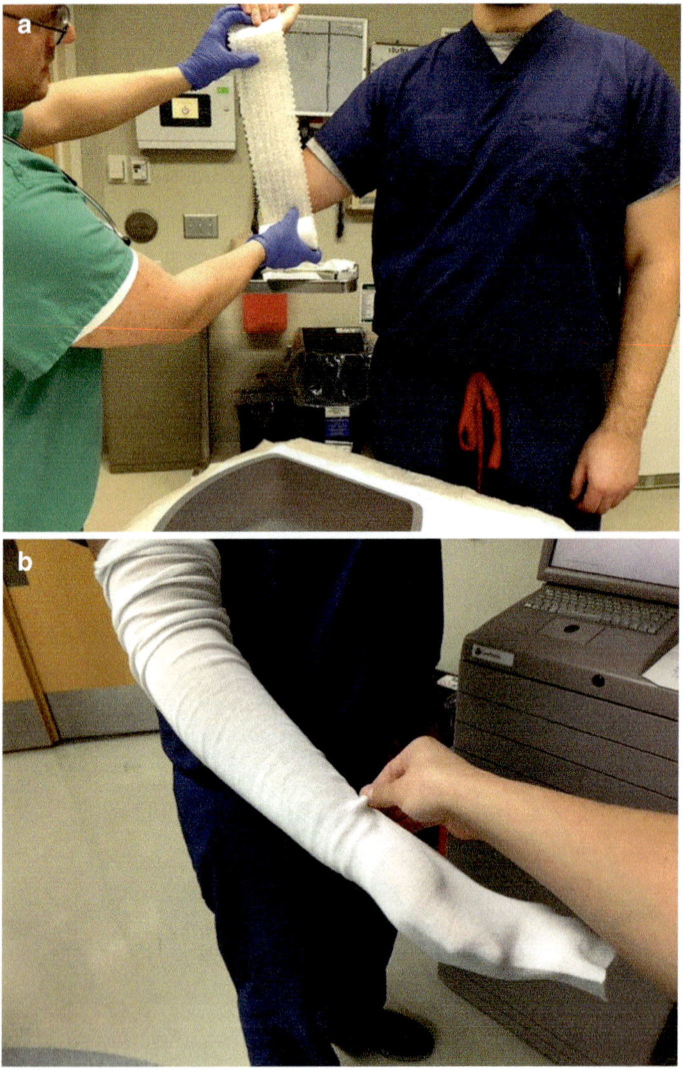

Figure 6.5 (**a**) "Plaster splint application – measurement – fold stockinette" – Measure the length of plaster needed for the splint, and roll out approximately 8–10 layers for upper extremity (UE) splints and 10–12 layers for lower extremity (LE). (**b**) For adults, generally 3–4 inch width stockinette will suffice for UE and 4–6 inch width for LE. It should extend at least 5 cm beyond the area to be splinted.

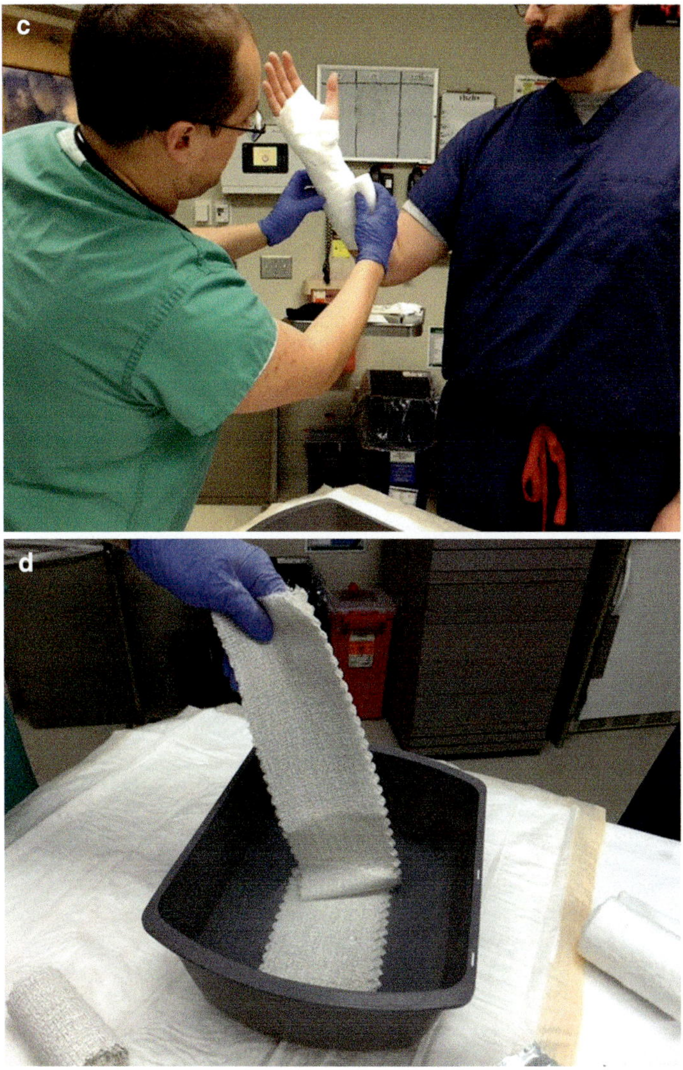

FIGURE 6.5 (continued) (**c**) "Plaster splint application – Webril" – apply 2–3 layers of Webril to the area to be splinted. Make sure to overlap layers by 25–50% and avoid wrinkles. (**d**) To avoid thermal injury, submerge the plaster in tepid water, no hotter than 24°C (75°F), as the plaster becomes warmer as it hardens

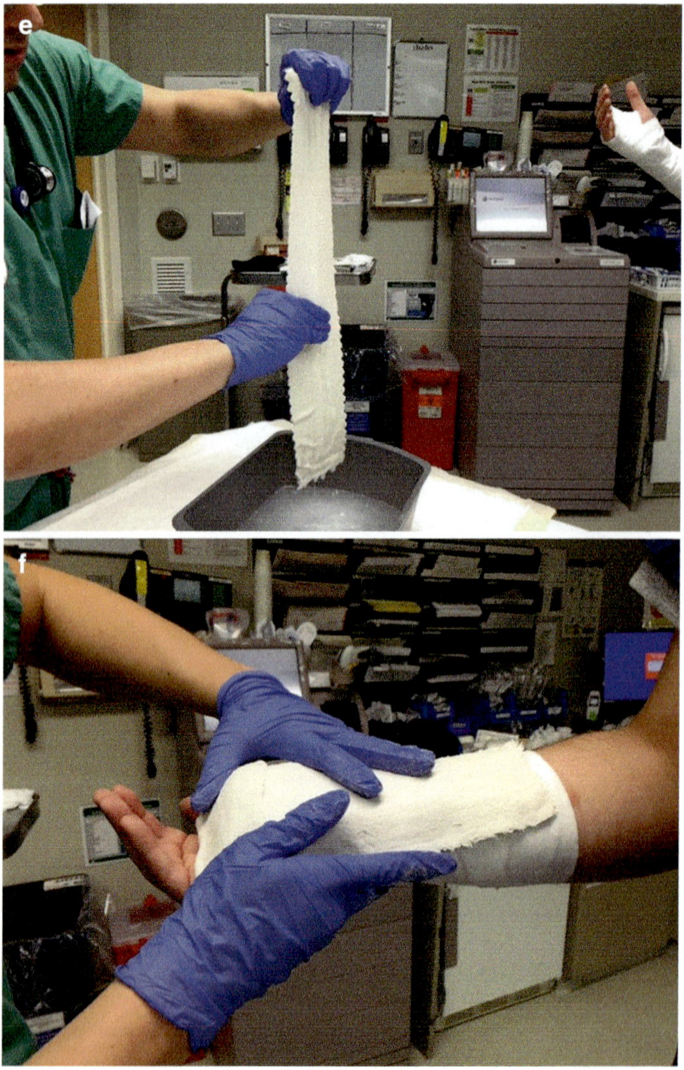

FIGURE 6.5 (continued) (**e**) "Plaster splint application – smooth plaster" – use your fingers to smooth out the plaster and ring out the excess water. Lay it on a flat surface to further eliminate wrinkles. (**f**) "Plaster splint application – apply splint" – apply the splint over the Webril. Avoid using your fingertips which can create indentations

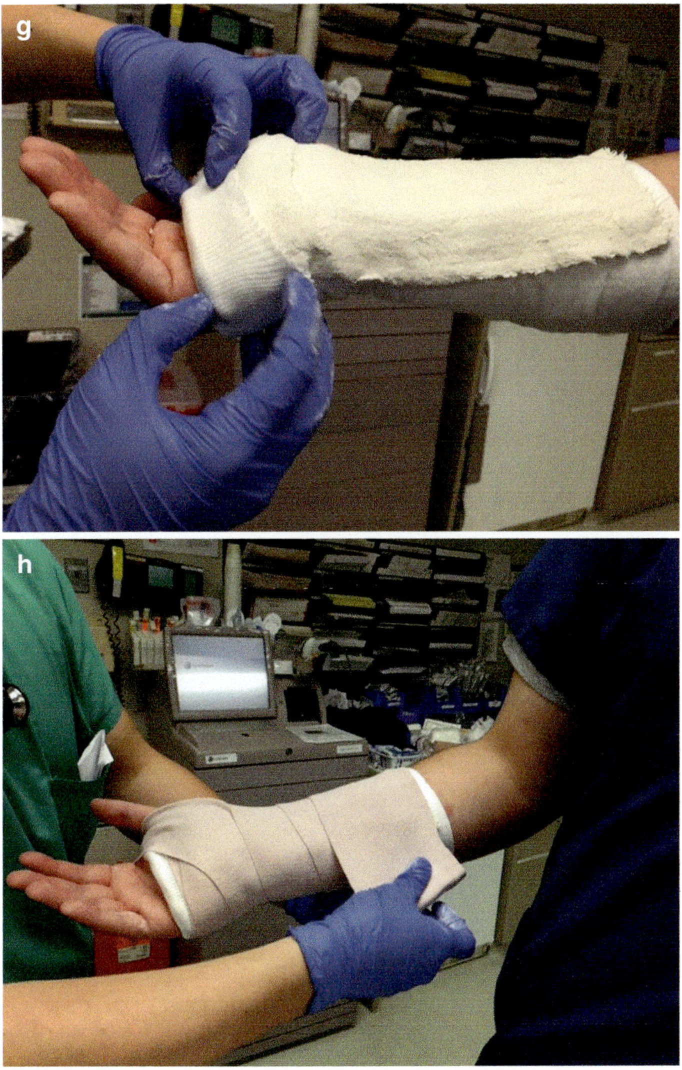

FIGURE 6.5 (continued) (**g**) "Plaster splint application – fold stockinette" – fold the stockinette back over the ends of the plaster and Webril to create smooth edges. (**h**) "Plaster splint application – secure splint" – use an elastic wrap to secure the splint

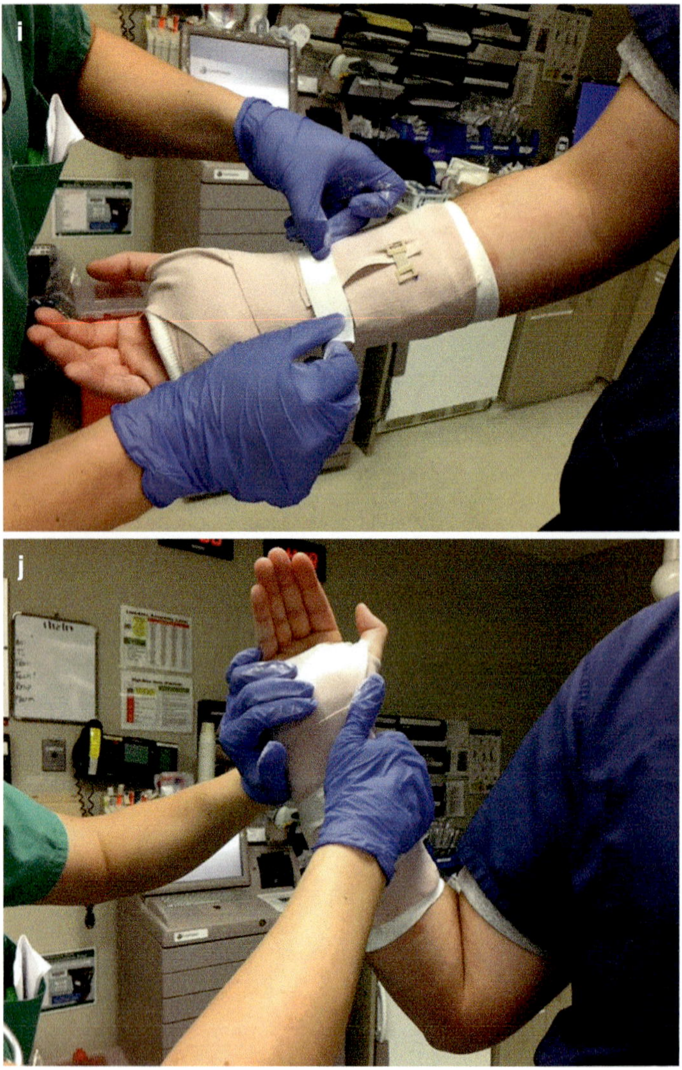

FIGURE 6.5 (continued) (**i**) "Plaster splint application – maintain splint" – add clips/tape to maintain immobilization. (**j**) "Plaster splint application – molding" – use only the palms to mold the splint into proper position

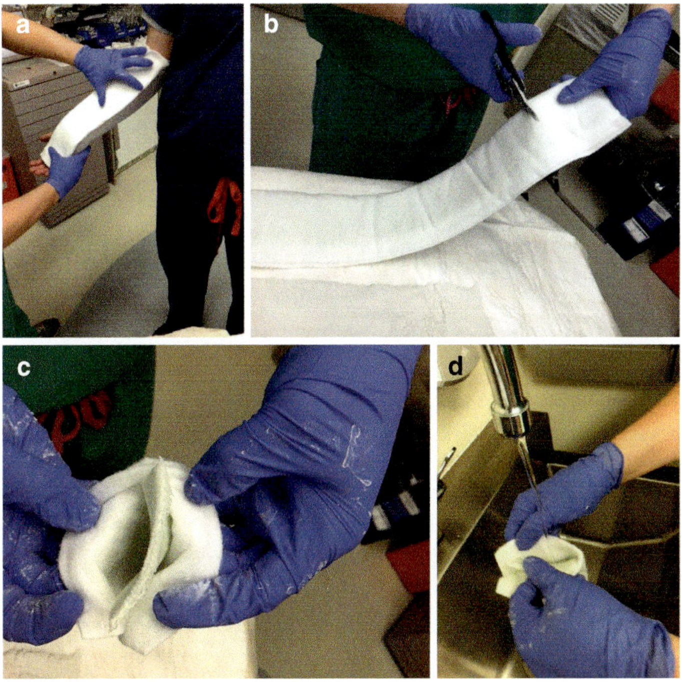

Figure 6.6 Prefabricated Fiberglass Splint Application – "measurement" – (**a**) measure the length of the fiberglass material required to immobilize the extremity (+/- stockinette). (**b**) "cutting" – use trauma shears to trim the ends to avoid sharp edges. (**c**) "stretching" – pull the cotton covering beyond the fiberglass edges to avoid direct contact with the skin. (**d**) "wetting" – open one end for water to enter and initiate the curing process. (**e**) "applying" – place splint on the extremity (fold back stockinette over edges if implemented). (**f**) "securing" – affix splint to the extremity

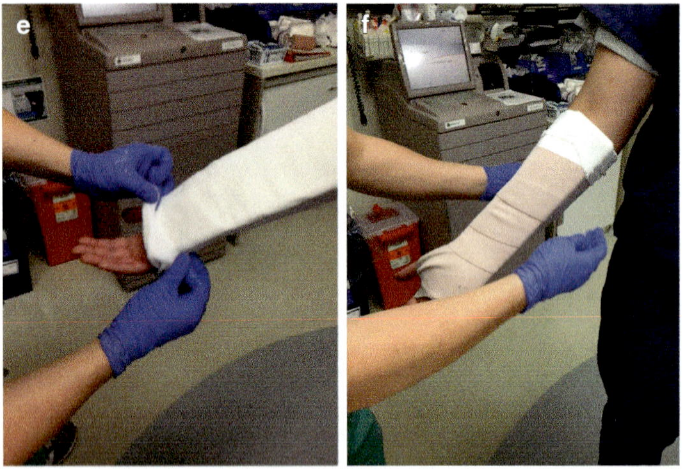

FIGURE 6.6 (continued)

2. Add water and eliminate excess by "milking" between fingers. Place on hard surface to remove wrinkles/ensure even saturation of all layers (See Figs. 6.7, 6.8, and 6.9).
3. Apply splint. Fold stockinette/padding back to create smooth edges, and mold to contours of extremity to facilitate/maintain "reduction" and ensure strict immobilization *(implement three-point fixation)* (See Figs. 6.10 and 6.11)
   *****Mold with palms only, three-point fixation to maintain reduction.*****

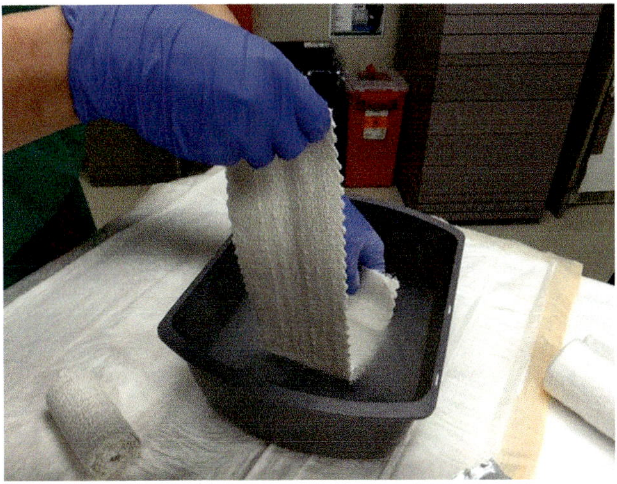

FIGURE 6.7 "Add water" – Pay attention to the temperature, as using water that is too hot can lead to thermal burns

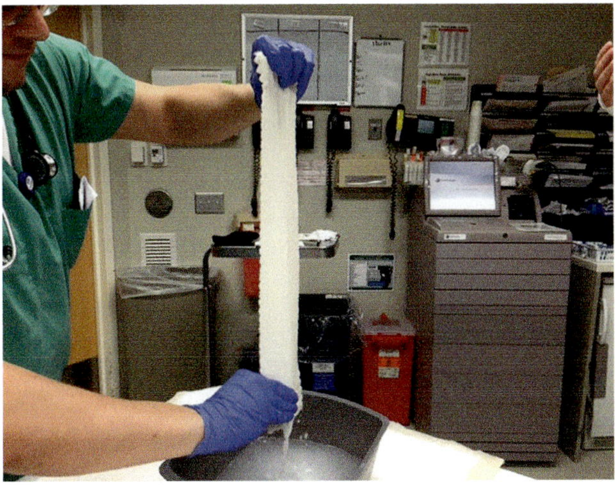

FIGURE 6.8 "Milking" – Adequate milking is required for optimal fixation and setting time

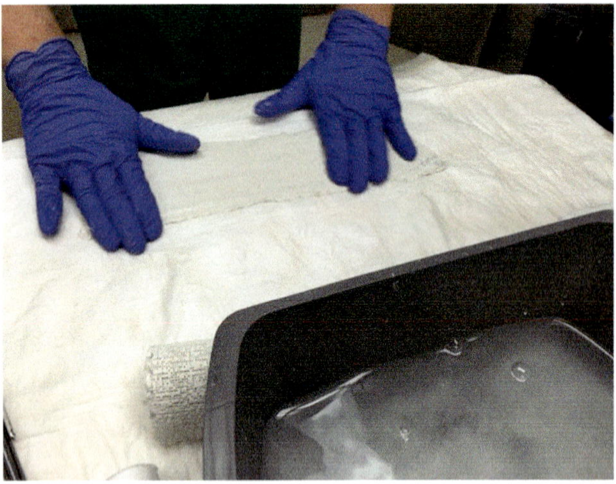

FIGURE 6.9 "Remove wrinkles" – will reduce risks of pressure injuries and decrease setting time by eliminating excess moisture

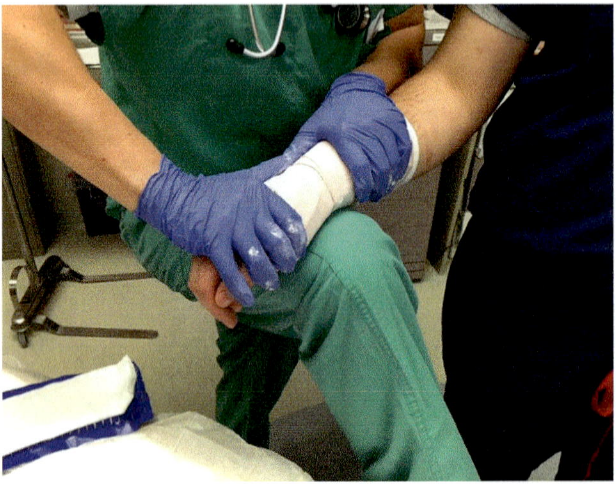

FIGURE 6.10 "Molding" – Use only the heels of the palm to implement 3-point fixation

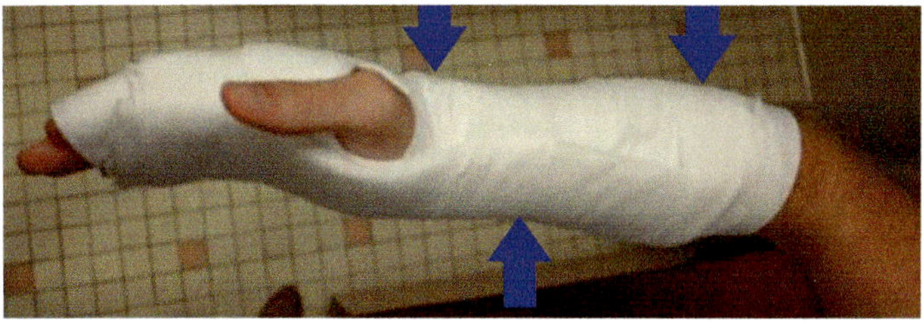

Figure 6.11 "3-point fixation" – molding pattern involving 3-points of pressure that will serve to facilitate/maintain reduction and ensure strict immobilization. (Reprinted from Alexandre V, Hodax JD. Splinting and casting techniques. In: Hodax J, Eltorai A, Daniels A, editors. The orthopedic consult survival guide. Cham: Springer International Publishing; 2017. p. 25–39. With permission from Springer Nature)

Casting

- Involves circumferential application of plaster/fiberglass: standard treatment for many closed, non-displaced, and/or unstable fractures/dislocations (e.g., trimalleolar fracture/dislocation).
- ****If implementing cast in acute injury period, consider "bi-valving" to accommodate swelling.****
- Bi-valving involves using the cast saw to create two incisions in the cast on opposite sides to facilitate pressure release (See Fig. 6.12).

A. *Advantages*

- Superior immobilization, definitive management for complex/unstable injuries
- Circumvents patient non-compliance issues
- *Fiberglass*, less heat generated versus *plaster* as it cures

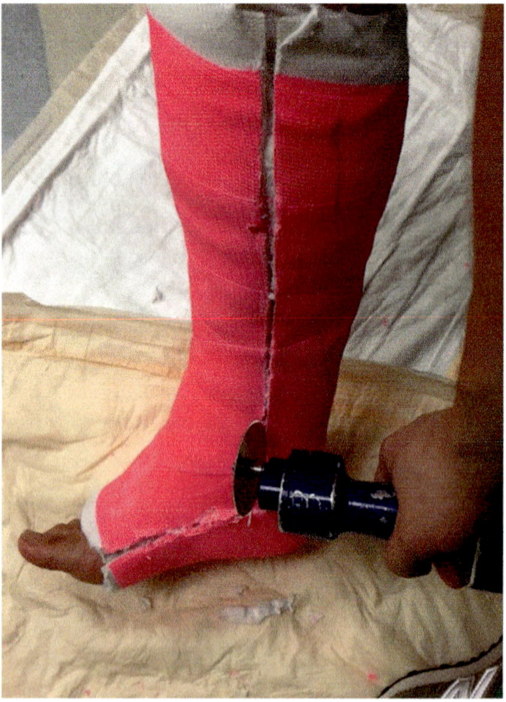

FIGURE 6.12 "Bi-valved" short leg cast: serves to diminish elevated compartment pressures by accommodating swelling in the acute injury period

B. Disadvantages

- Requires more skill/time for application (attention to deforming forces-gravity/muscle paramount for optimal application)
- Does not accommodate soft tissue swelling (heightened risk of thermal injuries/pressure sores, compartment syndrome, etc.)
- May experiences loss of reduction as swelling decreases/ padding compresses as patient regains mobility

C. Casting Technique

****Perform/document neurovascular exam prior to immobilization.****

****Arrange comfortable/appropriate position for patient/provider before cast application. ****

****Place extremity in "position of function" before and after padding/cast material application to avoid areas of excess wrinkling/pressure.****

1. Estimate length/apply stockinette to affected extremity (should extend ~5–10 cm beyond area of intended immobilization).
    - Upper extremity injuries require 3–4 inch width stockinette, lower extremity 4–6 inch width (See Fig. 6.13).

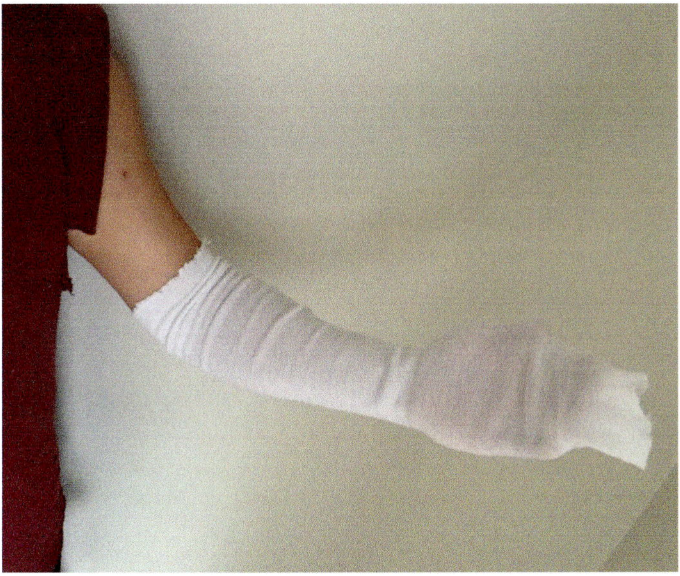

FIGURE 6.13 "Applying stockinette" – Note the extra length apportioned at each end

- Care should be taken to ensure stockinette is not constricting and there is absence of wrinkling over flexion points/bony prominences by smoothing/trimming as required (See Fig. 6.14).

2. Apply 2–3 layers of cotton padding (Webril) evenly, generating ~25–50% overlap and extending ~3–5 cm past intended cast length edges (See Figs. 6.15 and 6.16).

General recommendations:

- Hands/feet 2 inch width
- Upper extremity 3–4 inch width
- Lower extremity 4–6 inch width

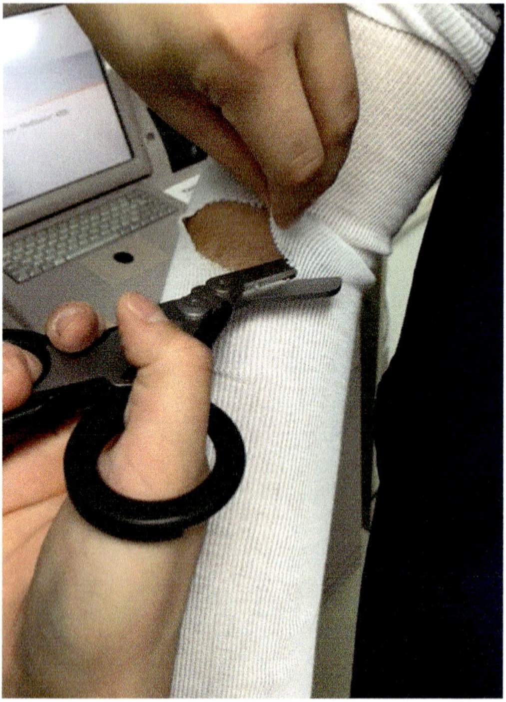

FIGURE 6.14 "Elimination of wrinkles" – use shears to eradicate wrinkles over areas of flexion

- Bony prominences/areas of substantial swelling require extra padding (e.g., radial/ulnar styloid, olecranon, patella, malleoli, and heel). Manipulate to allow for uniform application and avoid excessive stretching that can generate increased circumferential pressure (heightened risk of compartment syndrome).

3. Plaster/fiberglass material selected should also be implemented as above (even application, ~25–50% overlap, avoid wrinkles/excess tension, and remain within cotton padding/stockinette edges).

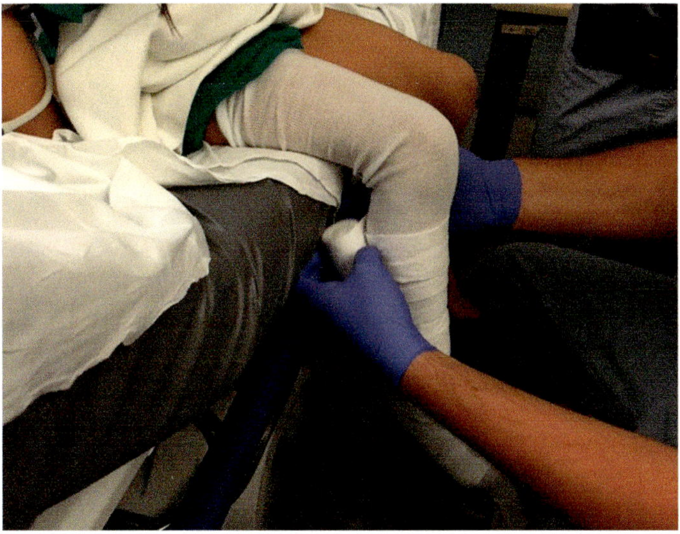

FIGURE 6.15 "Applying Webril to lower extremity" – Note the attention to proper tension/distance covered between subsequent turns

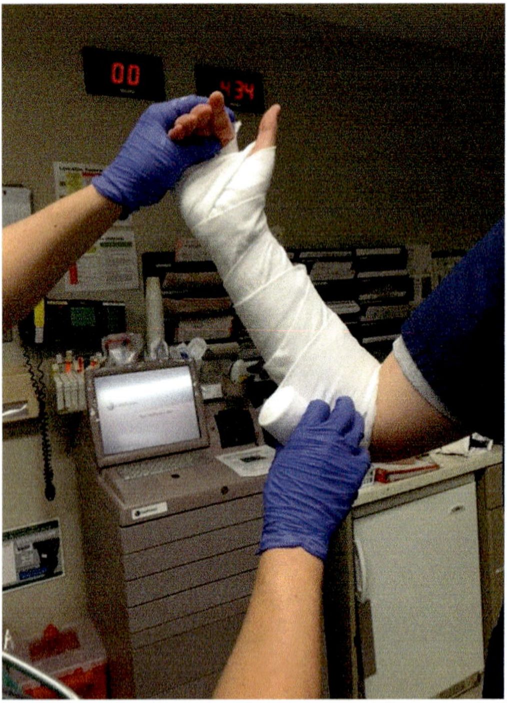

FIGURE 6.16 "Applying Webril to upper extremity"

4. Prior to application of final layer of casting material, fold back stockinette/cotton padding to ensure no free/sharp edges exist (See Fig. 6.17).

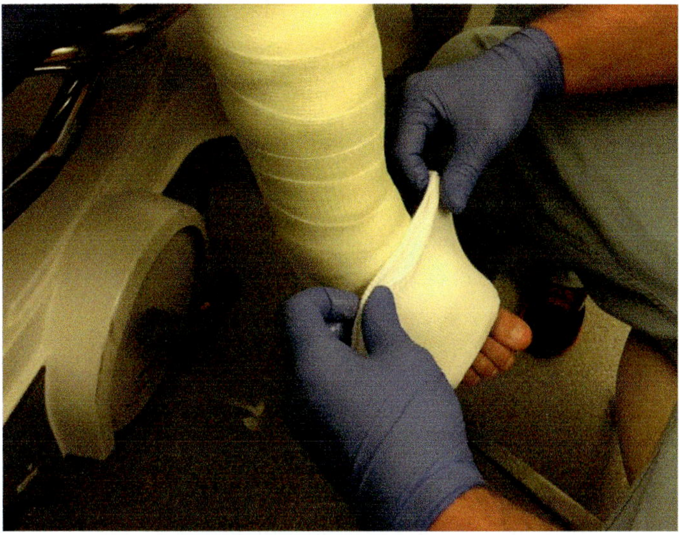

FIGURE 6.17 "Folding back stockinette" – fold back the stockinette before applying the final layer of casting material. This ensures a smooth edge around the ends of the cast

5. Mold with ***heels of palms only*** while still deformable, and employ ***3-point fixation*** (See Figs. 6.18 and 6.19)

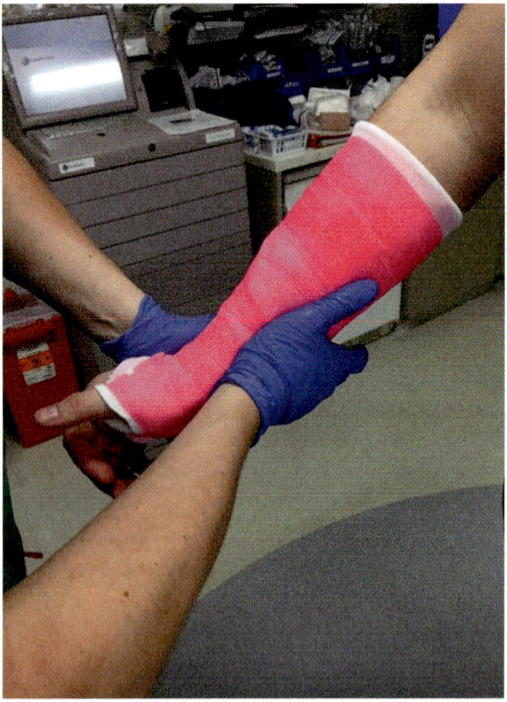

Figure 6.18 "Molding upper extremity" – note only the heels of the palms are implemented

D. Splint/Cast Aftercare

Get post-immobilization imaging

- Educate patients on appropriate splint/cast care; supply explicit verbal/written instructions on importance of injured extremity elevation, associated precautions, and warning signs of urgent need for re-evaluation (e.g., compartment syndrome).
- Most splints/casts require follow-up within 1 week after application.

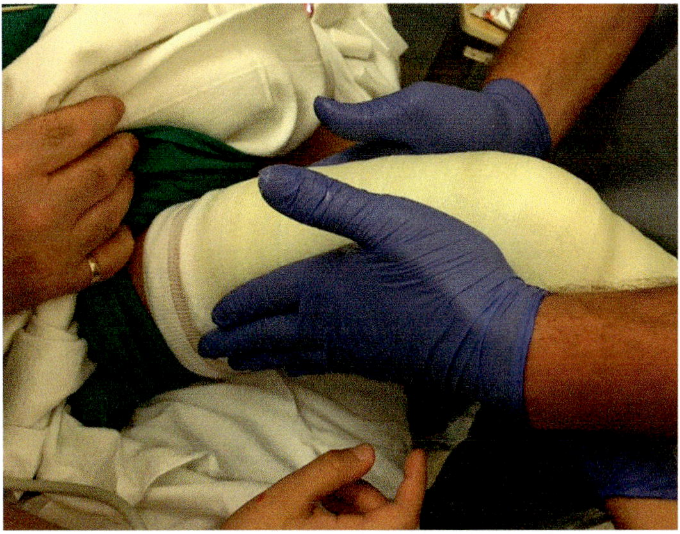

FIGURE 6.19 "Molding lower extremity" – note only the palms are employed for cast patterning

Immobilization Specifics

A. Upper Extremity

1. **Radial Gutter**

- *Indications:* non-displaced/non-rotated second and third metacarpal (MCP) or phalangeal injuries, associated soft tissue injuries that involve or extend over these joints.
- *Technique:* immobilization courses along the radial forearm→just beyond DIPJ of the index/middle fingers, leaving thumb free.
- *Position:* forearm neutral rotation; wrist slight extension; MCPJ ~70–90 degrees flexion; PIPJ/DIPJ ~5–10 degrees flexion ("intrinsic plus" protected position) (See Figs. 6.20 and 6.21).

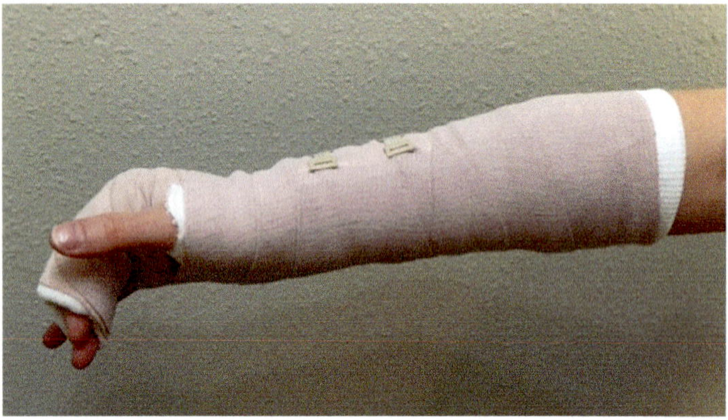

Figure 6.20 "Radial gutter plaster splint"

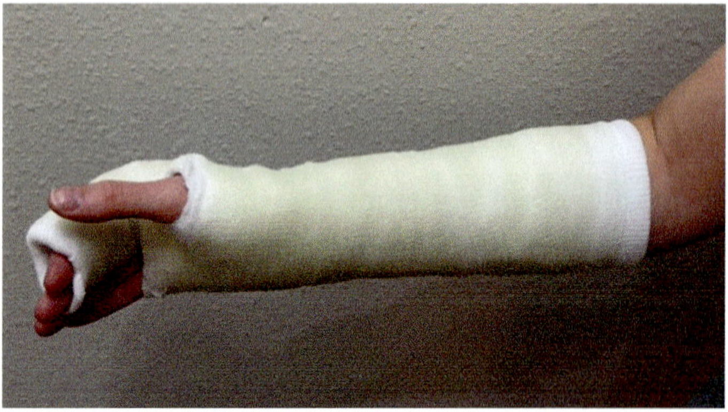

Figure 6.21 "Radial gutter cast"

2. **Ulnar Gutter**

   - *Indications:* non-displaced/non-rotated fourth and fifth MCP or phalangeal injuries, soft tissue injuries that involve or extend over these joints.
   - *Technique:* immobilization courses along the ulnar forearm→just beyond DIPJ of ring/little fingers.

- *Position:* forearm neutral rotation; wrist slight extension; MCPJ ~70–90 degrees flexion; PIPJ/DIPJ ~5–10 degrees flexion (See Figs. 6.22 and 6.23).

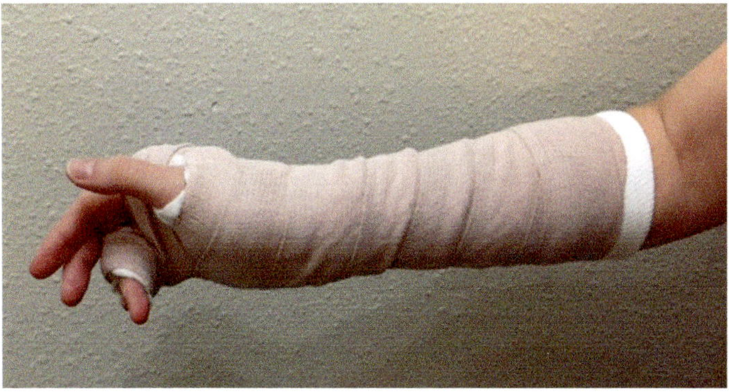

FIGURE 6.22 "Ulnar gutter plaster splint application"

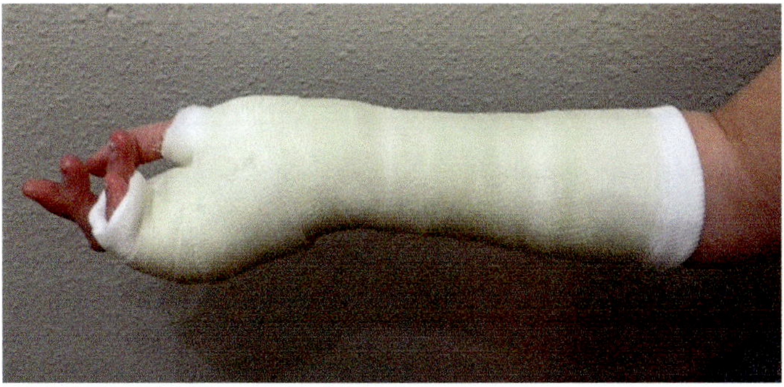

FIGURE 6.23 "Ulnar gutter cast application"

3. ***Thumb Spica***

- *Indications:* scaphoid/thumb injuries, first carpometacarpal (CMC) degenerative disease, ligamentous/tendon injuries (e.g., ulnar collateral ligament, De Quervain tenosynovitis) and/or associated soft tissue injuries that involve or extend over these joints.
- *Technique:* immobilization involves radial aspect of the ~ distal third forearm➔just distal to thumb interphalangeal joint (IPJ), encircling thumb.
- *Position:* forearm neutral rotation, wrist ~20 degrees extension, hand neutral/thumb in "position of function" (e.g., "holding soda can") (See Figs. 6.24 and 6.25).

4. ***Dorsal Block-Extension Splint (DBES)***

- *Indications:* selected proximal phalanx fractures, MCPJ/PIPJ dorsal dislocations (volar plate injury), dorsal soft tissue injuries/protection of flexor tendon repairs.
- *Technique:* immobilization applied to dorsal surface of distal forearm (proximal dorsal MCPJ for pure finger injuries)➔dorsal DIPJ.

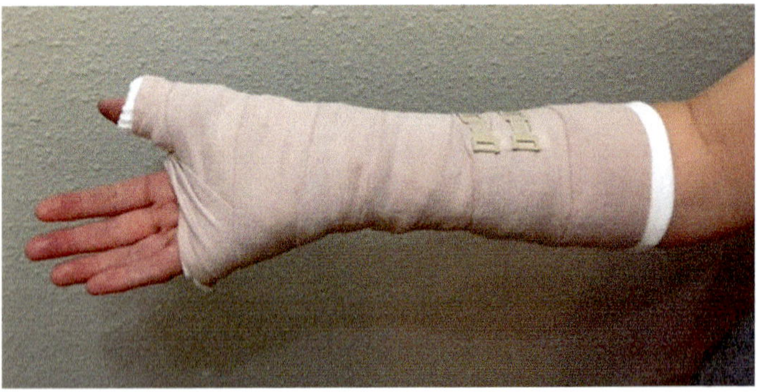

Figure 6.24 "Thumb spica plaster splint"

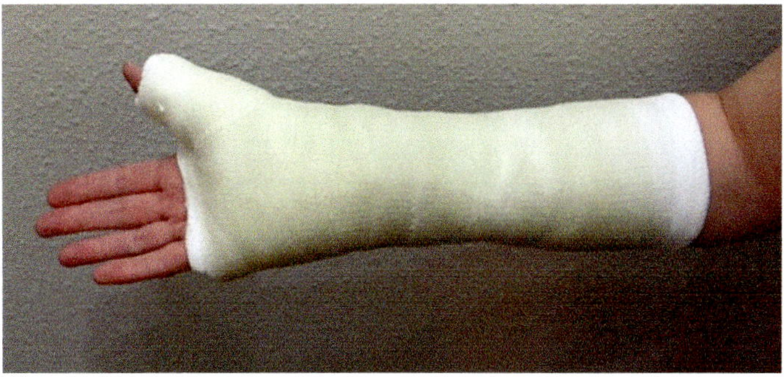

FIGURE 6.25 "Thumb spica cast"

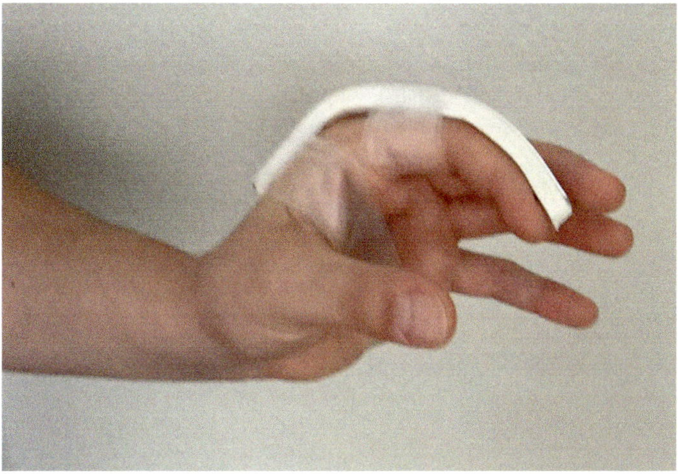

FIGURE 6.26 "Isolated digital DBES" – Note the digit is able to flex, but is limited in extension

- *Position*: forearm neutral rotation, wrist ~30 degrees extension, MCPJ ~90 degrees flexion
  ****PIPJ should be able to flex freely, yet be limited in extension.**** (See Fig. 6.26)

5. ***Volar Wrist Splint***

- *Indications:* soft tissue injuries of hand/wrist, carpal bone injuries (e.g., lunate/peri-lunate dislocation, pisiform fracture), second to fifth metacarpal fractures, protection of extensor tendon repairs. Immobilization for RA/carpal tunnel symptomatology.
- *Technique:* immobilization begins at the volar mid-forearm→distal palmar crease.
- *Position:* forearm neutral rotation, wrist ~20 degrees extension, hand "intrinsic-plus position."
- ***Allows full elbow flexion, forearm pronation/supination; not recommended for distal radial/ulna fractures.*** (See Fig. 6.27)

6. ***Sugar Tong***

- *Indications:* distal radius/ulna fractures (prevents forearm pronation/supination by controlling elbow motion).

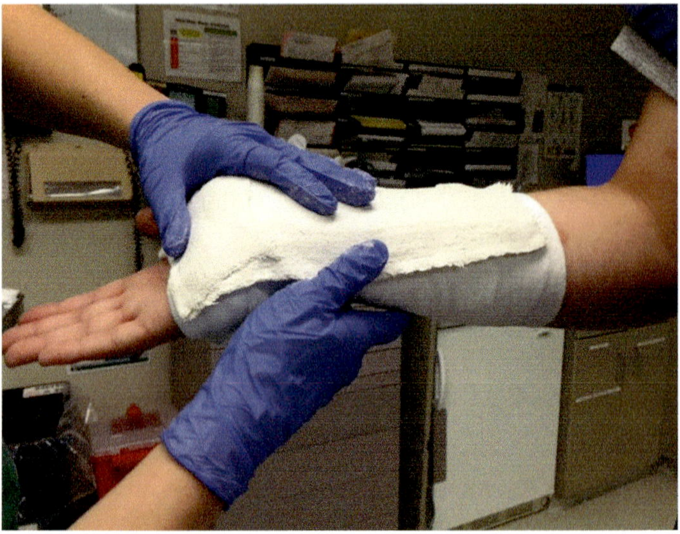

FIGURE 6.27 "Volar wrist plaster splint"

- *Technique:* immobilization begins at the volar proximal palmar crease and proceeds along the volar forearm toward the elbow, courses behind, and then returns distally just proximal to the MCPJ. *****Do not extend immobilization past volar proximal palmar crease/dorsal MCPJs, or it can initiate "irreversible" hand stiffness.*****
- *Position:* elbow 90 degrees flexion, forearm neutral rotation, wrist slight extension (~20 degrees), and hand in "protected "position (thumb free) (See Fig. 6.28).

7. ***Long Arm Posterior Splint***

- *Indications:* humeral shaft/proximal forearm fractures (e.g., elbow dislocation): *controls flexion/exten-*

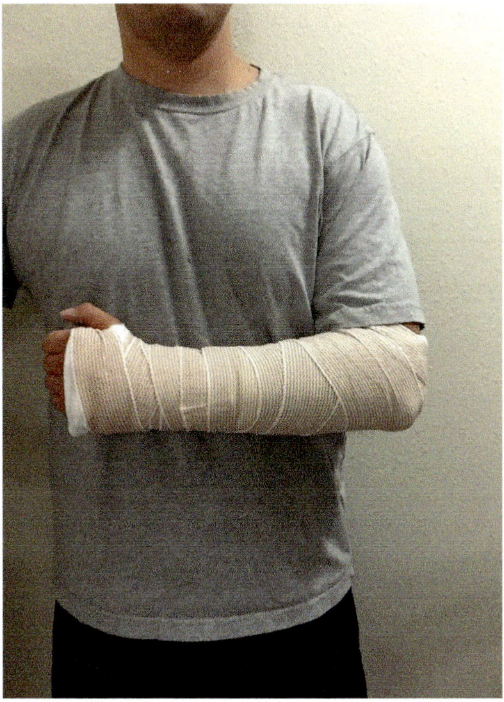

FIGURE 6.28 "Sugar tong splint"

sion at the elbow, but not forearm pronation/supination; thus not appropriate for distal forearm injuries.

- *Technique:* immobilization begins on posterior aspect of proximal humerus and continues distally along ulnar aspect of forearm/hand, to the level of proximal palmar crease.
- *Position:* forearm neutral rotation, wrist slight extension, and hand neutral, "position of function" (See Fig. 6.29).

8. ***Coaptation Splint***

- *Indications:* initial management of proximal humerus/humeral shaft fractures *(e.g., transverse/short oblique fracture patterns that can suffer from distraction/*

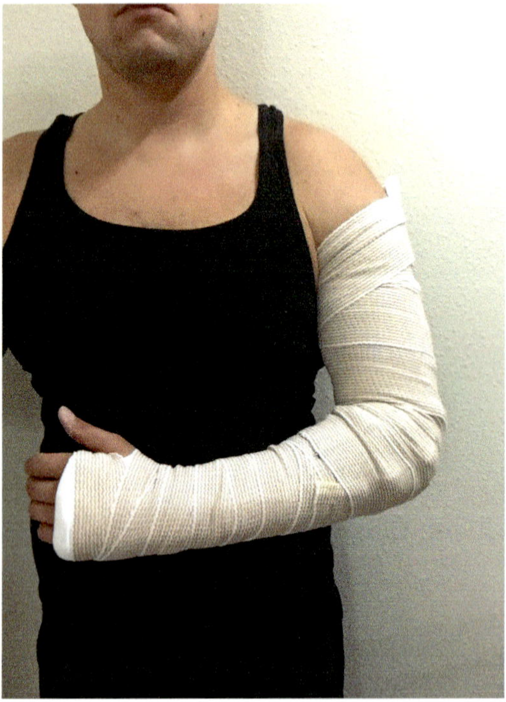

FIGURE 6.29 "Posterior long arm splint"

increased risk for non-union if placed in "hanging cast" immobilization).

- *Technique:* immobilization begins proximally above the deltoid, courses around the elbow, and ends just below the axillary region ***(entire length of the humerus should be immobilized/must extend above area of injury to avoid motion through fracture site)***.
- *Position:* elbow 90 degrees flexion, forearm neutral rotation.
  ****Can cause irritation to axillary region, may be difficult to apply/maintain in obese patients and persons with ample breast tissue.**** (See Fig. 6.30)

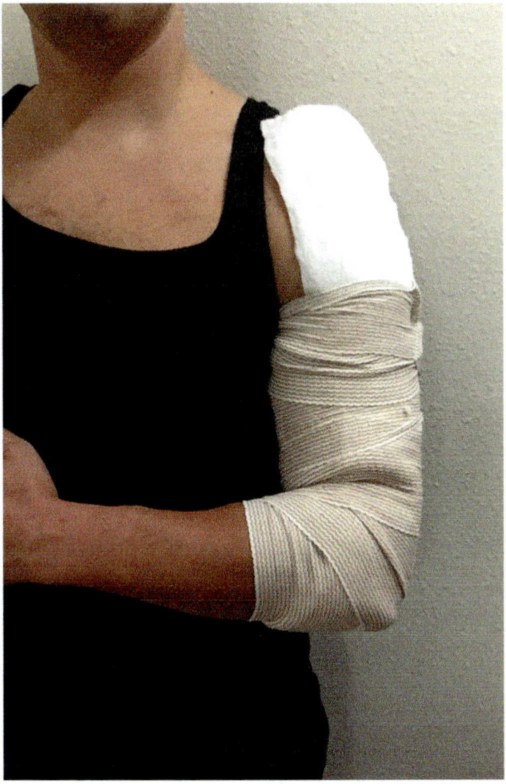

FIGURE 6.30 "Coaptation splint" – immobilization should extend above fracture site medially/laterally

B. Lower Extremity

- *Preformed Immobilization*

1. ***Ankle Stirrup:*** *Prefabricated Splint (Readily Available/ Easy Application)*
   - *Indications:* ankle sprains (e.g., lateral ligament complex), associated soft tissue strains (e.g., posterior tibialis/peroneal tendon pathology)
   - Specific ankle fracture patterns: isolated distal fibula or Weber A classification injuries (fracture line below syndesmosis)
   - Ankle joint pain/weakness (e.g., degenerative disease/inflammatory disorders; post-traumatic injury/ deformity for heightened support) (See Figs. 6.31 and 6.32)

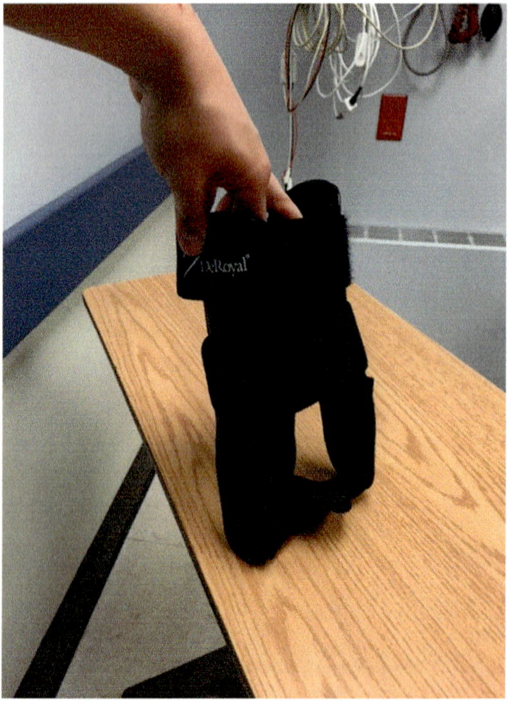

FIGURE 6.31 "Ankle stirrup brace"

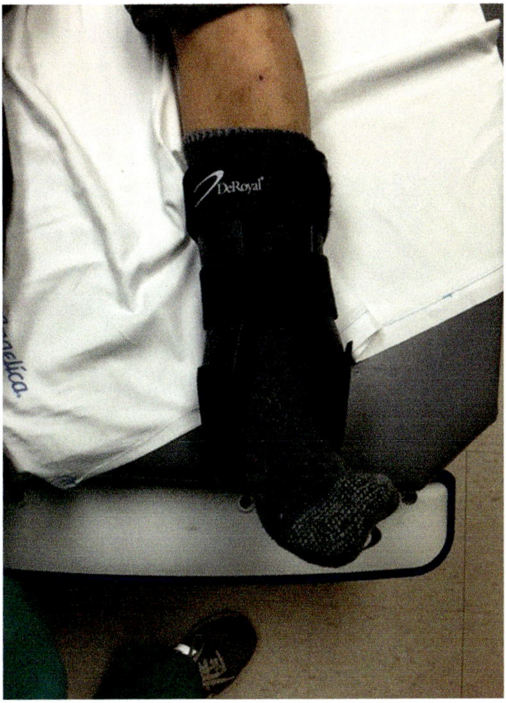

FIGURE 6.32 "Ankle stirrup application"

2. ***Knee Immobilizer (KI):*** *Prefabricated (Static Versus Dynamic)*

Indications:

- Knee ligamentous injuries/postoperative care, (e.g., MCL sprain, ACL repair)
- Pre/post-operative immobilization for select distal femur, proximal tibia and patella fractures

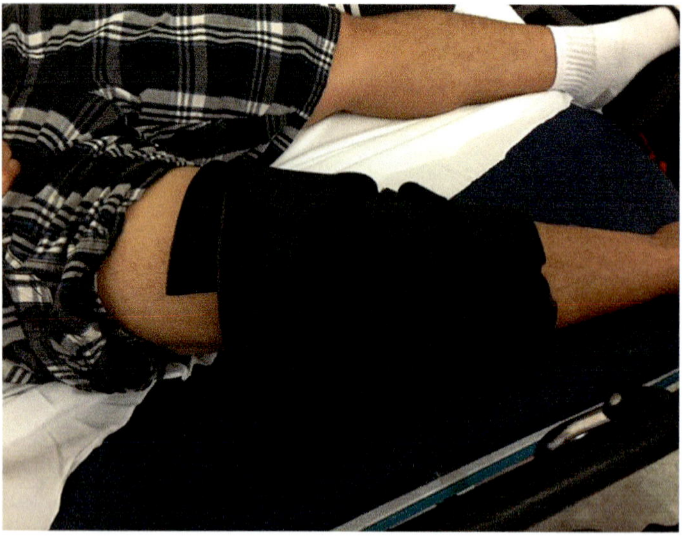

FIGURE 6.33 "Static KI"

- Following patella/posterior hip dislocation reduction
- Protection and support of quadriceps/patellar tendon (extensor mechanism) injuries
- Following repair/protection of complex soft tissue injuries that involve or extend to knee joint surface (See Figs. 6.33 and 6.34)

- ***Splinting***

1. ***Posterior Ankle Splint***

- *Indications:* rotationally stable ankle injuries (isolated non-displaced fibula **OR** medial malleolar fractures), ankle/foot sprains and strains, metatarsal/tarsal bone

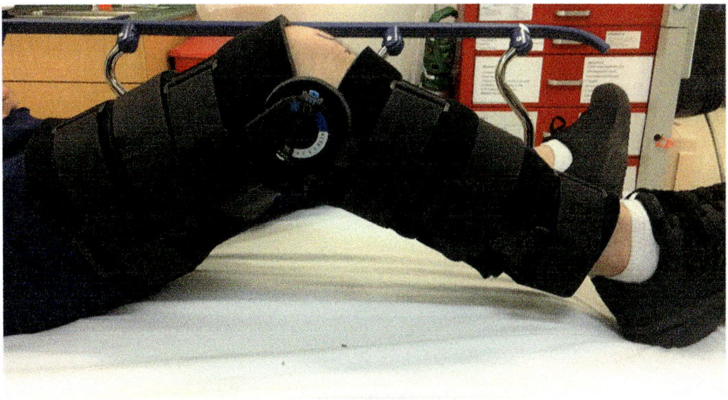

FIGURE 6.34 "Dynamic KI: hinged brace"

fractures, Achilles tendinopathy/rupture, and protection of soft tissue injuries.

- *Technique:* immobilization begins at the distal phalangeal/tarsal region depending upon injury/desire for toe plate extension and extends to the posterior mid-calf region (just below level of the fibular head).
- *Position:* ankle, neutral rotation, 90 degrees flexion (neutral).

  Irrespective of Achilles tendon ruptures (want tendon ends to re-approximate), avoid excessive ankle plantarflexion to avoid Achilles tendon (equinus) contractures that can lead to subsequent decreased dorsiflexion range/power. ** (See Fig. 6.35)

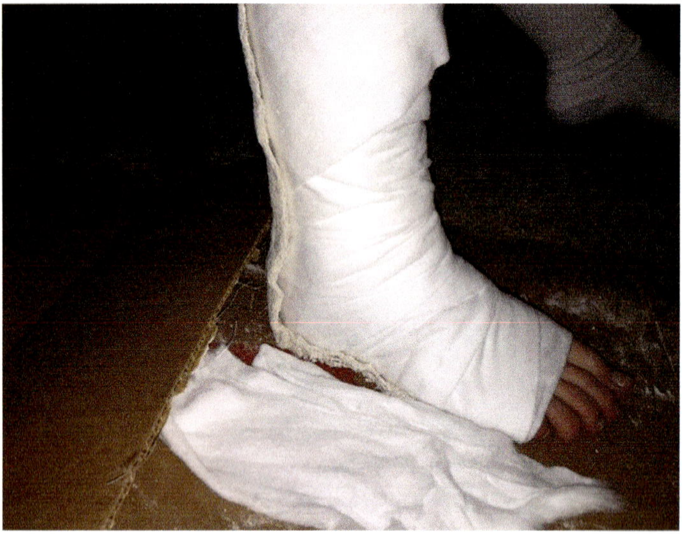

FIGURE 6.35 Posterior ankle splint made with plaster

2. ***Posterior Ankle/Stirrup Splint***

- *Indications:* unstable/post-reduction ankle fractures and/or dislocations.
- *Technique:* **(a)** ***posterior portion*** begins at the distal phalangeal/tarsal region depending upon injury/desire for toe plate extension and extends to the posterior mid-calf region (just below level of the fibular head). **(b)** ***Stirrup portion*** begins below level of fibular head

and courses distally, under plantar surface of foot, and returns to an equal height on opposite side.
*Posterior portion of splint is always applied first.*

- *Position:* ankle, neutral rotation, 90 degrees flexion (neutral) (See Fig. 6.36).

3. ***Long Leg Posterior Splint (+/− Side Slabs for Rotational Control)***
   *****Side slabs should be ~ five layers versus the posterior portion that should be ~ 10 layers.*****

- *Indications:* distal femur/proximal tibia fractures, extensor mechanism/knee injuries, following repair/

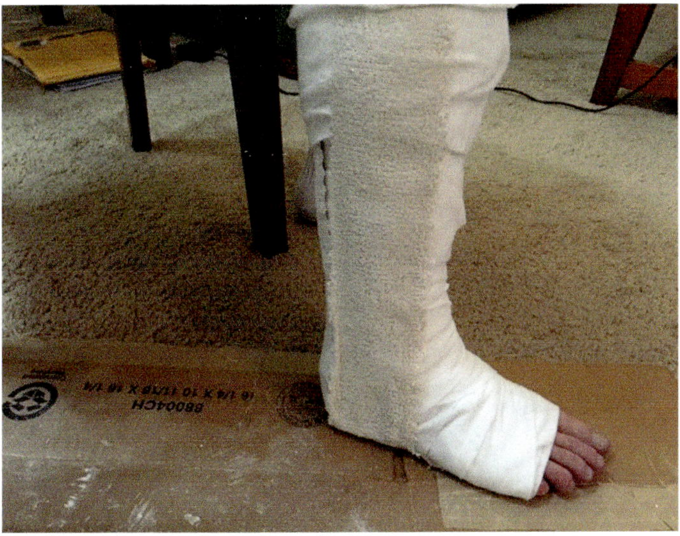

FIGURE 6.36 Posterior + Stirrup splint (Posterior "U")

protection of complex soft tissue injuries that involve or extend to joint surface.

****Can be extended distally for more distal injuries (e.g., tibial shaft fractures/ankle with addition of stirrup component)*****

- *Technique:* initiated just below gluteal crease and extends to just proximal to the malleoli.
- *Position:* knee joint should be maintained in ~15–20 flexion to prevent delayed loss of ROM and/or residual stiffness (See Fig. 6.37).

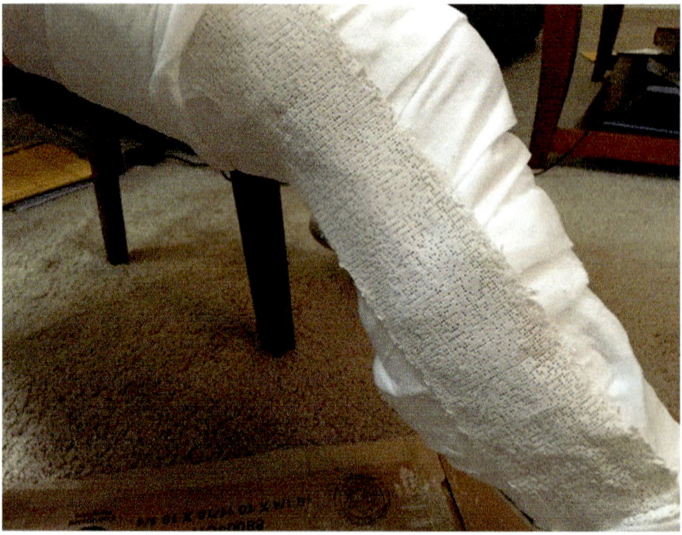

Figure 6.37 Long-leg posterior splint with addition of side slabs for rotational control

- ***Casting***

1. ***Short Leg Cast***

- *Indications:* definitive treatment of ankle/foot injuries (non-displaced/"reduced" fractures)/soft tissue injuries (e.g., posterior tibialis/peroneal/Achilles tendon pathology).
- *Technique:* immobilization begins at metatarsal heads and ends ~2 inches distal to fibular head.
- *Position:* supine/upright or prone with knee flexed (relaxes gastrocnemius muscle) and ankle in neutral flexion.

The ankle should be placed in plantarflexion for Achilles tendon ruptures to allow for tendon apposition. (See Figs. 6.38 and 6.39)

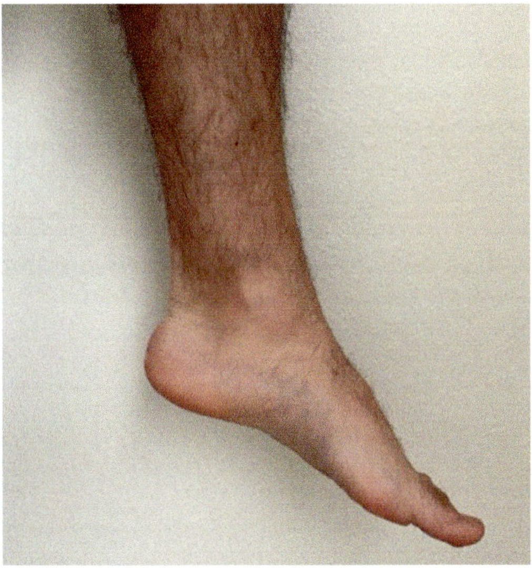

FIGURE 6.38 Plantarflexion/gravity equinus position: ankle positioning for initial Achilles tendon rupture treatment

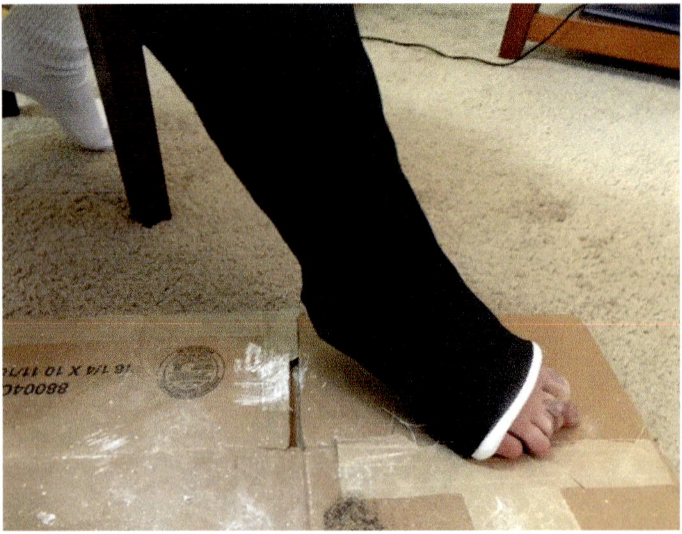

FIGURE 6.39 "Casting of Achilles tendon rupture" – ankle/foot casted in plantarflexion/gravity equinus position for initial Achilles tendon rupture treatment

(a) Measure from the metatarsal heads to ~ knee; cut stockinette to length.

*****Allow extra room to fold back before application of final layer of casting material; smooth away wrinkles/folds (trim crease at anterior ankle).*****

(b) Wrap cast padding over stockinette; ensure padding extends from metatarsal heads to level just distal to fibular head.

*****Gently wind cast padding around foot→ankle in figure-of-eight pattern; ensure edges do not cut into 90 degree bend of the ankle.*****

*****Apply extra padding to the metatarsal heads, heel, malleoli, proximal fibula, and anterior tibia.*****

(c) Wet cast material; wrap foot/ankle using moderate tension, implementing technique as above.

(d) Perform preliminary mold to ensure neutral ankle flexion/medial longitudinal arch of foot is restored.

(e) Fold stockinette back over edges of casting material, and then apply one final layer to incorporate stockinette/cotton padding edges.

(f) Mold posterior aspect of cast to assume a ~triangular shape (convex at anterolateral/medial borders, flat over anterior/posterior compartments and medial surfaces) (See Figs. 6.40 and 6.41).

Pearls:

- Ensure foot is at 90° (orthogonal) to lower leg; ankle equinus (foot plantarflexion) for an extended period of immobilization can lead to an irreversible Achilles tendon contracture.

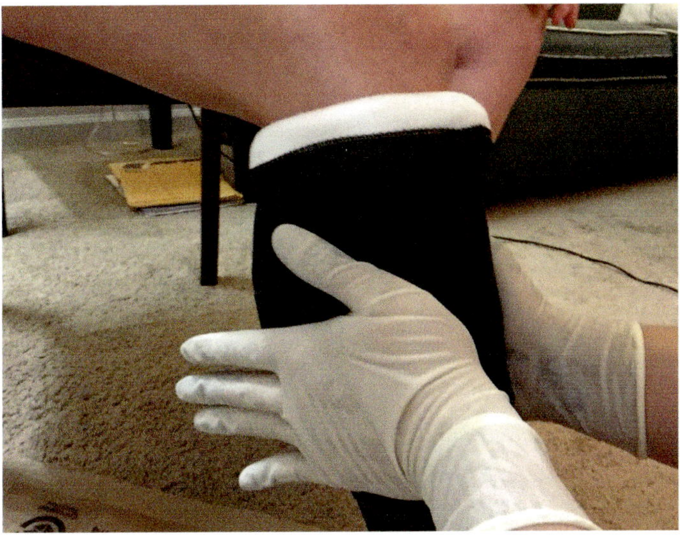

FIGURE 6.40 Molding short leg cast

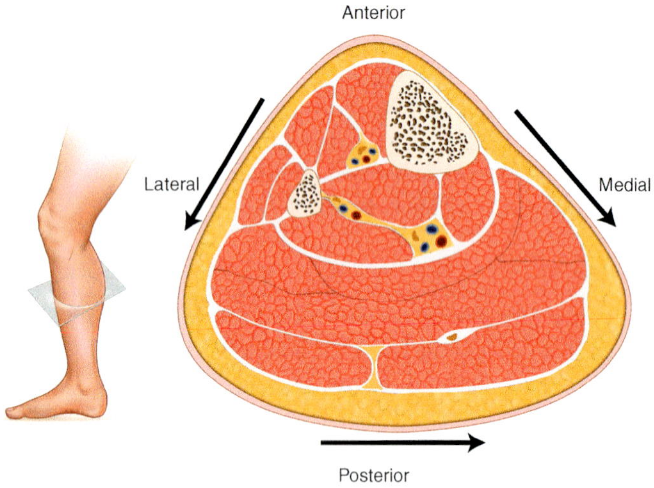

FIGURE 6.41 "Triangular shape" – desired when molding a short leg cast; note the flattening over the anterior/posterior/medial surfaces with intervening convex regions

- Maintain position of function of immobilized joint throughout casting process; stockinette and/or associated padding can create wrinkling/pressure points upon repositioning.
- Avoid applying cast too high posteriorly (can irritate popliteal space).

2. ***Long Leg Cast:*** Definitive treatment for select distal femur and proximal tibia fractures

   - *Technique:* immobilization begins distally at the metatarsal heads, with the proximal edge slightly below the greater trochanter on the lateral side, and just inferior to the groin on the medial side.
   - *Position:* knee joint should be maintained in ~15–20 flexion to prevent delayed loss of ROM and/or residual stiffness.

     *****First apply short leg section as described above, and then construct long leg portion.*****

(a) Apply additional cast padding over areas as outlined above, in addition to the patella and fibular head/neck region to protect against potential pressure points and areas susceptible to neurapraxia.
(b) Extend knee joint until ~10–15 degrees short of full extension, and apply cotton padding/cast material as above.
(c) While cast is curing, mold gently to conform to the normal curvature of the tibia and circumferentially about the knee; "supracondylar" molding will help control rotation and overall length of limb.
Ensure foot is plantigrade. If necessary, apply/maintain gentle pressure to sole of forefoot. (See Figs. 6.42–6.51)

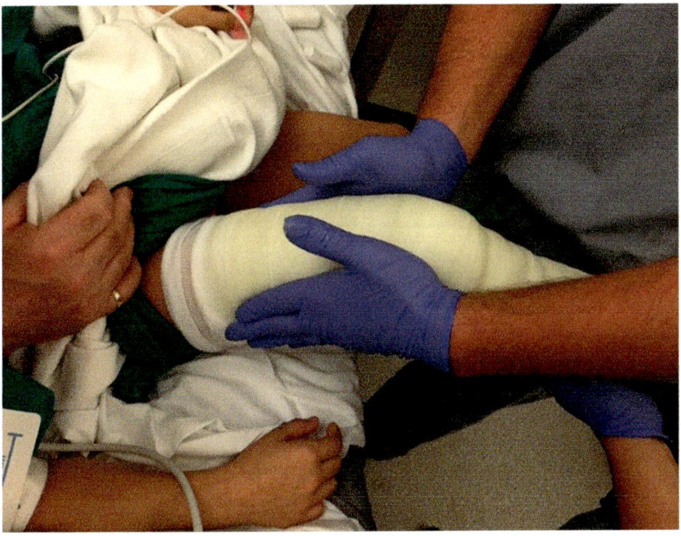

FIGURE 6.42 "Supracondylar mold" – note sculpting at the level of the medial/lateral epicondyles

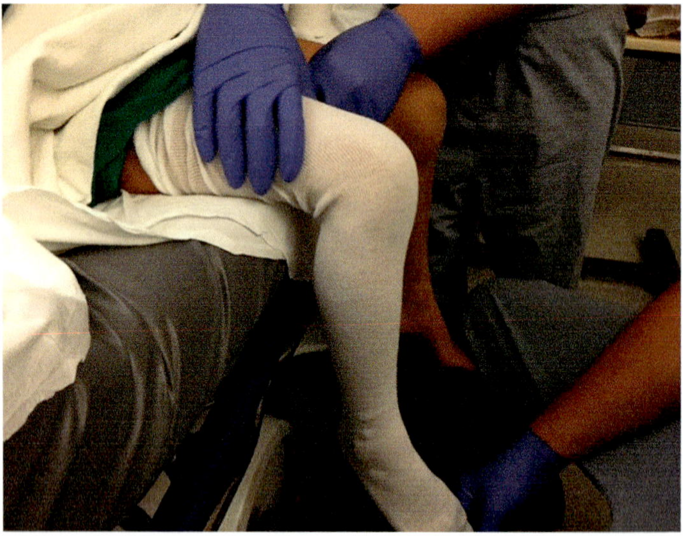

FIGURE 6.43 "Long leg cast sequence" – placement of patient in proper position prior to cast application

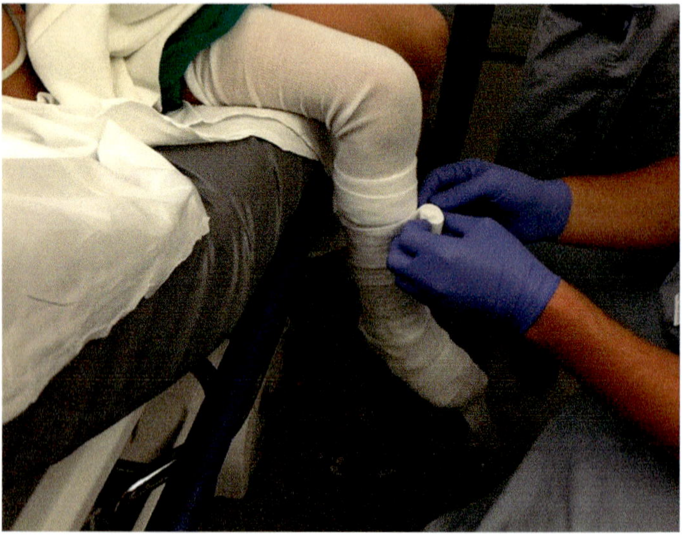

FIGURE 6.44 "Long leg cast sequence" – application of Webril

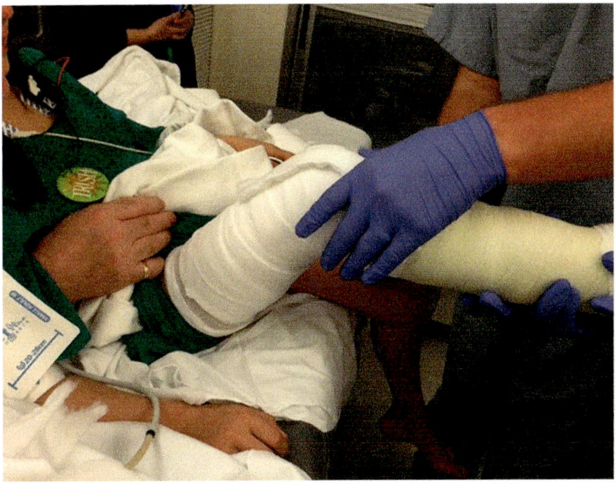

FIGURE 6.45 "Long leg cast sequence" – application of extra padding to bony prominences (ex: patella)

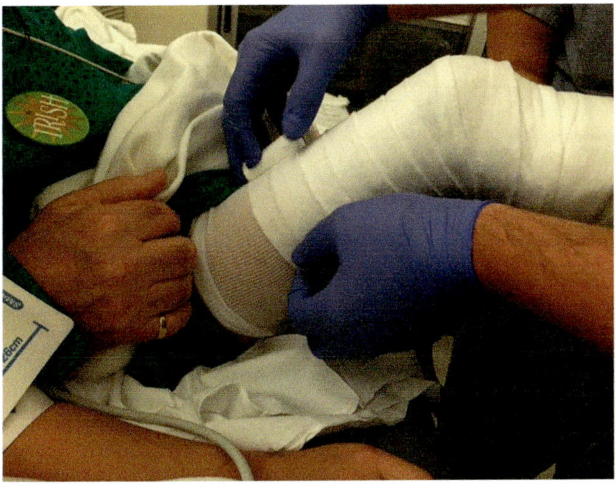

FIGURE 6.46 "Long leg casting sequence" – application of upper leg portion after lower leg section completed

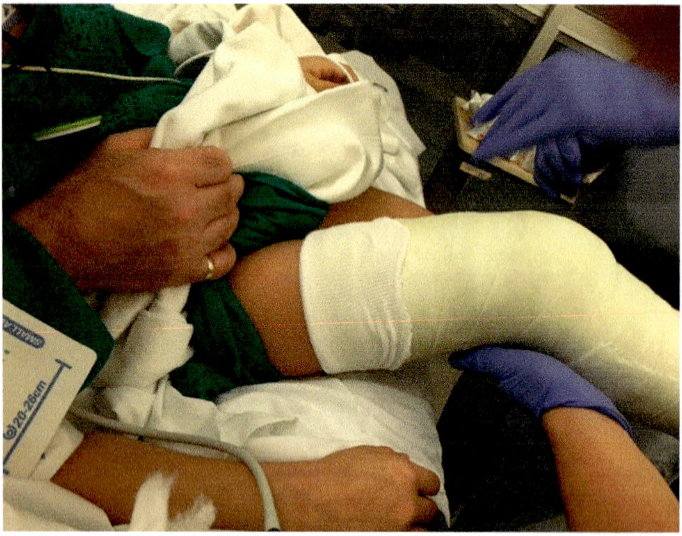

FIGURE 6.47 "Long leg casting sequence" – folding over of stockinette to ensure smooth ends prior to application of the final layer of casting material

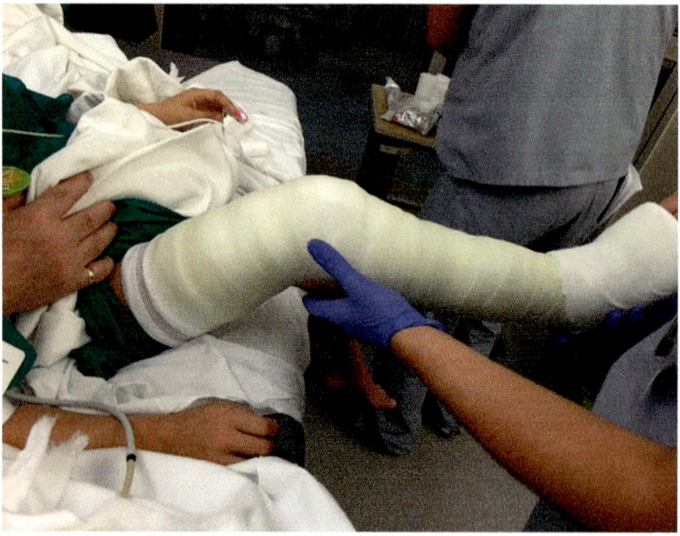

FIGURE 6.48 "Long leg cast sequence" – proper positioning of patient prior to final cast molding

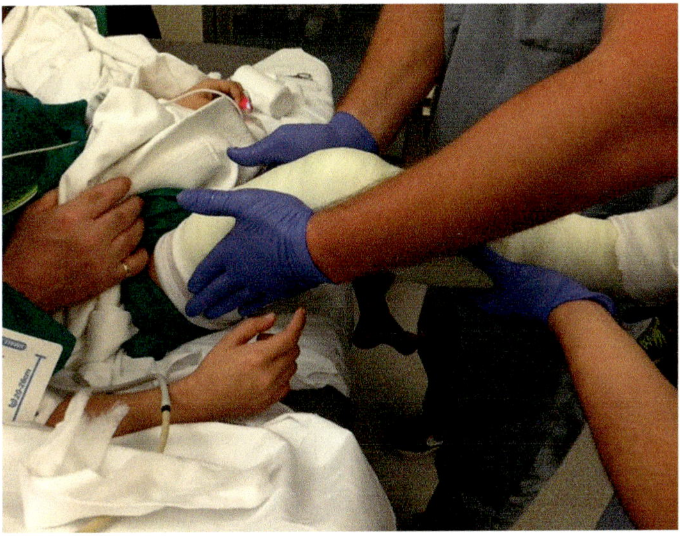

FIGURE 6.49 "Long leg cast sequence" – supracondylar molding

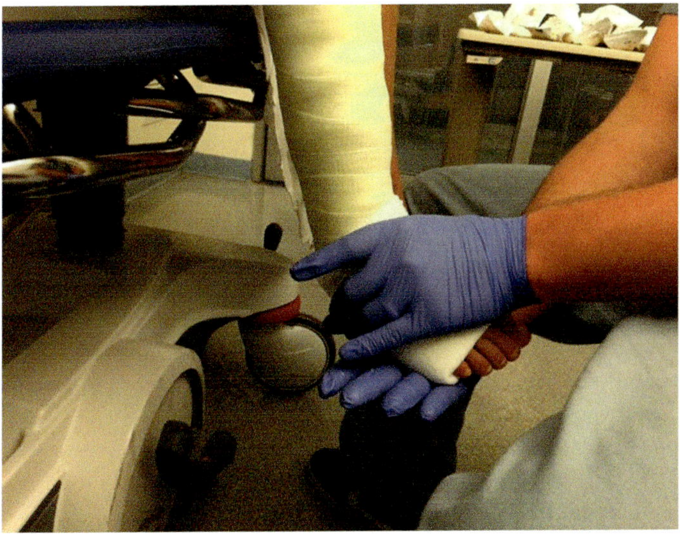

FIGURE 6.50 "Long leg cast sequence" – maintaining the ankle in neutral position

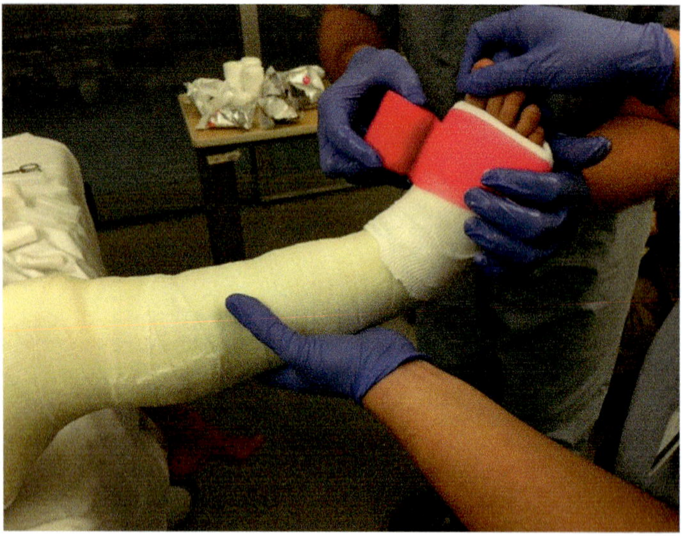

FIGURE 6.51 "Long leg cast sequence" – application of the final layer of cast material

Tips for Immobilization Success

- Patient education regarding swelling, signs of vascular compromise, and recommendations for reassessment is paramount to avoid potential complications of extended immobilization.

  ****All displaced fractures should be "reduced" to minimize pain/patient discomfort, decrease risk of neurovascular injury, minimize soft tissue complications, etc. (including those that will require operative intervention).*****

- Patients with non-traumatic musculoskeletal disorders (e.g., gout/infections/burns) may also benefit from short-term immobilization.

- Adequate analgesia and muscle relaxation are critical for optimal outcome.
- Reduction maneuvers are generally specific to certain fracture patterns and/or locations.
- Attempt to correct/restore length, rotation, and angulation of fracture fragments.
- Three-point contact (molding) is necessary to maintain "closed" reduction: involves application of pressure at site of fracture, as well as proximal/distal.
- Consider immobilization of joint above/below injury to help maintain overall bony alignment.
- Immobilization position for wrist/hand fractures ("intrinsic plus" position) (See Fig. 6.52).

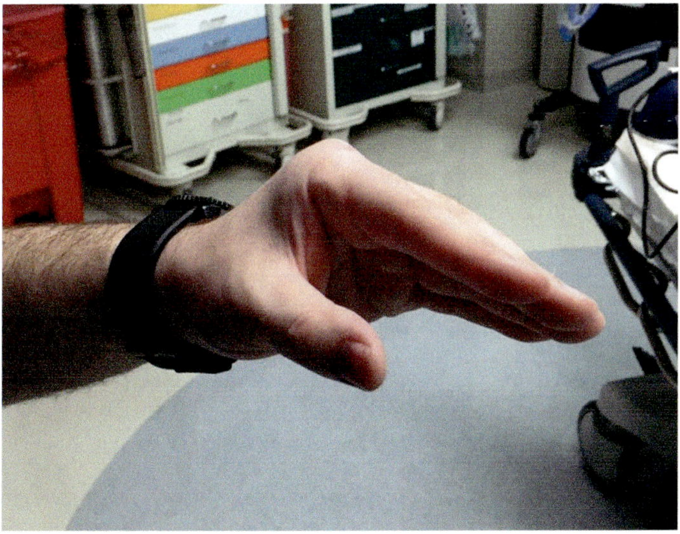

FIGURE 6.52 "Intrinsic plus" position

Immobilization Complications to Avoid

A. *Compartment Syndrome*

- It is less common with usage of splints versus circumferential casting. ***However***, can occur with splint implementation from constricting/excess padding.
- ***Management:*** remove all constricting bandages/splint material, and initiate early surgical consultation with respect to potential need for operative intervention.

B. Heat Injury/Pressure Sores

- It results from stockinette/cast padding wrinkles, indentions in plaster/fiberglass (using fingers to mold), poor padding practices (insufficient padding over bony prominences), etc. (See Fig. 6.53).
- Heat generated is ***inversely*** proportional to the setting time and ***directly*** proportional to the number of layers of casting material implemented.
- Dip water temperature/cast thickness: factors most strongly associated with cast-related burns (risk of thermal injury significantly increases when dip water temperature is too hot and the casting material is too thick).

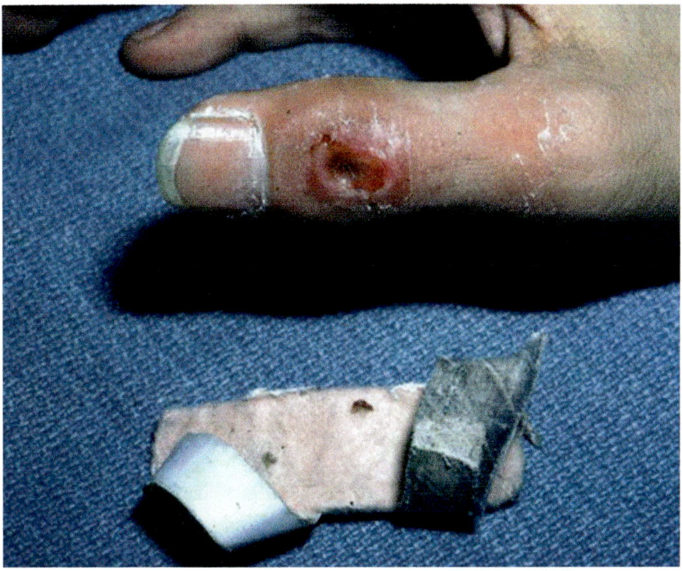

FIGURE 6.53 "Pressure sore" – Note that poor cast application (failure to remove wrinkles, provide adequate padding of bony prominences) can lead to pressure sores and neurovascular injury. (Image reproduced with permission from Roy A Meals, MD, University of California, Los Angeles, David Geffen School of Medicine, published by Medscape Drugs & Diseases (https://emedicine.medscape.com/), Mallet Finger, 2017, available at https://emedicine.medscape.com/article/1242305-overview)

C. Cast Saw Burns

- ***Use strong caution when removing casts.*** Cast saws are designed to cut hard casting material, not softer surfaces (e.g., padding/skin), but complications can still exist (e.g., burns/abrasions) (See Fig. 6.54).

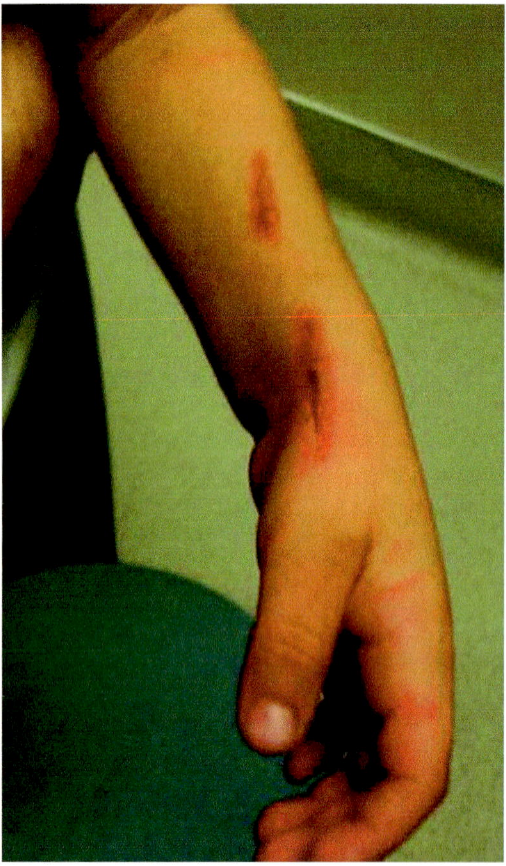

Figure 6.54 "Cast saw burns" – Avoid excess pressure while using cast saw to remove casting material. (Reprinted from Abdelgawad A, Naga O. Casts, splints, and braces. In: Abdelgawad A, Naga O, editors. Pediatric orthopedics. New York: Springer; 2014. p. 493–501. With permission from Springer Nature)

Medical Record Documentation

- Note indication for immobilization.
- Describe any wounds/location under immobilization.

- Document neurovascular exam findings (***Before and After*** application).
  ****Indicate type/temporal guidelines regarding re-evaluation of the injury.****
  ****Certain subsets of patients are at higher risk for immobilization-related complications.****
  – Patients with an inability to effectively communicate (e.g., obtunded/comatose multi-trauma patient).
  – Patients with impaired sensation at baseline (e.g., spinal cord injury, DM).
  – Patients with disorders that include increased tone/spasticity (usually associated with poor communication skills/poor nutrition, etc.).

Suggested Readings

1. Baecher NB. Volar splinting. Medscape. 14, 2018. Retrieved from: https://emedicine.medscape.com/article/109769-overview.
2. Boyd A, et al. Principles of splinting & casting. Am Fam Physician. 2009a;79(1):16–22.
3. Boyd A, et al. Splints & casts: indications & methods. Am Fam Physician. 2009b;80(5):491–9.
4. Chapman M, et al. Chapman's orthopaedic surgery. 2000.
5. Chundnofsky CR, Byers SE. Splinting techniques. In: Roberts JR, Hedges J, editors. Clinical procedures in emergency medicine. 4th ed. Philadelphia: Saunders Elsevier; 2004. p. 909–21.
6. Egol K, Koval K, Zuckerman J. Part I. In: Handbook of fractures. 4th ed: Lippincott and Williams; 2010.
7. Fitch M. Basic splinting techniques. NEJM. 2008;359:32–7.
8. Griggs SM, Weiss AP. Bony injuries of the wrist, forearm, and elbow. Clin Sports Med. 1996;15(2):373–400.
9. Hak DJ, Golladay GJ. Olecranon fractures: treatment options. J Am Acad Orthop Surg. 2000;8(4):266–75.
10. Halanski MA, et al. Thermal injury with contemporary cast-application techniques and methods to circumvent morbidity. J Bone Joint Surg Am. 2007;89(11):2369–7.
11. Halanski M, et al. Cast and splint immobilization: complications. J Am Acad Orthop Surg. 2008;16(1):30–40.

12. Lee SG, Jupiter JB. Phalangeal and metacarpal fractures of the hand. Hand Clin. 2000;16(3):323–32.
13. Leggit J, Meko CJ, et al. Acute finger injuries: part I. Tendons and ligaments. Am Fam Physician. 2006;73:210–6.
14. Roberts DM, Stallard TC. Emergency department evaluation and treatment of knee and leg injuries. Emerg Med Clin North Am. 2000;18(1):67–84.
15. Simon RR, Sherman SC, editors. Emergency orthopedics: the extremities. 6th ed. China: The McGraw-Hill Companies; 2007. p. 16.
16. Smith G, et al. Fiberglass cast application. Am J Emerg Med. 2005;23(3)
17. Tintinalli J, et al. Chapter 263. Initial evaluation and management of orthopedic injuries. In: Tintinalli's emergency medicine: a comprehensive study guide., 8e. McGraw-Hill Education / Medical: New York, NY.
18. Zemel NP. Metacarpophalangeal joint injuries in fingers. Hand Clin. 1992;8(4):745–54.

Chapter 7
Distal Radius

Daniel Purcell and Bryan A. Terry

Introduction

- Distal radius injuries are extremely common; thus it is imperative to possess a thorough understanding of their evaluation and treatment.
- Injuries not recognized/managed incorrectly can lead to heightened patient morbidity (cosmetically and functionally), initiating potential for long-term disability.

A. ***ANATOMY***

- *Distal surface* is biconcave, containing facets that allow articulation with the proximal carpal row (scaphoid and lunate).
- *Medial surface* (sigmoid notch of radius) forms semicircular region that articulates with head of the ulna, allowing forearm pronation/supination.

D. Purcell (✉)
Emergency Department, New York University Langone Medical Center Brooklyn, New York, NY, USA
e-mail: daniel.purcell@nyumc.org

B. A. Terry
The Brooklyn Hospital Center, Brooklyn, NY, USA

D. Purcell et al. (eds.), *Emergency Orthopedics Handbook*,
https://doi.org/10.1007/978-3-030-00707-2_7

- *Lateral surface* elongates into prominent styloid process, providing insertion for the brachioradialis muscle.
- Metaphyseal widening of the distal radius (composed primarily of trabecular/cancellous bone) begins ~ 2 cm proximal to the radio-carpal joint; this decreased cortical support enhances risk of fracture based upon inferior loading characteristics.

B. *RADIOGRAPHIC EVALUATION*

- ***Normal Radiographic Values***

1. ***Radial Length or Height:*** distance between one line perpendicular to long axis of the radius passing through distal tip of radial styloid and a second line intersecting the distal articular surface of the ulnar head; normal range ~ 10–13 mm
2. ***Radial Inclination or Angulation:*** angle between one line connecting the radial styloid tip/ulnar aspect of the distal radius and a second line perpendicular to the longitudinal axis of radius; normal range between 21° and 25° (See Fig. 7.1)

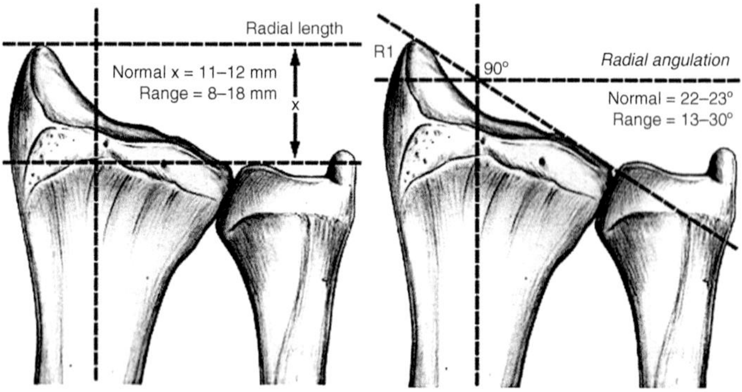

FIGURE 7.1 Posteroanterior (PA) view. (Reprinted from Berger, et al. Extra articular distal radius fractures. In: Berger RA, Weiss APC, editors. Hand surgery. Philadelphia: Lippincott Williams & Wilkens; 2004. With permission from Wolters Kluwer Health)

3. ***Palmar (Volar) Tilt:*** angle between one line drawn along the distal radial articular surface and a second line perpendicular to the longitudinal axis of the radius at the joint margin; normal average ~ 11°–12° (See Fig. 7.2)

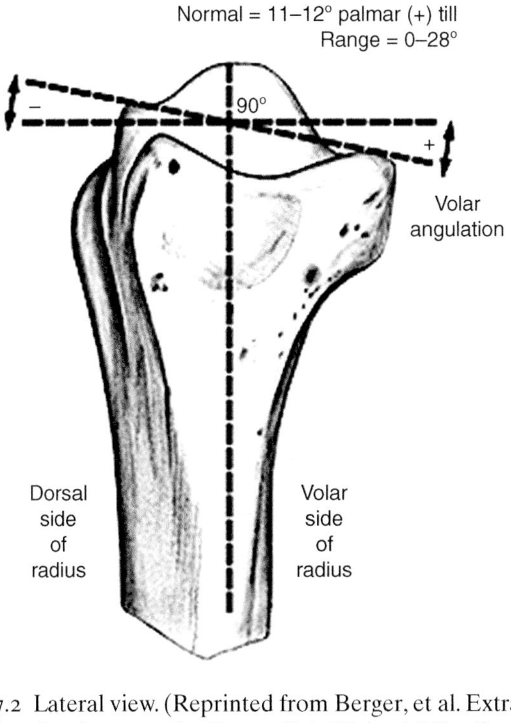

FIGURE 7.2 Lateral view. (Reprinted from Berger, et al. Extra articular distal radius fractures. In: Berger RA, Weiss APC, editors. Hand surgery. Philadelphia: Lippincott Williams & Wilkens; 2004. With permission from Wolters Kluwer Health)

C. *DISTAL RADIUS FRACTURES*

- Incidence increases with age; readily comparable to the rise in hip fractures.
- Causally related to decreasing bone quality (osteopenia/"fragility fractures"), unexpected falls/ trauma, functional decreases in strength/dexterity, alterations in gait, and overall proportional increase in the elderly population subset.
- Despite their high frequency, indications for surgical intervention and method of treatment still remain relatively subjective.
- Most common mechanism of injury involves fall on an outstretched hand (FOOSH): (See Fig. 7.3)

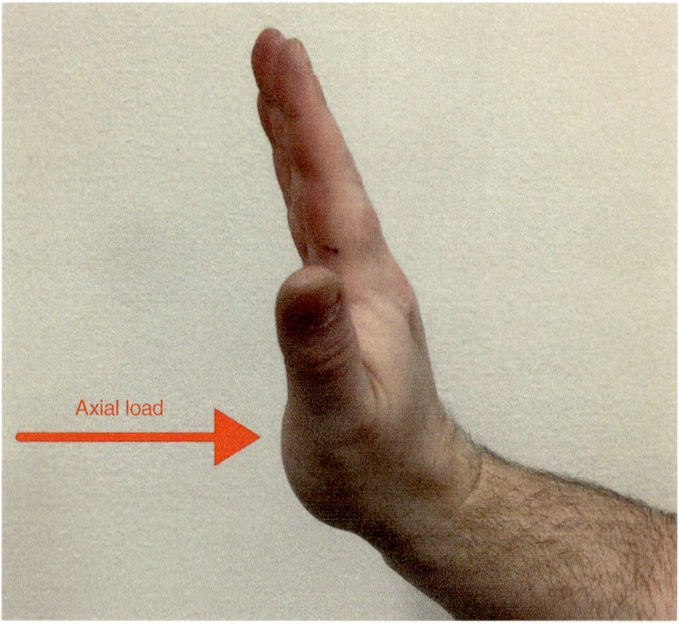

FIGURE 7.3 Fall on outstretched arm (FOOSH) produces an axial load onto the distal radius

Patient bodyweight is transmitted along longitudinal axis of radius, resulting in massive bending forces, eventually leading to metaphyseal collapse.

- Volar cortex fails under tension, while the dorsal cortex cannot withstand the heightened compressive forces; mechanical penetration of the stiffer, more proximal, diaphyseal cortex also contributes to injury.
- Diagnosis/treatment of distal radius fractures involves:
  - Understanding biomechanics of the fracture
  - Differentiating between intra/extra-articular injuries
  - Appreciation of dorsal/volar cortex comminution
  - Recognition of severity/direction of fracture displacement (angulation) and/or shortening
  - Assessment of the DRUJ and surrounding soft tissue integrity
  - Determining "physiologic age" of the patient

These variables help determine the *stability* of the fracture pattern, generally the most important factor in formulating a treatment plan. Patient handedness, activity requirements, patient expectations, etc. must also be considered.

- ***COMMON FRACTURE PATTERNS***

1. ***Colles Fracture ("Dinner Fork" Deformity)*** (See Fig. 7.4a–c)

   - Comprise >90% of distal radius fractures; patient lands with wrist hyperextended, experiencing a pronation force across the wrist as the body rotates away from the arm (See Fig. 7.5).

2. ***Smith Fracture ("Garden Spade" Deformity)*** (See Fig. 7.6a, b)

   - Demonstrates opposite mechanism, clinical and radiographic appearance to Colles fractures ("*reverse Colles*"); patient lands with wrist flexed, experiencing supination force as body rotates toward the arm (See Fig. 7.7).

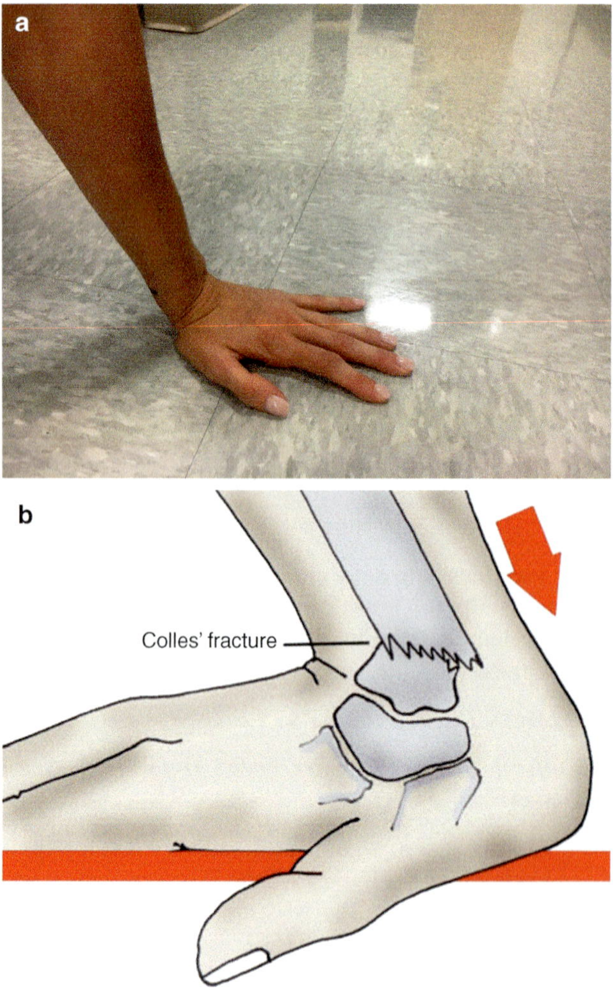

FIGURE 7.4 Colles fracture: (**a**) injury mechanism, (**b**) pathology, (**c**) "dinner fork" deformity. (**b**: Reprinted from Mesplié G, Lemoine S. Recent Fractures of the Inferior Extremity of the Radius. In: Hand and Wrist Rehabilitation. Cham: Springer; 2015: 147–169. With permission from Springer Nature. **c**: Reprinted from https://commons.wikimedia.org/wiki/File:Poignet_Gauche_suite_a_fracture_type_Pouteau_Colles.jpg. With permission from Creative Commons License: https://creativecommons.org/publicdomain/zero/1.0/deed.en)

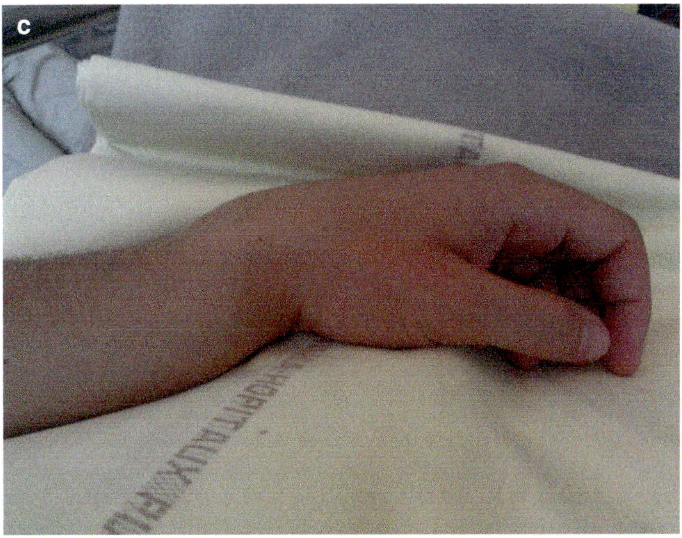

FIGURE 7.4 (continued)

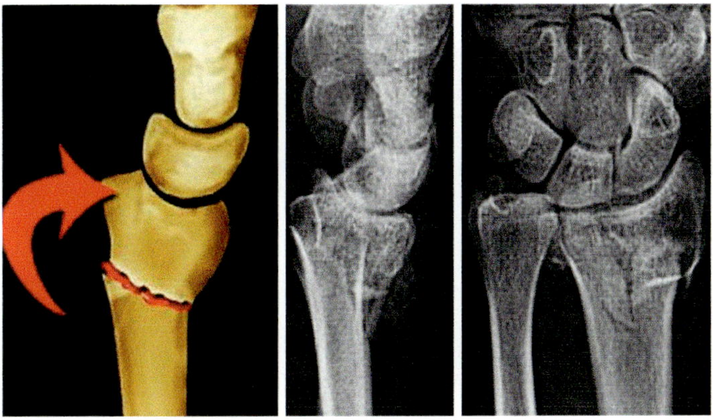

FIGURE 7.5 Apex volar/dorsal angulation pattern (dorsal displacement of distal fracture fragment) seen in Colles fractures. (Reprinted from http://rad.desk.nl/en/p476a23436683b/wrist-fractures.html. With permission from Robin H.M. Smithuis)

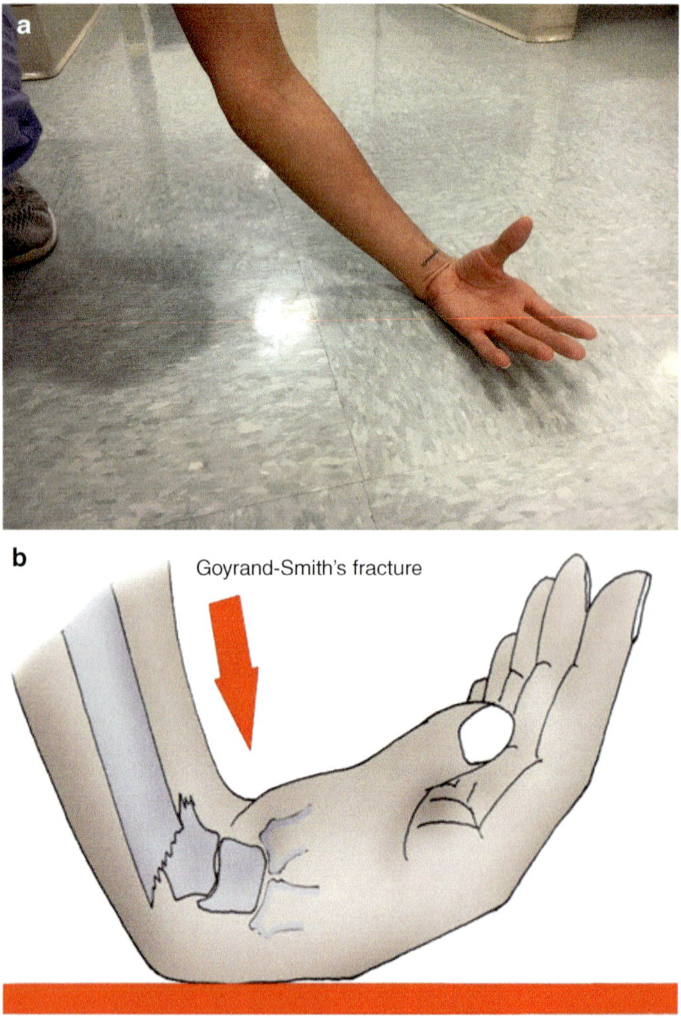

FIGURE 7.6 Smith fracture: (**a**) injury mechanism, (**b**) pathology. (**b**: Reprinted from Mesplié G, Lemoine S. Recent fractures of the inferior extremity of the radius. In: Hand and wrist rehabilitation. Cham: Springer; 2015: 147–169. With permission from Springer Nature)

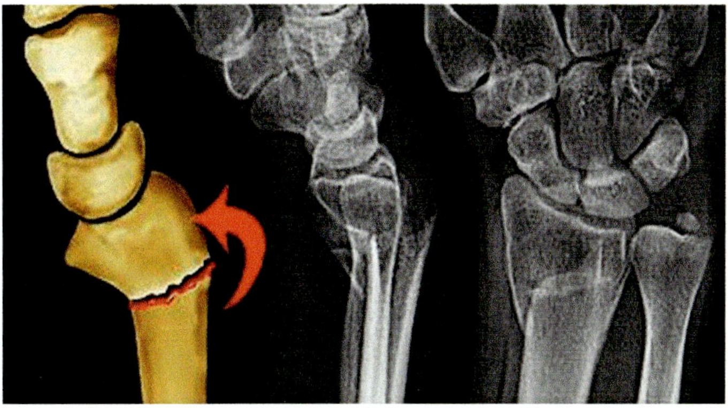

FIGURE 7.7 Apex dorsal/volar angulation pattern (volar displacement of distal fracture fragment) seen in Smith fractures. (Reprinted from http://rad.desk.nl/en/p476a23436683b/wrist-fractures.html. With permission from Robin H.M. Smithuis)

3. ***Barton Fracture***

- Dorsal/Volar (more common) distal radius rim disruption; occurs secondary to shear forces acting upon distal articular radial surface.
- Highly unstable injury, with significant tendency for repeat displacement following manipulation ***(almost always requires operative treatment)*** (See Figs. 7.8, 7.9, and 7.10)

4. **Radial Styloid Fracture (Chauffer's Fracture)**

- Avulsion fracture of radial styloid process by extrinsic wrist ligaments
- Generally involves abutment of scaphoid against the styloid with the wrist positioned in dorsiflexion and ulnar deviation
- Usually part of comminuted, intra-articular fracture or intercarpal ligamentous injury (e.g., scapholunate disruption) (See Fig. 7.11)

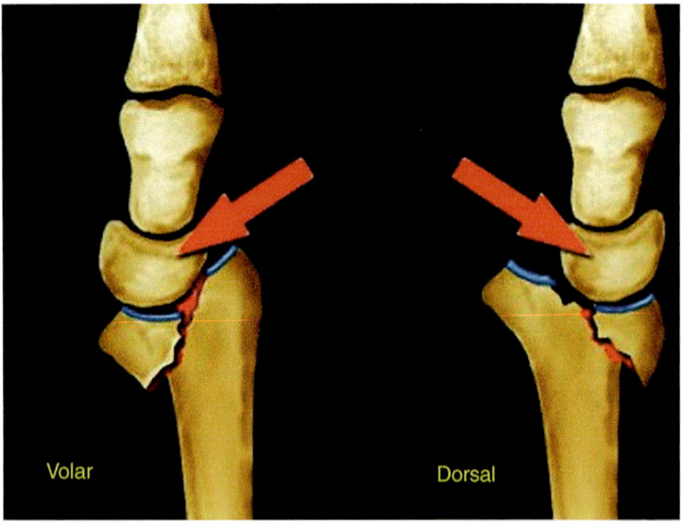

FIGURE 7.8 Barton fractures. (Reprinted from http://rad.desk.nl/en/p476a234366 83b/wrist-fractures.html. With permission from Robin H.M. Smithuis)

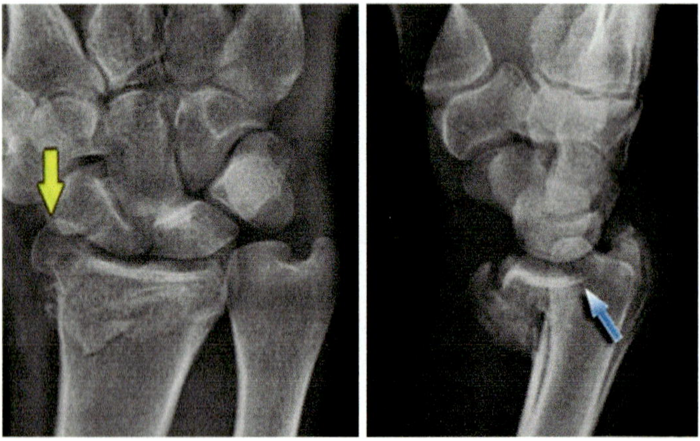

FIGURE 7.9 Volar Barton fracture: volar rim maintains its relationship with carpus despite being displaced proximally (blue arrow); there is also a radial styloid fracture leading to loss of radial inclination (yellow arrow). (Reprinted from http://rad.desk.nl/en/p476a234366683b/wrist-fractures.html. With permission from Robin H.M. Smithuis)

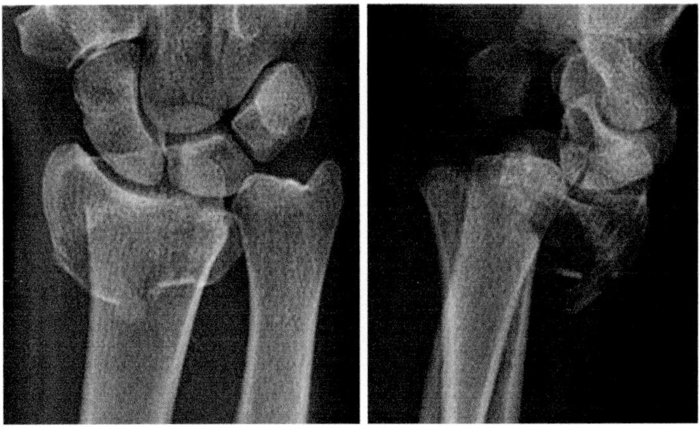

FIGURE 7.10 Dorsal Barton fracture: note dorsal rim of radius and carpus are displaced proximally and dorsally. (Reprinted from http://rad.desk.nl/en/p476a23436683b/wrist-fractures.html. With permission from Robin H.M. Smithuis)

D. *CLINICAL EVALUATION*

- Comprehensive history and physical examination should be performed prior to administering anesthetic and/or any attempts at fracture reduction ***(unless neurovascular compromise/threat to skin integrity exists)***.
- Special attention should be paid to median nerve function, documenting any evidence of diminished neuromotor function (See Fig. 7.12 and 7.13).
- Perfusion status should also be assessed, along with detailed examination of flexor/extensor tendon function.
- Examination of the forearm, elbow, and shoulder is critical to avoid missing subtle, more proximal injuries, while distal carpal/phalangeal injuries also need to be excluded.
- Multiple ligamentous attachments cross the distal radial region, helping to assist in fracture reduction via "ligamentotaxis" (application of longitudinal distraction force, allowing surrounding soft tissue envelope to help realign bony fragments, maintain fracture length, and facilitate reduction).

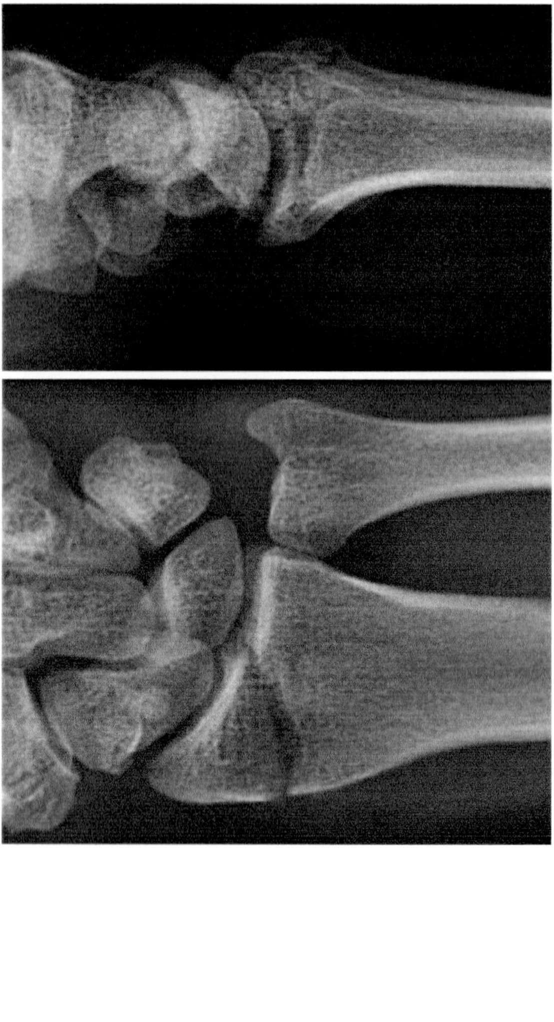

FIGURE 7.11 Isolated radial styloid fracture. (Reprinted from http://rad.desk.nl/en/p476a23436683b/wrist-fractures.html. With permission from Robin H.M. Smithuis)

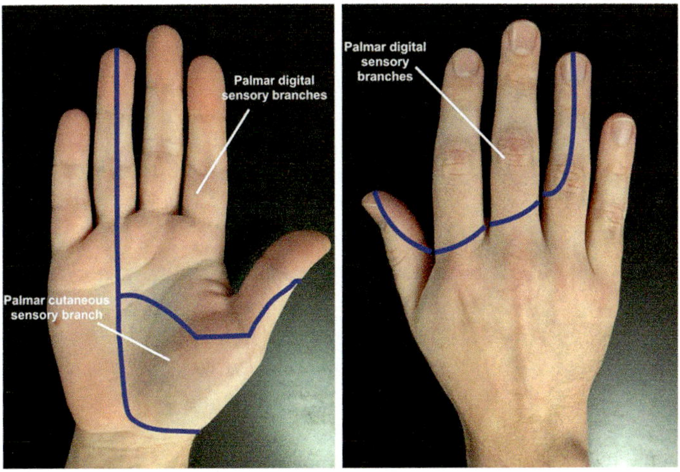

FIGURE 7.12 Median nerve sensory distribution

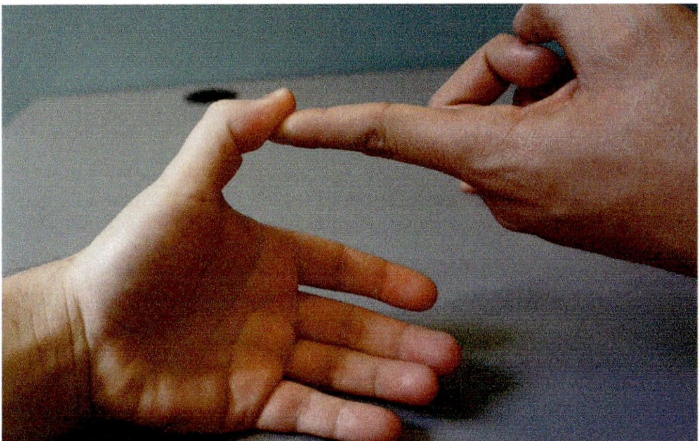

FIGURE 7.13 Testing median nerve/AIN function: resisted thumb IPJ flexion

- ***All grossly displaced fractures, especially those with neurovascular compromise, require timely reduction (irrespective of potential need for future surgical intervention).***
- ***"Anatomic" reduction is the goal for every patient; however, it is not "possible" nor required in every patient to achieve satisfactory functional outcome; patient demographics (age, handedness)/expectations, bone quality/associated clinical characteristics, social needs, etc. must also be considered; some clinical scenarios require higher levels of specialization and/or surgical intervention regardless of the best of efforts.***
- Despite the relationship between "anatomic" reduction and functional wrist capacity, many patients maintain "normal" wrist function and/or experience minimal pain, despite clear radiographic evidence of residual deformity.

E. ***REDUCTION TECHNIQUE(S) FOR DORSALLY DISPLACED FRACTURES (COLLES FRACTURES)***

Method 1 (No Equipment Necessary)

- Relies on direct manipulation of distal fracture fragment.

  1. Employs both hands to disimpact fracture fragments by the application of ***longitudinal traction and extension forces*** across the wrist.
  2. While maintaining traction, apply flexion and ulnar deviation forces to "reduce" distal fragment.
  3. Fracture then maintained in "reduced" position by applying pronation, flexion, and ulnar deviation forces during immobilization application (See Fig. 7.14a–c).

Method 2 (Requires "Finger Traps")

- Helpful for both "reduction" and application of immobilization when no assistant available.
- Relies on longitudinal traction through ligamentotaxis and assistance of gravity (See Fig. 7.15).

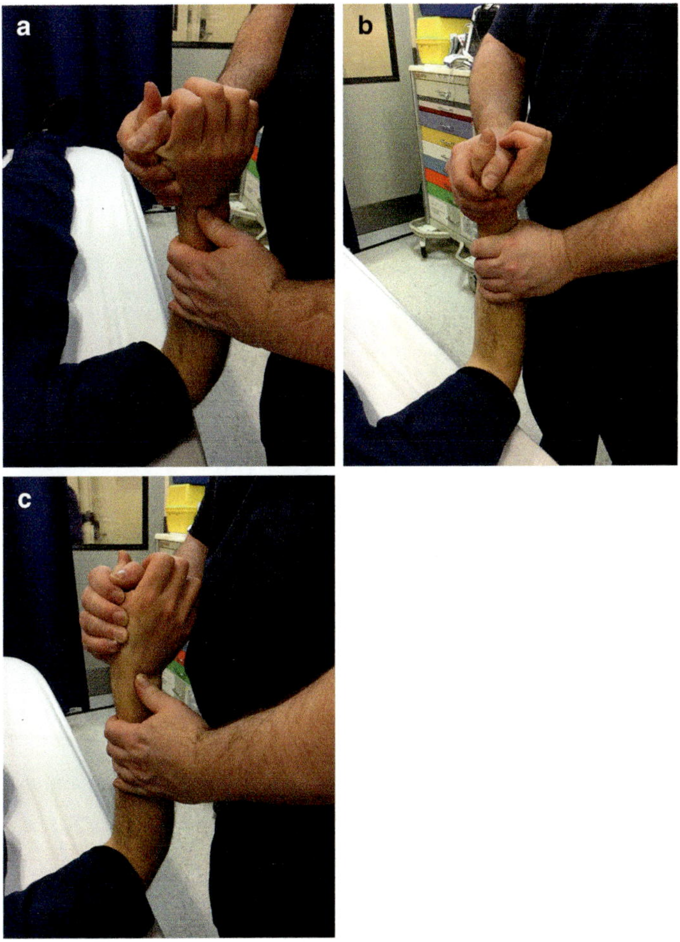

FIGURE 7.14 Longitudinal traction method for displaced Colles fracture: (**a**) initial positioning with firm grip of patient hand with palpation of fracture site, (**b**) fracture deformity reproduced while wrist extended, (**c**) distal fracture fragment moved in volar/ulnar direction

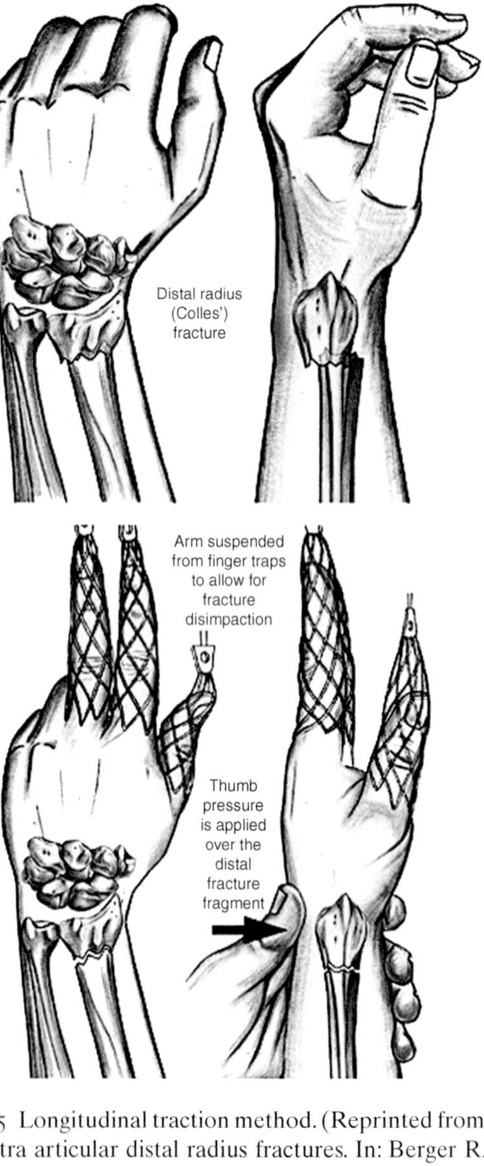

FIGURE 7.15 Longitudinal traction method. (Reprinted from Duncan S, et al. Extra articular distal radius fractures. In: Berger RA, Weiss APC, editors. Hand surgery. Philadelphia: Lippincott Williams & Wilkens; 2004. With permission from Wolters Kluwer Health)

Immobilization: Sugar-Tong Splint (See Fig. 7.16)

- Volar aspect should allow full metacarpophalangeal joint flexion; incorporation of elbow prevents forearm rotation (less risk of fracture fragment displacement) (See Fig. 7.17).
- Appropriate position of immobilization: hand/wrist placed in slight flexion/ulnar deviation.
- Excessive wrist flexion can result in the development of median nerve dysfunction *(acute carpal tunnel syndrome)* versus lack of wrist flexion can result in late fracture displacement.
- ***Prediction of poor outcome following attempted "closed" reduction:***
  - Radial shortening >5 mm compared to contralateral side
  - Radial inclination <15°
  - Loss of palmar tilt >10° (neutral tilt acceptable)
  - Intraarticular step-off >2 mm
  - DRUJ articular incongruity >2 mm

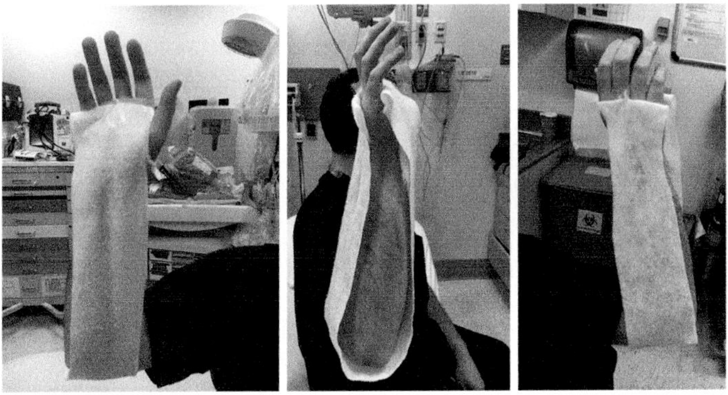

FIGURE 7.16 Sugar-tong splint: note the distal aspect allows for full MCPJ flexion

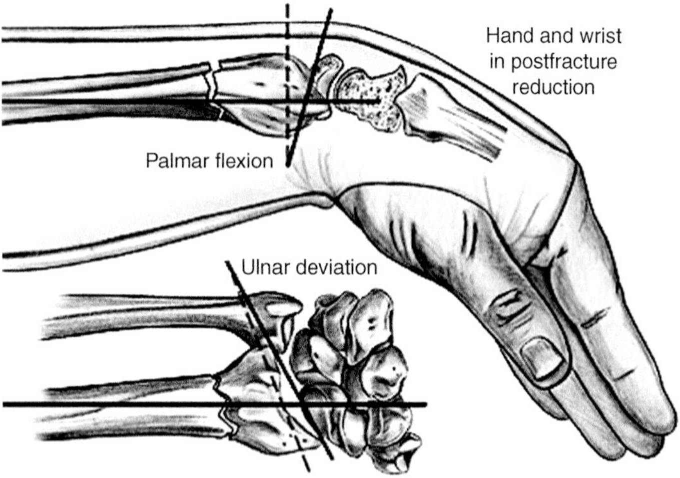

FIGURE 7.17 Immobilization position. (Reprinted from Duncan S, et al. Extra articular distal radius fractures. In: Berger RA, Weiss APC, editors. Hand surgery. Philadelphia: Lippincott Williams & Wilkens; 2004. With permission from Wolters Kluwer Health)

- ***Factors affecting repeat displacement following "closed" reduction:***
  - Greater amount of initial displacement implies greater energy imparted to cause primary translation.
  - Age of patient/associated bone quality: older individuals with osteopenic bone have greater tendency to experience repeat displacement.
  - Larger metaphyseal defects contribute to diminished bony support (buttress) to maintain alignment and articular congruity.

F. **COMPLICATIONS**

1. ***Non-union:*** uncommon based upon vast blood supply.
2. ***Malunion:*** more common complication that can lead to functional alteration of inherent wrist biomechanics; most commonly manifests as excessive dorsal angulation,

increased radial shortening, and/or loss of radial inclination.

Radiographic evidence of malunion is exceedingly more common than clinically symptomatic malunion.

3. ***Post-traumatic Arthritis:*** may encompass cosmetic deformity, pain/discomfort, and/or associated functional deficits (>2 mm incongruity of articular surface may be the most important factor in its development).

   Can still occur despite "anatomic" fracture reduction

Pearls:

- Always evaluate for *ipsilateral proximal forearm, elbow, and shoulder* injuries based upon FOOSH mechanism.
- All grossly displaced fractures should undergo closed reduction *regardless of future need/desire for surgical management*; offers pain relief, diminishes post-injury swelling/risk of development of *compartment syndrome* and relieves potential stress on median nerve *(acute carpal tunnel syndrome).*
- If median nerve dysfunction/ACTS development occurs, *immediately* relieve constriction, remove immobilization, and observe for relief of symptoms; if no improvement exhibited, potential surgical exploration with carpal tunnel release should be considered (appropriate consulting team should be notified promptly).
- **Always *educate, document discussion, and provide written discharge instructions* regarding potential for development of compartment syndrome/ACTS.**
- ***Ulnar Styloid Process fracture:*** usually associated with distal radius fractures, *rarely isolated.*
- ***Lateral Elbow X-Ray:*** line drawn through center of radial head/neck should always bisect humeral capitellum (capitulum) regardless of elbow position (degree of flexion) (See Fig. 7.18a, b).
- **Galeazzi Fracture/Dislocation:** involves a fracture of the middle-distal third radial diaphysis with an associated disruption of the DRUJ (See Fig. 7.19).

- Don't overlook isolated ***radio-carpal dislocation*** or one associated with a *distal radius fracture*; it can produce severe, permanent consequences the longer it remains displaced *(e.g., median nerve dysfunction/ACTS)* (See Fig. 7.20).

a

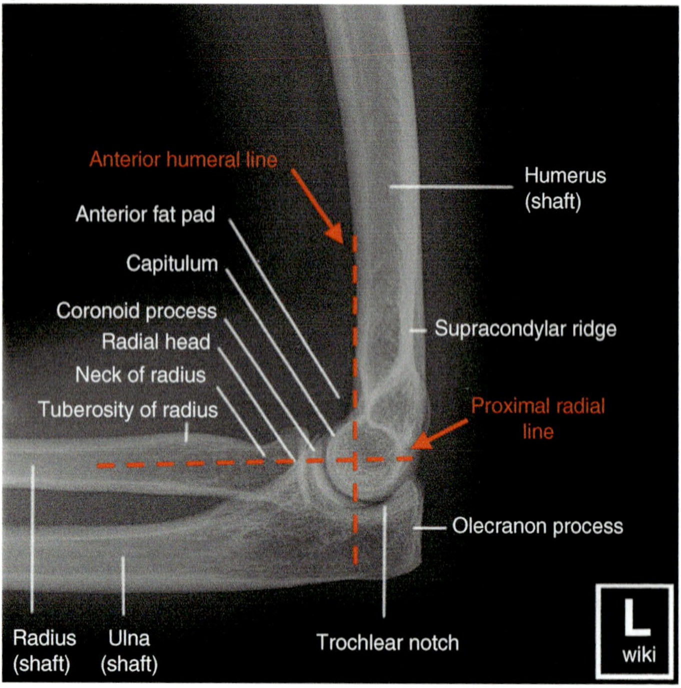

FIGURE 7.18 (**a**) Annotated lateral elbow X-ray with depiction of anterior humeral and proximal radial line, (**b**) joint movement pivots around the intersection of these lines. (**a**: Reprinted with permission from wikiRadiography.net: http://www.wikiradiography.net/page/Elbow+Radiographic+Anatomy. **b**: Reprinted from Haugstedyt J. Dissociations of the Radius and Ulna: Surgical Anatomy and Biomechanics. In: Berger RA, Weiss APC (eds). Hand Surgery. Philadelphia: Lippincott Williams & Wilkens; 2004. With permission from Wolters Kluwer Health)

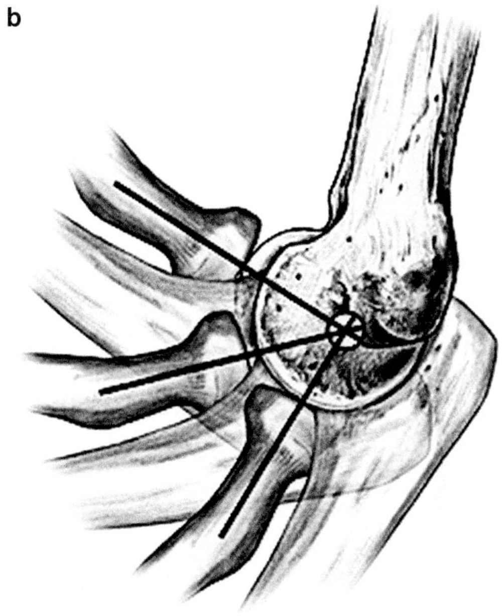

FIGURE 7.18 (continued)

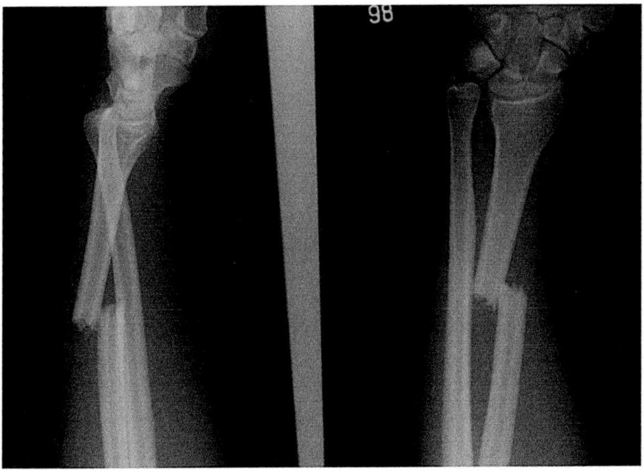

FIGURE 7.19 Galeazzi fracture. (Reprinted with permission from Northwestern University, Feinberg School of Medicine, Department of Emergency Medicine)

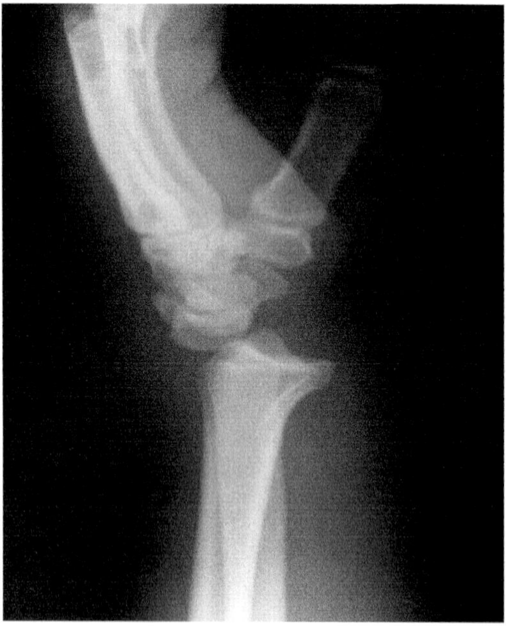

FIGURE 7.20 Dorsal radio-carpal dislocation. (Reprinted from Dumontier C, Meyer zu Reckendorf G, Sautet A, Lenoble E, Saffar P, Allieu Y. Radiocarpal dislocations: classification and proposal for treatment. J Bone Joint Surg Am. 2001;83(2):212. With permission from Wolters Kluwer Health, Inc.)

Suggested Reading

1. Adams B, et al. Ch 19: Distal radioulnar joint instability. In: Hand surgery. 1st ed. Philadelphia, PA: Lippincott Williams & Wilkens; 2004. p. 337–54.
2. Bowers WH. The distal radioulnar joint. In: Green DP, editor. Operative hand surgery. New York: Churchill Livingstone; 1982. p. 743–69.
3. Bronstein AJ, et al. The effects of distal radius fracture malalignment on forearm rotation: a cadaveric study. J Hand Surg. 1997;22:258–62.
4. Catalano LW, et al. Displaced intra-articular fractures of the distal aspect of the radius. J Bone Joint Surg. 1997;79:1290–302.

5. Cooney WP, et al. Fractures and dislocations of the wrist. In: Rockwood CA, Green DP, Bucholz RW, et al., editors. Rockwood and greens fractures in adults. Philadelphia: Lippincott Williams & Wilkins; 1996. p. 745–867.
6. Davis DI, Baratz M. Soft tissue complications of distal radius fractures. Hand Clin. 2010;26(2):229–35.
7. Diaz-Garcia RJ, et al. A systematic review of outcomes and complications of treating unstable distal radius fractures in the elderly. J Hand Surg Am. 2011;36(5):824–35.
8. Duncan S, et al. Ch 15: Extraarticular fractures of the distal radius. In: Hand surgery; Philadelphia, PA: Lippincott Williams & Wilkens. p. 247–73.
9. Fernandez DL, et al. Fractures of the distal radius. In: Green's operative hand surgery. 4th ed. New York: Churchill Livingstone; 1999. p. 929–85.
10. Fernandez D, et al. Fractures of the distal radius. 2nd ed. New York: Springer; 2002. isbn:0-387-95195-4.
11. Földhazy Z, et al. Long-term outcome of non-surgically treated distal radius fractures. J Hand Surg [Am]. 2007;32(9):1374–84.
12. Geissler WB, et al. Distal radioulnar joint injuries associated with fractures of the distal radius. Clin Orthop. 1996;327:135–46.
13. Goldfarb A, et al. Wrist fractures: what the clinician wants to know. Radiology. 2001;219:11–28.
14. Hanel DP, et al. Wrist fractures. Orthop Clin North Am. 2002;33(1):35–57.
15. Henry MH. Distal radius fractures: current concepts. J Hand Surg [Am]. 2008;33(7):1215–27.
16. Jupiter J. Ch 16: Intraarticular distal radius fractures. In: Hand surgery; Philadelphia, PA: Lippincott Williams & Wilkens. p. 277–94.
17. Kleinman WB. Distal radius instability and stiffness: common complications of distal radius fractures. Hand Clin. 2010;26(2):245–64.
18. Knirk JL, et al. Intra-articular fractures of the distal end of the radius in young adults. J Bone Joint Surg Am. 1986;68:647–59.
19. Louis DS. Barton's and Smith's fractures. Hand Clin. 1988;4:399–402.
20. Makhni EC, Ewald TJ, Kelly S, Day CS. Effect of patient age on the radiographic outcomes of distal radius fractures subject to nonoperative treatment. J Hand Surg [Am]. 2008;33(8):1301–8.
21. Metz VM, et al. Imaging techniques for distal radius fractures and related injuries. Orthop Clin North Am. 1993;24(2):217–28.
22. Nicolaidis SC, et al. Acute injuries of the distal radioulnar joint [review]. Hand Clin. 2000;16:449–59.

23. Trumble TE, et al. Factors affecting functional outcome of displaced intraarticular distal radius fractures. J Hand Surg. 1994;19:325–40.
24. Turner RG, et al. Complications of distal radius fractures. Orthop Clin North Am. 2007;38(2):217–28.
25. Wright T. Chapter 18: Malunion of the distal radius & ulna. In: Hand surgery; Philadelphia, PA: Lippincott Williams & Wilkens; 2004. p. 321–34.
26. Wheeless' Textbook of Orthopaedics. Trauma and Fractures Menu. Data Trace Internet Publishing, LLC. Retrieved from: http://www.wheelessonline.com/ortho/trauma_fractures_index.
27. "The Treatment of Distal Radius Fractures: Guideline and Evidence Report." Dec 2009, American Academy of Orthopaedic Surgeons. Retrieved from: www.aaos.org/guidelines

Chapter 8
Wrist

Daniel Purcell and Bryan A. Terry

Introduction

- Anatomic bridge from forearm to the hand.
- Assists in force transmission, helps generate and execute powerful/coordinated movements of the hand, and provides strict stabilization during performance of fine motor activities.
- Methodical approach is key to appropriately diagnosing and managing these fragile, yet often complex injuries.

Wrist (Carpal) Anatomy

- Formed by eight carpal bones, roughly arranged in two rows, with numerous ligamentous attachments that assist in maintaining stability and coordinating movement.

D. Purcell (✉)
Emergency Department, New York University Langone Medical Center Brooklyn, New York, NY, USA
e-mail: daniel.purcell@nyumc.org

B. A. Terry
The Brooklyn Hospital Center, Brooklyn, NY, USA

D. Purcell et al. (eds.), *Emergency Orthopedics Handbook*,
https://doi.org/10.1007/978-3-030-00707-2_8

- ***Bony Anatomy:***
  1. *Proximal row (radial → ulna direction):* scaphoid (spans both rows), lunate, triquetrum, and pisiform; only scaphoid and lunate articulate with the distal radius.
  2. *Distal row:* trapezium, trapezoid, capitate and hamate; these bones articulate with metacarpal bones of the hand (See Fig. 8.1).
- It is also composed of several joints:
  1. ***Distal radioulnar joint (DRUJ)****:* acts as a pivot point to generate forearm pronation/supination.

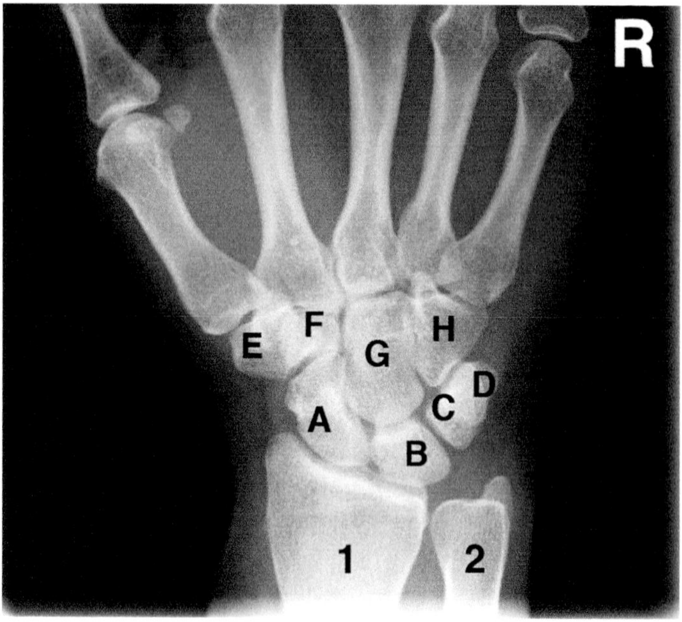

FIGURE 8.1 Carpal bones: A (scaphoid), B (lunate), C (triquetrum), D (pisiform), E (trapezium), F (trapezoid), G (capitate), H (hamate), 1 (radius), 2 (ulna). (Reprinted with permission from Dr. Jochen Lengerke. Retrieved from https://commons.wikimedia.org/wiki/File:Xray_hand_with_color.jpg)

2. ***Radio-carpal joint:*** region between radius and proximal carpal row; this articulation permits wrist flexion/extension and radial/ulnar deviation.
3. ***Midcarpal joint:*** area between the two carpal rows; considered a "functional" rather than "anatomical" unit, as it does not contain an uninterrupted ("classic") articular surface (See Fig. 8.2).

- ***Carpal Tunnel:*** fibro-osseous passageway on palmar aspect of the wrist; transmits median nerve and nine extrinsic flexor tendons to the hand. Median nerve compression can lead to paresthesias, pain, numbness, and/or weakness within its anatomic distribution (See Fig. 8.3).
- ***Guyon's Canal:*** structural space created on ulnar aspect of the wrist that transmits ulnar artery/nerve from forearm to the hand (See Fig. 8.4).

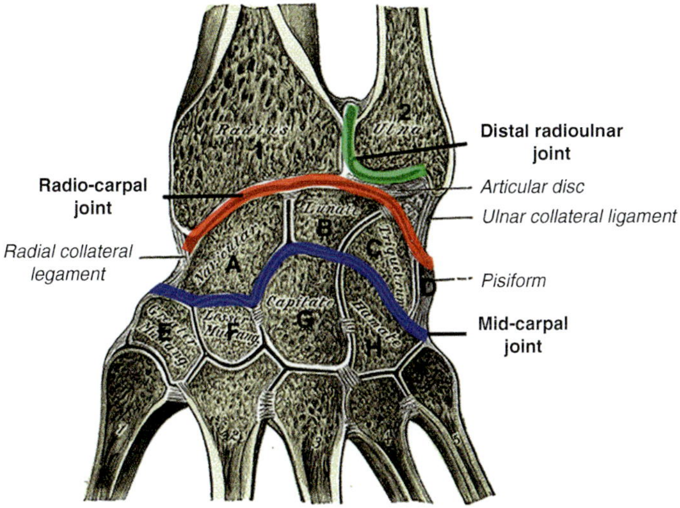

FIGURE 8.2 Joints of the wrist. (Adapted with permission from https://commons.wikimedia.org/wiki/File:Gray336.png)

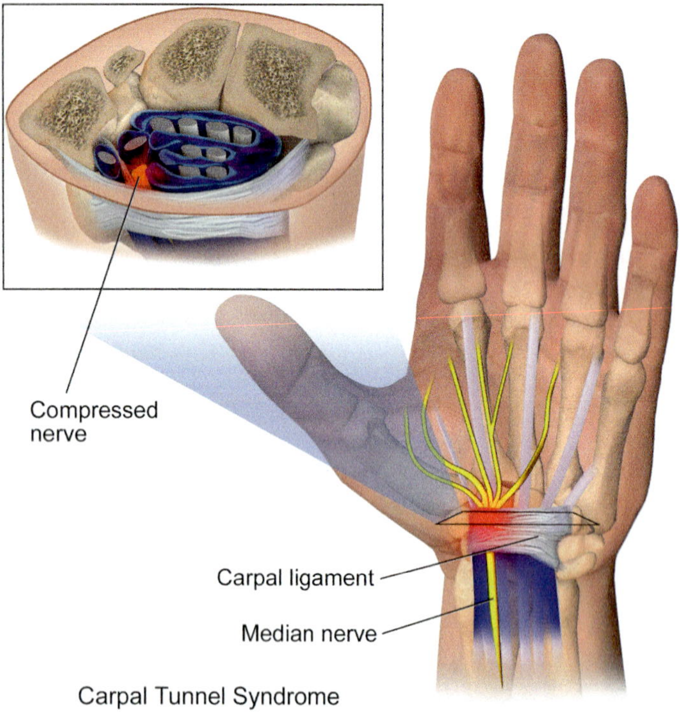

FIGURE 8.3 Carpal tunnel syndrome. (Reprinted from Blausen.com staff. Medical gallery of Blausen Medical 2014. WikiJournal of Medicine. 2014;1(2). doi:https://doi.org/10.15347/wjm/2014.010. ISSN 2002-4436. https://commons.wikimedia.org/wiki/File:Carpal_Tunnel_Syndrome.png. With permission from Bruce Blaus)

- ***Extensor Tendon Compartments:*** dorsal side wrist tunnels that transport extrinsic extensor tendons to their digital insertion sites; tendons held firmly in place by extensor retinaculum and travel in synovial tendon sheaths to facilitate their excursion over dorsal wrist surface.
- ***Anatomic Snuffbox:*** triangular structural deepening on the radial/dorsal aspect of the hand; contains radial artery, cephalic vein, and dorsal cutaneous branch of radial nerve

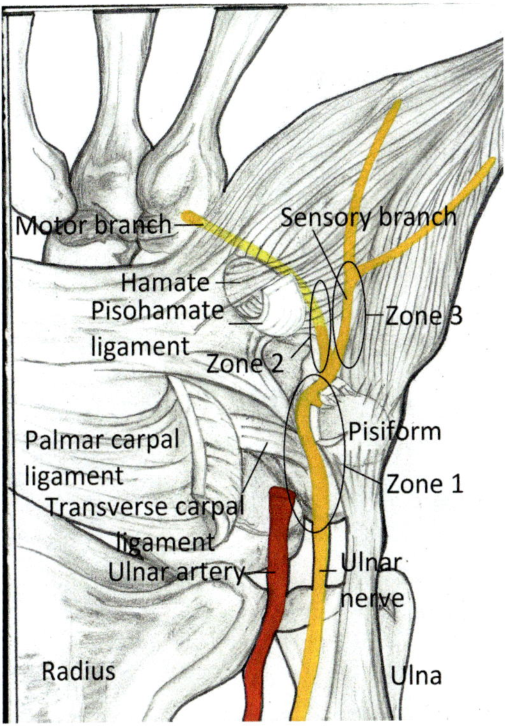

FIGURE 8.4 Guyon's canal: labeled "Zone 1" floor (transverse carpal ligament), roof (palmar carpal ligament), ulnar border (pisiform), radial border (hook of hamate). (Reprinted from http://www.ehealthstar.com/anatomy/guyons-canal. With permission from Ehealthstar.com)

(superficial radial nerve). Borders accentuated with *thumb extension*.

- ***Lister's Tubercle:*** palpable prominence on dorsal distal radius; serves as pulley for EPL tendon and reference landmark for wrist joint arthrocentesis (See Fig. 8.5a, b).
- ***Ulnar Styloid Process:*** distal ulna bony prominence that serves as attachment point for triangular fibrocartilage

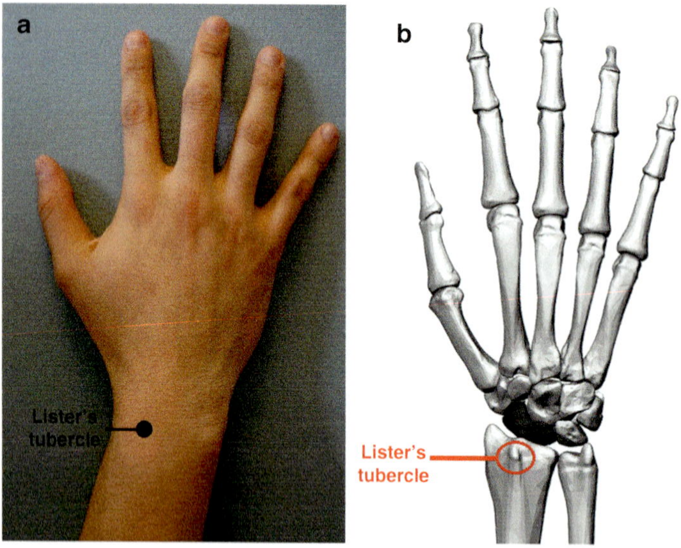

FIGURE 8.5 Lister's tubercle: (**a**) surface anatomy, (**b**) skeleton. (**b**: Adapted from https://commons.wikimedia.org/wiki/File:Left_hand_dorsal_view_Arabic_YM.png with permission from Creative Commons License: https://creativecommons.org/licenses/by-sa/4.0/deed.en)

complex (TFCC); disruption may signal damage to TFCC, instability of DRUJ, or concomitant distal radius injury (See Fig. 8.6).

Wrist/Hand Blood Supply:

- Contains rich vascular network supplied by radial/ulnar arteries; these vessels branch to perfuse distal digits while also coalescing to form overlapping collateral circulation through formation of two major palmar arches.

  1. ***Superficial palmar arch:*** distal to deep arch; supplied predominately by *ulnar artery*.
  2. ***Deep palmar arch:*** supplied principally by deep branch of *radial artery* (See Fig. 8.7).

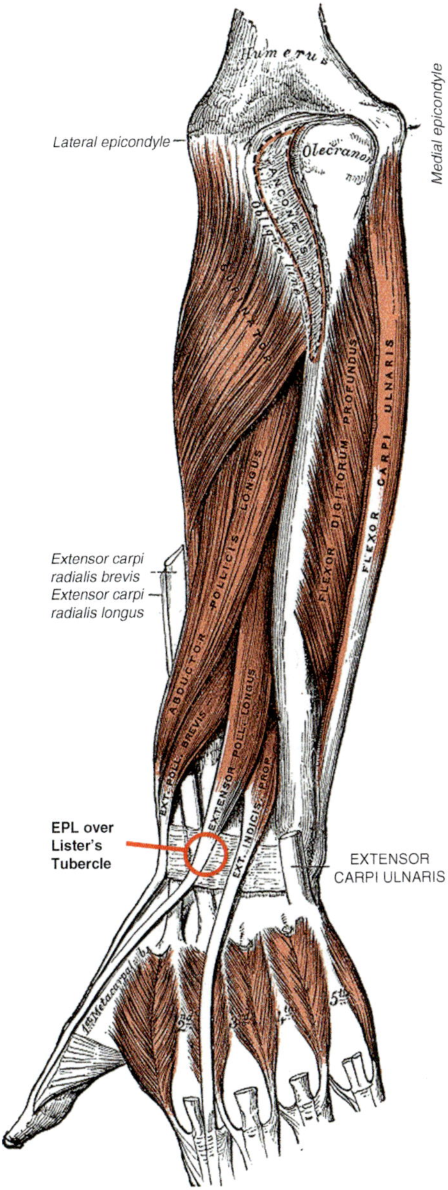

FIGURE 8.6 EPL and Lister's tubercle: anatomic relationship. (Adapted from with permission from https://commons.wikimedia.org/wiki/File:Gray419.png)

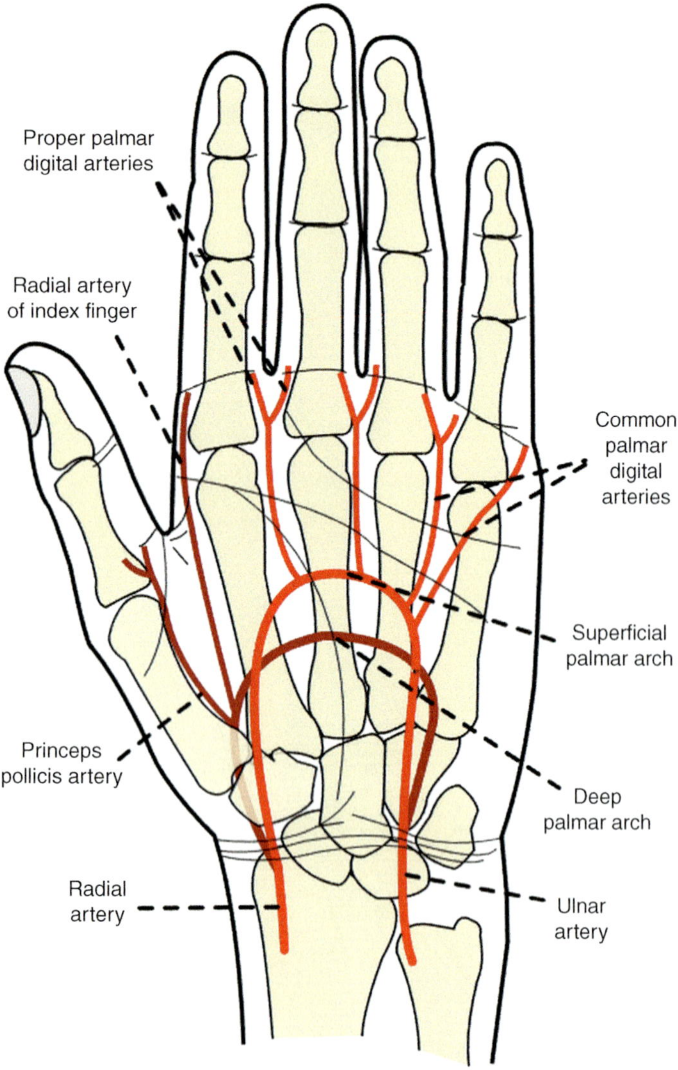

FIGURE 8.7 Blood supply of the hand. (Reprinted with permission from https://commons.wikimedia.org/wiki/File:Gray1237.svg)

Clinical Assessment

- ***History:***
  - Determine the timing/mechanism of injury, previous/associated injuries, loss of function *(neuromotor/perfusion deficits)*, position of the wrist at time of injury, activities and/or motion(s) that alleviate/exacerbate patient discomfort, previous treatment, etc.
  - Be sure to document hand dominance, employment-specific requirements, and/or recreational /professional activity needs (e.g., surgeon, musician, etc.)

- ***Physical Examination:***
  - Visual inspection-note evidence of swelling, ecchymosis, associated skin changes, and/or positional deformity.
  - Measure passive/active ROM (compare with contralateral wrist).
  - Palpate bony prominences (Lister's tubercle, scaphoid tubercle, ulnar styloid, etc.) and any areas of communicated patient discomfort.
  - Assess overall appearance, temperature alterations/differences in handedness, pulse strength, digital capillary refill, and consider systemic disease that may affect healing and/or contribute to future potential complications (e.g., DM, peripheral vascular disease, etc.).
  - Evaluate potential neuromotor deficits and record results of overall strength, functional capacity, and neurologic assessment.

- ***Plain Radiographic Examination:*** (See Fig. 8.8a–c)

  A. ***Carpal bone alignment:*** standard joint spacing is suggested when carpal bones are visualized in parallel when examined in profile; physical overlap can be suggestive of abnormal tilting, dislocation, and/or carpal fracture.

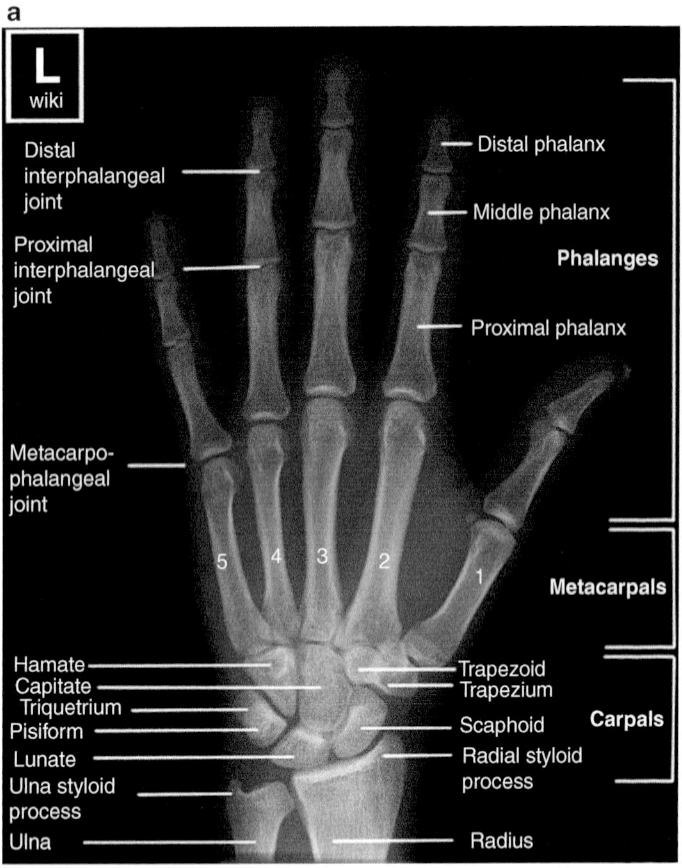

FIGURE 8.8 Hand X-ray: (**a**) PA, (**b**) lateral, (**c**) oblique A–C. (Used with permission from http://www.wikiradiography.net/page/Hand+Radiographic+Anatomy)

b

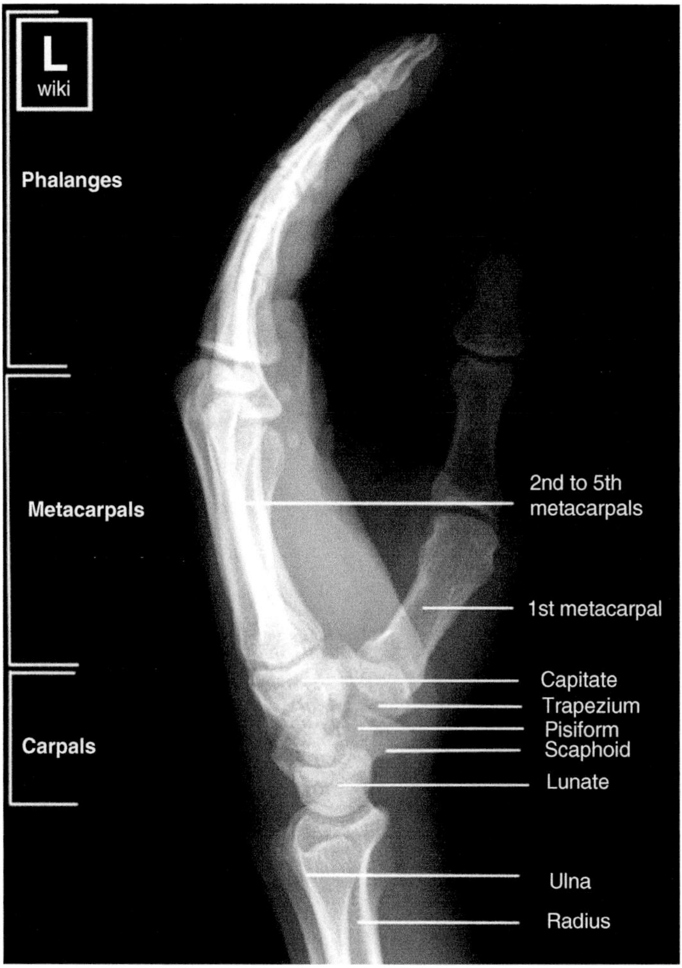

FIGURE 8.8 (continued)

c

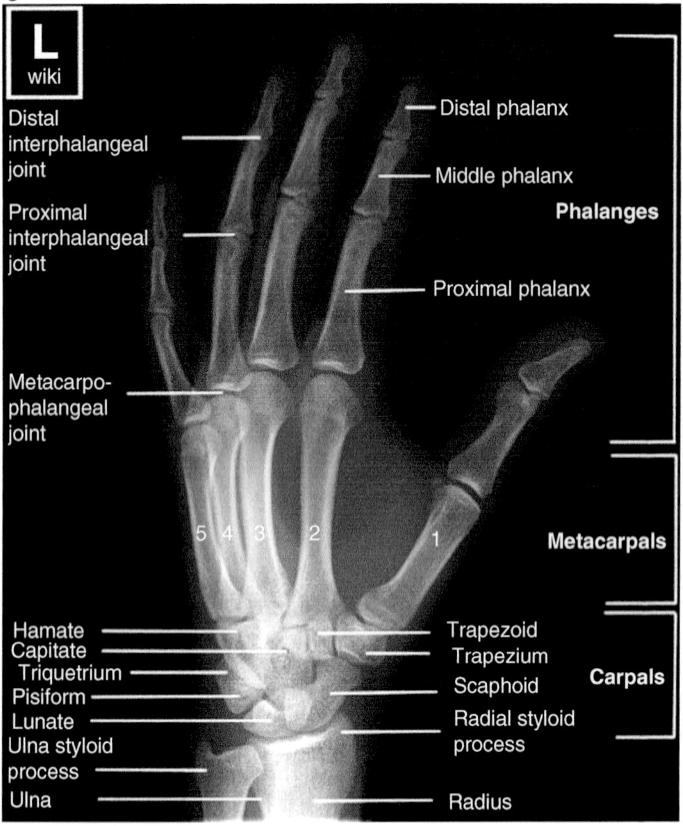

FIGURE 8.8 (continued)

B. ***Carpal (Gilula) arcs:*** three smooth, continuous arcs should be identified on PA view.

I. ***First arc:*** outlines proximal surfaces of the scaphoid, lunate, and triquetrum.
II. ***Second arc:*** traces their distal surfaces.
III. ***Third arc:*** follows proximal curvatures of the capitate and hamate (See Fig. 8.9).

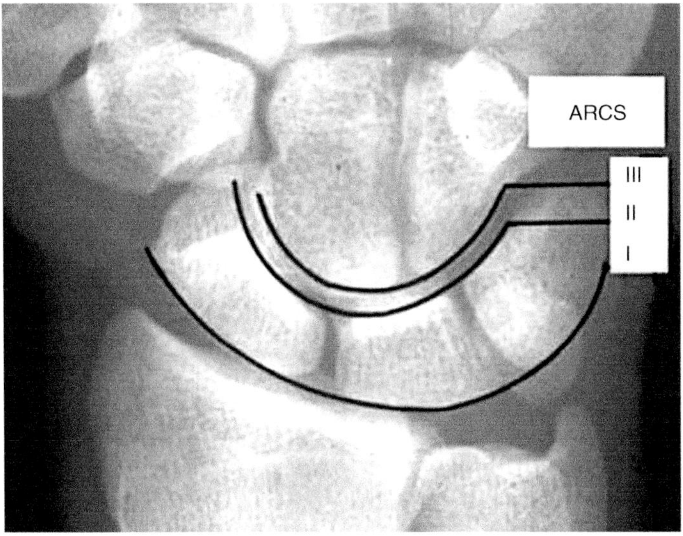

FIGURE 8.9 Carpal arcs. (Reprinted from http://www.radiologyassistant.nl/en/p42a29ec06b9e8/wrist-carpal-instability.html. With permission from Robin Smithuis)

An arc is disrupted if it cannot be traced smoothly and continuously; disruption is generally indicative of ligamentous tear and/or fracture.

1. ***First arc:*** radio-carpal row; disruption is suggestive of *lunate dislocation.*
2. ***Second arc:*** mid-carpal row; disruption is suggestive of *peri-lunate dislocation.*
3. ***Third arc:*** outlines proximal surface of distal carpal row.

Selected Individual Bones

A. ***Scaphoid (navicular):*** second largest carpal bone; *most commonly fractured carpal bone.*

- ***Shape:*** changes with wrist movement; lengthens in extension/ulnar deviation, yet shortens with flexion/

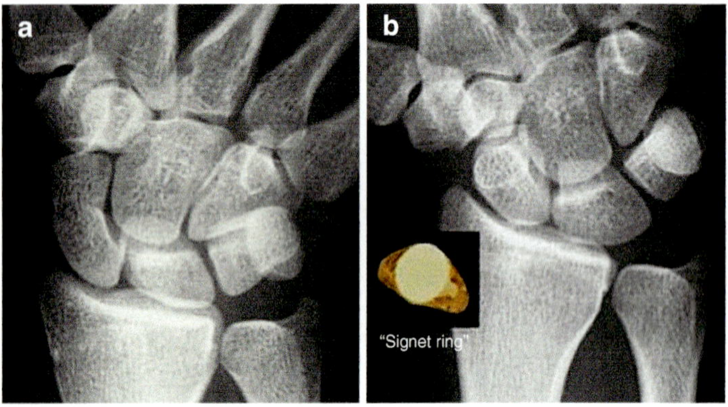

Figure 8.10 Scaphoid: (**a**) extension/ulnar deviation, (**b**) flexion/radial deviation ("signet ring" sign). (Reprinted from http://www.radiologyassistant.nl/en/p42a29ec06b9e8/wrist-carpal-instability.html. With permission from Robin Smithuis)

radial deviation, displaying a "signet ring" cortical appearance (See Fig. 8.10)

- Contains three anatomic regions: proximal pole, distal pole (tubercle), and the waist (mid-portion that separates the two poles)
- Functions as link across the mid-carpal joint, providing functional continuity between the proximal and distal carpal rows
- Approximately 80% of its surface is covered in cartilage, leaving only a small area for arterial blood supply; this reduces its capacity for periosteal healing and leads to an increased risk of delayed, malunion, and/or nonunion.

- ***Blood Supply:***

  1. ***Dorsal carpal branch of radial artery:*** provides ~ 70–80% of vascular supply, entering slightly distal to scaphoid waist at the dorsal ridge; provides perfusion to proximal aspect of scaphoid in retrograde fashion

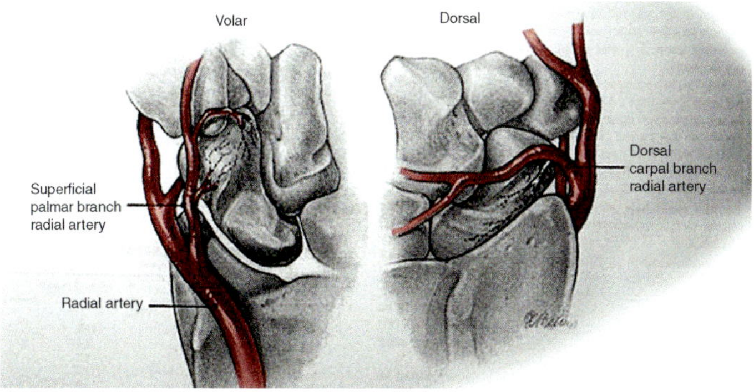

FIGURE 8.11 Blood supply of scaphoid: Majority of perfusion occurs in retrograde fashion in a distal to proximal direction. More proximal fractures thus have higher rates of nonunion due to a diminished blood supply. (Reprinted from http://morphopedics.wikidot.com/scaphoid-fractures with permission from Creative Commons License: https://creativecommons.org/licenses/by-sa/3.0/)

2. ***Palmar and superficial palmar branches (scaphoid branches):*** enter at distal tubercle and accounts for remaining vascular supply *(none of which reaches the proximal pole)* (See Fig. 8.11).
   Generally accepted that with proper treatment (immobilization), nearly 100% of tuberosity/distal third fractures and 80–90% of waist fractures will heal uneventfully; however, it has been reported that only 60–70% of proximal pole fractures heal free of complication(s).

- ***Injury Mechanism:*** Similar to distal radius fractures, a fall on an outstretched hand (FOOSH injury) transmits a large hyperextension force across the wrist joint; *however*, unlike distal radius fractures, scaphoid fractures are more common among young men, with a peak incidence in the second and third decades.

A. Extreme ***hyperextension*** locks scaphoid into the distal radial scaphoid fossa, with the capitate acting as a fulcrum for fracture generation.
B. **"Punch"** ***mechanism:*** involved metacarpal delivers a palmar-directed shear force across distal scaphoid.

   - Kinematic effect(s) of an "unstable" scaphoid fracture essentially describes a loss of functional continuity between the carpal rows.

- ***Clinical Evaluation/Treatment:*** (See Figs. 8.12 and 8.13)

  - Anatomic snuffbox tenderness, described as "classic" physical finding, may be "overly sensitive" with false-positive results elicited through compression of superficial radial nerve; tenderness at the scaphoid tubercle is also quite limited in detecting scaphoid fractures when implemented in isolation.
  - ***Compression test:*** involves loading scaphoid via axial compression of the thumb along the line of the first metacarpal (See Fig. 8.13).
  - Preceding provocative maneuvers, along with "scaphoid series," should minimize possibility of missing an acute scaphoid fracture.
    ****Never Rely on Imaging Alone****
  - Estimated as much as 30% of all scaphoid fractures might not be detected on initial X-rays *(even with perfect radiographic technique and an experienced physician interpreting the films).*
    *****Cortical disruption may not be radiographically evident in acute injury period*****
    *****Any clinical suggestion of fracture, despite negative imaging analysis, should prompt immobilization in thumb spica splint/cast*****
    *****If left untreated, there is a heightened risk of nonunion/AVN and associated future potential complications*****

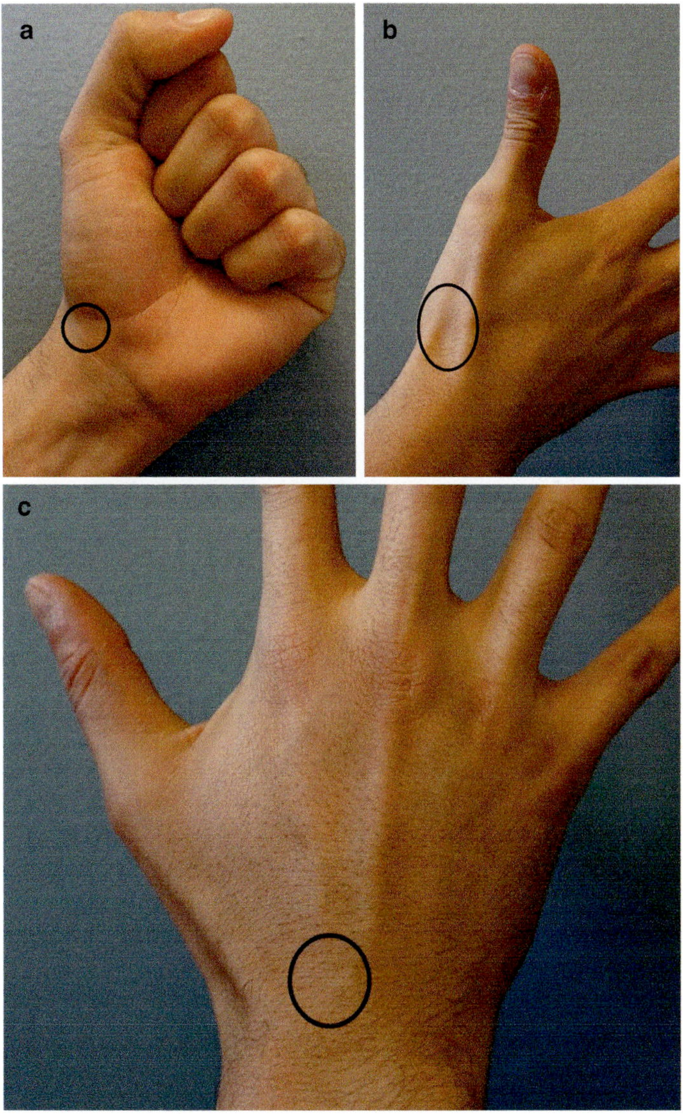

FIGURE 8.12 Locations to palpate scaphoid: (**a**) tubercle, (**b**) anatomical snuff box, (**c**) proximal pole

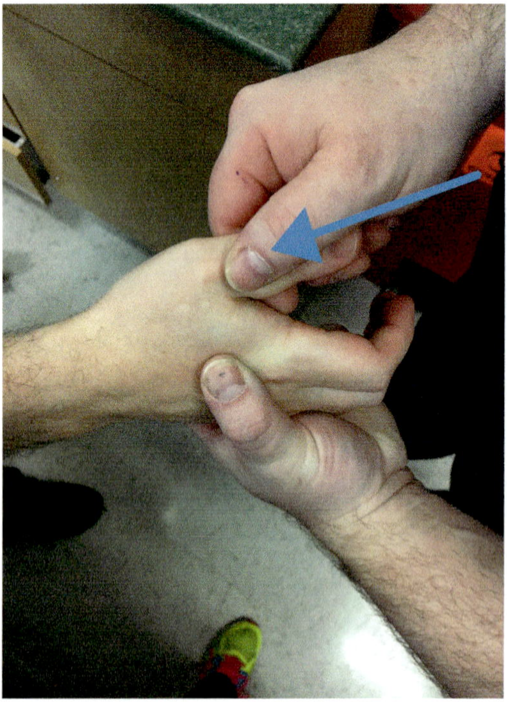

FIGURE 8.13 Scaphoid compression test: axial compression of the scaphoid

- Based upon its high sensitivity/specificity, *MRI* is considered "gold standard" in diagnosis of occult scaphoid fractures; however, in many instances, MRI is neither practical nor available. Thus, adequate clinical follow-up and repeat imaging should lead to detection.
- Average time for healing of non-displaced scaphoid fracture treated with immobilization, free of complication(s), is ~8 to 12 weeks.
- Common post-traumatic complications include pain, arthritic degeneration, functional deficits, delayed union, malunion, and/or nonunion.

- ***Preiser's disease (scaphoid osteonecrosis):*** development of osteonecrosis (AVN) of scaphoid with no previous history of substantial trauma; etiology secondary to repetitive microtrauma and/or side effects of medications (e.g., steroids/chemotherapy) in conjunction with existing defective vascular perfusion; most commonly involves proximal pole.

B. ***Lunate:***

- "Keystone" of proximal carpal row, yet ***most commonly dislocated carpal bone.***
- Isolated injuries are rare and often overlooked on routine imaging secondary to superimposed structures. Slightly oblique X-ray imaging may better delineate suspected fractures, or CT should be considered.
- ***Shape:*** normally appears trapezoidal; if becomes tilted, can appear triangular ("piece-of-pie" sign), which may indicate ligamentous injury and/or potential dislocation (See Fig. 8.14a, b).
- ***Lunate dislocation:*** radio-lunate articulation disrupted, as the residual carpus remains stable.
- ***Peri-lunate dislocation:*** radio-lunate articulation is maintained, while the remaining carpus becomes displaced.
- *****Lunate dislocation:*** **can mimic *peri-lunate dislocation,* especially on PA projection –> lateral imaging is *key* to make this distinction.**** (See Figs. 8.15a, b and 8.16)

  A. ***Lunate Dislocation:*** *Lunate tilted out, while capitate and residual carpus remains centered over radius.*
  B. ***Peri-lunate Dislocation:*** *Lunate remains centered over distal radius, while capitate and remaining carpus are displaced.*

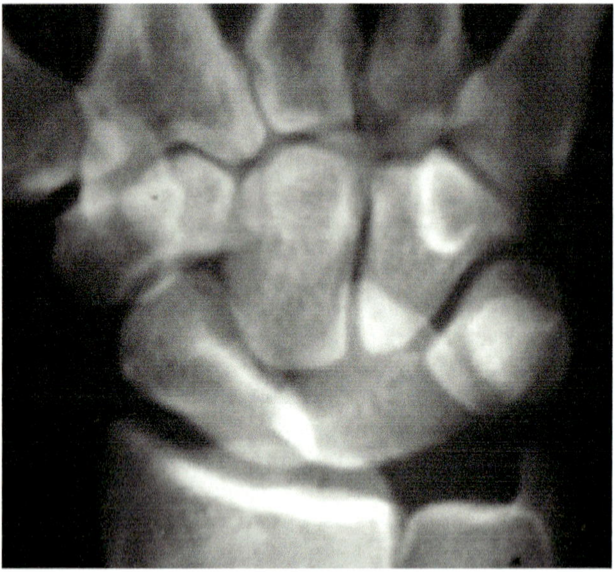

FIGURE 8.14 Lunate dislocation: PA clenched fist view; note the pie-shaped lunate and loss of parallelism. (Reprinted from http://www.radiologyassistant.nl/en/p42a29ec06b9e8/wrist-carpal-instability.html. With permission from Robin Smithuis)

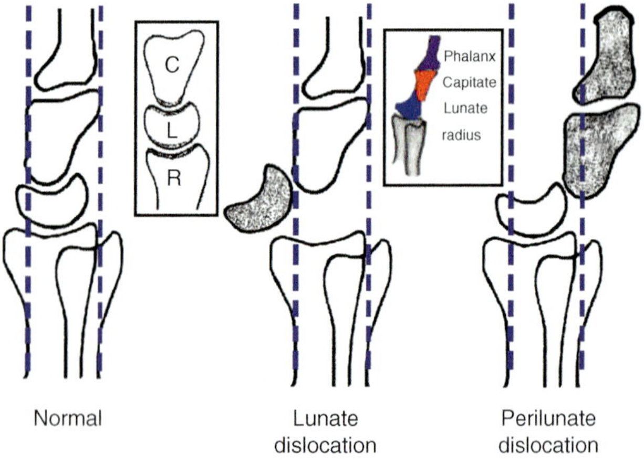

FIGURE 8.15 Wrist and carpal alignment: note aligned axis of distal radius, lunate, and capitate. (Image reprinted with permission from Medscape Drugs & Diseases (http://emedicine.medscape.com/), 2017, available at: http://emedicine.medscape.com/article/397035-overview)

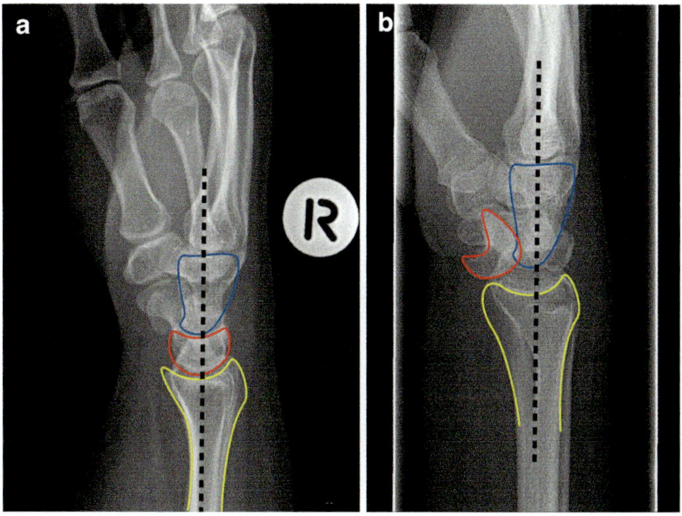

FIGURE 8.16 Lateral wrist X-ray: (**a**) normal alignment (yellow, radius; red, lunate; blue, capitate), (**b**) lunate dislocation – note the "spilled teacup" sign of the lunate. (Reprinted from http://www.emcurious.com/blog-1/2015/7/8/1ftadghymctqd2flw27ao4zwl1m6tb with permission from Creative Commons License: https://creativecommons.org/licenses/by/4.0/)

****Imaging Clues to Lunate Dislocation:***

1. PA: break in Gilula's arc (smooth contour), lunate/capitate overlap, and/or lunate appears triangular ("piece-of-pie" sign).
2. Lateral: loss of colinearity of radius, lunate and capitate ("spilled teacup" sign); capitate not positioned within distal articular cup of lunate.

****Imaging Clues to Peri-lunate Dislocation:***

A. ***PA View:*** disruption of expected smooth carpal arcs. Can also see "piece-of-pie" sign.
B. ***Lateral View:*** *usually* demonstrates dorsal peri-lunate dislocation *(lunate maintains normal relationship to distal radius, while capitate and remaining carpus are displaced dorsally)* (See Fig. 8.17a–c).

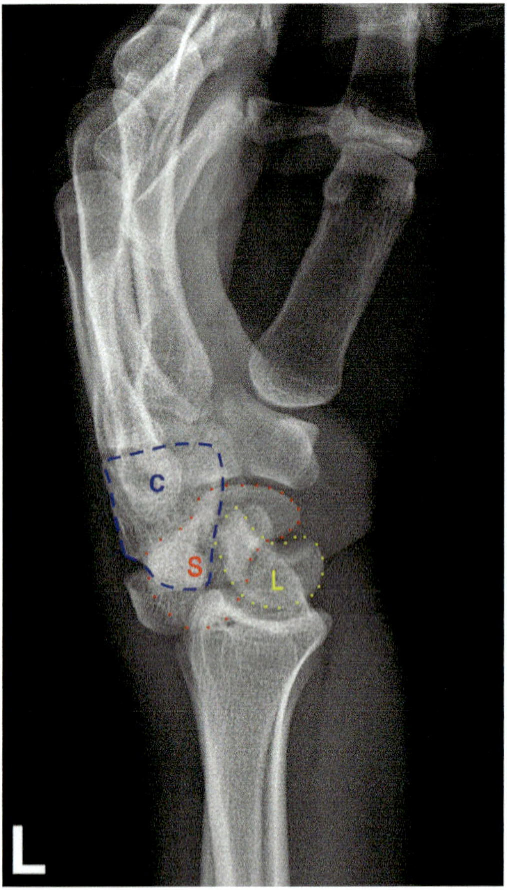

FIGURE 8.17 Peri-lunate dislocation X-ray: Lunate (yellow) remains centered over radius while capitate (blue) dislocates dorsally – scaphoid (red). (Used with permission from http://www.wikiradiography.net/page/Lunate+and+Perilunate+Dislocations)

- ***Injury mechanism:*** axial loading of the wrist in hyperextended/ulnar-deviated position.
- Dislocation can occur through greater arc (bone), lesser arc (ligaments), and/or combination of both.
- ***Sequence of injury:*** usually begins radially, with destabilization through body of scaphoid (fracture) and/or

through scapho-lunate interval (pure dislocation); *scaphoid bridges proximal and distal carpal rows; thus with dislocation between rows, the scaphoid must either rotate and/or fracture.*

Definitive Treatment Options

- ***Closed reduction and splinting/casting:*** despite initial success, usually generates poor long-term outcomes, with many patients experiencing functional deficit and/or recurrent dislocation.
- ***Closed reduction and percutaneous pin fixation.***
- ***Open reduction*** with ligamentous repair and/or percutaneous pin fixation.

*****CLOSED REDUCTION TECHNIQUE*****

- Place upper extremity in longitudinal traction, with the elbow at 90 degrees of flexion for ~10–15 min.
- Add 5–10 lbs of additional traction if possible to heighten distraction forces.
- **Dorsal peri-lunate dislocations are reduced through application of volar pressure to the carpus, with a counter-force applied to the lunate.**
- Palmar flexion then allows for reduction of the capitate into the concavity of the lunate (See Fig. 8.18).

*****If closed reduction is achieved/verified, interim operative intervention is still generally necessary to achieve enduring carpal stabilization.*****

*****If closed reduction cannot be obtained, the patient should be taken promptly to the OR for open reduction.*****

- Damage to ***median nerve*** is the most common associated injury; however, the associated *skin* can also become ischemic from the impinging radius/carpus.
- ***Fractures:*** typically follow hyperextension injury (FOOSH mechanism). Avulsions of dorsal pole are common in scapho-lunate dissociations (SLD), while fractures of ulnar aspect of palmar pole are associated with peri-lunate dislocations.

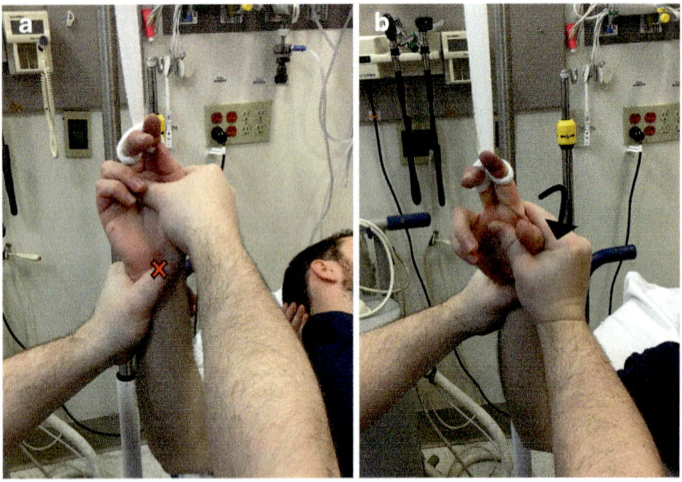

FIGURE 8.18 Lunate reduction: (**a**) The wrist is extended with the thumb placed over the proximal palmar lunate "X" to maintain concavity-up alignment, while the remaining fingers provide an opposing force to the residual carpus. (**b**) While maintaining manual longitudinal traction and applying pressure to palmar lunate, gradually flex the wrist to reduce the capito-lunate joint (arrow)

Treatment/Outcome:

- Most lunate fractures can be treated conservatively with immobilization. However, all fractures require serial imaging, ideally consisting of advanced imaging (MRI) to more definitively assess healing/revascularization, as there is a high incidence of nonunion, osteonecrosis, and potential for carpal collapse
- ***Kienbock's disease: (avascular necrosis lunate)*** probably no single cause – its origin may involve multiple factors (blood supply (arteries), blood drainage (veins), skeletal variations, and/or acute or repetitive trauma).

C. ***Triquetrum:*** located on medial side wrist, just distal to TFCC; articulates with lunate through luno-triquetral ligament (See Figs. 8.19 and 8.20a, b)

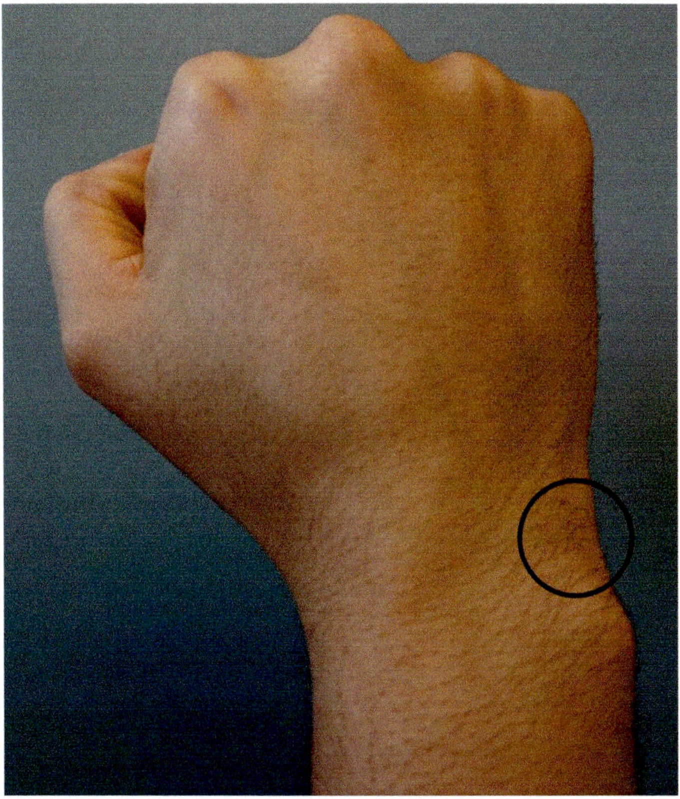

FIGURE 8.19 Triquetrum: just distal to ulnar styloid

- ***Fractures:*** most common mechanism of injury involves an impingement shear-type fracture, with the ulnar styloid contacting the dorsal aspect of the triquetrum with the wrist in extension and ulnar deviation.
- Physical examination generally reveals localized tenderness over dorsum of the wrist, just distal to the ulnar styloid.
- Frequently, only seen as ***dorsal chip*** fracture on the lateral projection, as the pisiform generally obscures the triquetrum on the frontal view (See Fig. 8.21a, b).

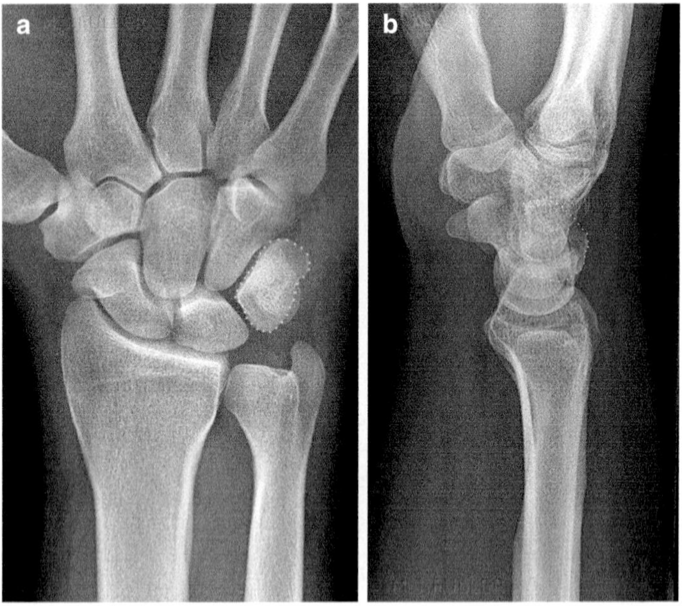

Figure 8.20 Triquetrum X-ray: (**a**) PA view, (**b**) lateral view. (**a**, **b**: Used with permission from http://www.wikiradiography.net/page/Triquetral+Fractures)

Treatment/outcome: generally depends upon location and amount of fracture displacement.

- Non-displaced/dorsal chip fractures *(non-articular injuries)* can usually be treated conservatively with immobilization (ulnar gutter splint/cast or volar splint).
- Rarely, more displaced fractures (>1 mm) or injuries that remain symptomatic despite significant healing time may ultimately require fragment excision.
- Triquetrium has abundant vascular supply, thus delayed/nonunion exceptionally rare.

D. ***Pisiform:*** sesamoid bone contained within the flexor carpi ulnaris (FCU) tendon; increases the moment arm (torque force) of the FCU muscle at its tendon traverses over the pisiform surface.

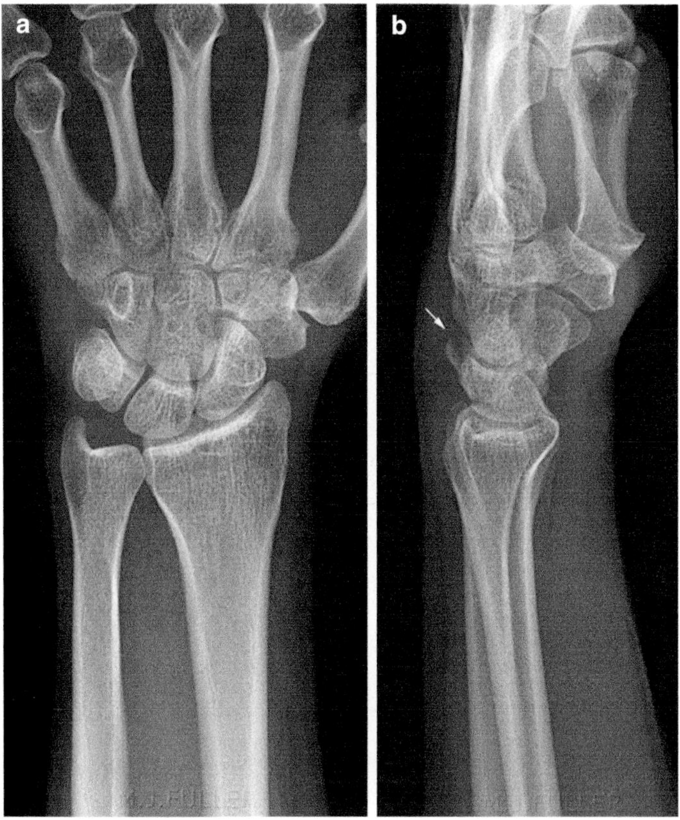

FIGURE 8.21 Triquetral fracture X-ray: (**a**) PA view, (**b**) lateral view, arrow points to pathognomonic dorsal chip fracture. (**a**, **b**: Used with permission from http://www.wikiradiography.net/page/Triquetral+Fractures)

- Delineates ulnar border of Guyon's canal, thus injuries to pisiform can also involve concomitant damage to ulnar nerve (See Fig. 8.22).
- ***Fractures:*** most sports-related, but injury may also occur following FOOSH mechanism. Diagnosis: can be difficult and they are easily missed upon initial examination.

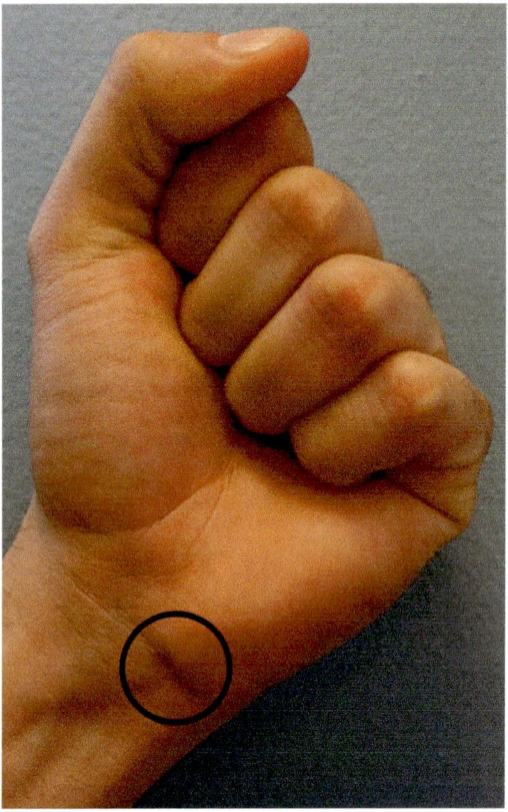

FIGURE 8.22 Pisiform

- Detection may require special imaging views such as an ~20–45° oblique image (wrist in radial deviation/mild supination) or "carpal tunnel" view (See Fig. 8.23a, b).
- *CT may also be required for diagnosis of occult fractures.*

Treatment/outcome: Most fractures heal with conservative measures, and patients are often treated with splint/cast immobilization.

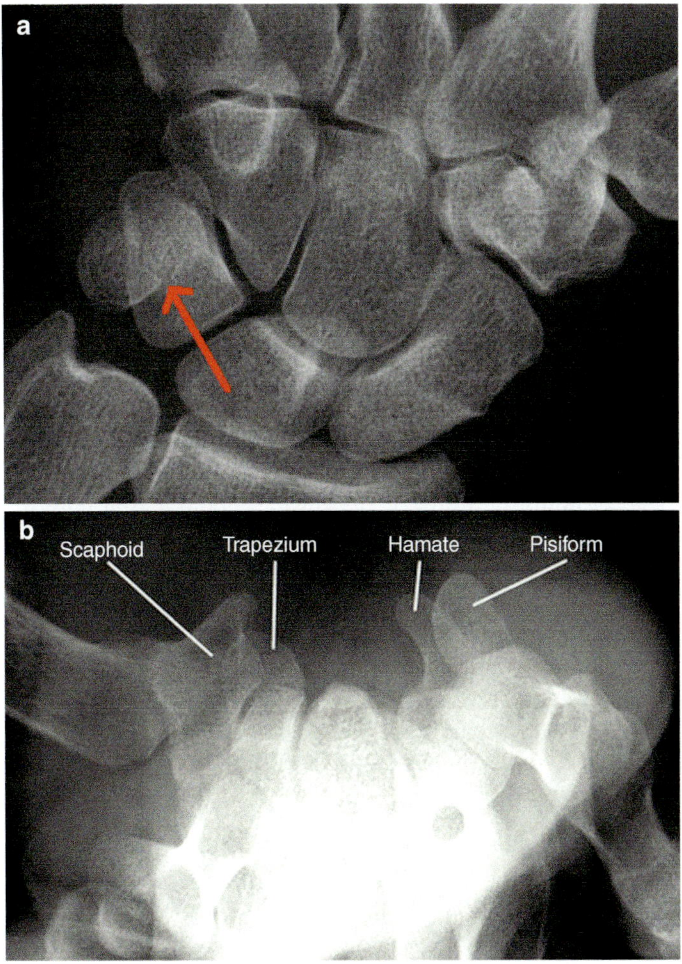

FIGURE 8.23 Pisiform X-ray: (**a**) oblique view showing fracture (arrow), (**b**) carpal tunnel view (no fracture). (**a**: Used with permission from Northwestern University, Feinberg School of Medicine, Department of Emergency Medicine. **b**: Reprinted from Watanabe A, Souza F, Vezeridis PS, et al. Ulnar-sided wrist pain. II. Clinical imaging and treatment. Skeletal Radiol. 2010;39(9):837–857. With permission from Springer Nature)

- However, some patients will continue to experience chronic discomfort despite adequate healing time. This occurs secondary to accelerated degenerative changes and may eventually require surgical excision *(usually associated with minor loss of grip strength).*

E. ***Hamate:***

- Roughly triangular-shaped bone composed of both a body and "hook-like" process projecting from its volar surface; situated in distal carpal row, at extreme ulnar border of wrist.
- The "hook" serves as distal, lateral border of Guyon's canal; thus injury may signal potential ulnar artery and/or nerve involvement (See Fig. 8.24).
- ***Fractures:*** overall quite rare, with the body much less commonly injured than its accompanying "hook" (may require oblique images to demonstrate pathology).
- Physical examination findings are generally non-specific and quite often absent. If symptoms are present, evaluation typically reveals discrete point tenderness over "hook," diminished grip strength, and/or paresthesias in ulnar nerve distribution.
- Two mechanisms that account for most "hook" fractures:

  - Repetitive microtrauma during sports activities (e.g., swinging clubs, bats, or racquets). Eventually leads to stress fracture development and often occurs in non-dominant hand.
  - Direct trauma during sport-specific activities, whereby equipment rests directly on hamate, with force directly transmitted to the bone.

- Fracture of the "hook" most commonly occurs at or near its base.

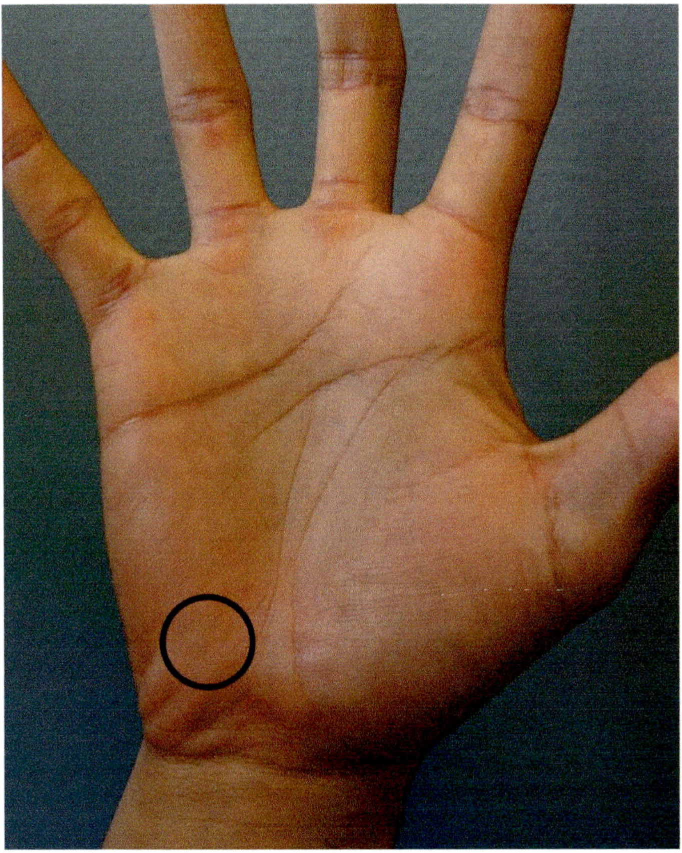

FIGURE 8.24 Hamate

- Similar to pisiform fractures, a *carpal tunnel view/CT may be necessary* to diagnose injury, with excision reserved for prolonged symptomatic injuries *(painful nonunion)*.
- Treatment involves immobilization if discovered early, yet many injuries are initially overlooked; this leads to

decreased healing potential based upon multifactorial contribution (fragment displacement, poor vascular supply, etc.).

- ***Pearls:***

A. ***Scapho-lunate (SL) dissociation ("Terry Thomas" sign):*** most common traumatic etiology of carpal instability; can occur in isolation or with wrist fractures.

   - Both the direction of traumatic force and the relatively weaker dorsal ligaments contribute to dorsal carpal displacement (FOOSH mechanism) (See Fig. 8.25).

Treatment:

1. ***Acute Tears:*** patients with partial tears and no evidence of carpal instability may be treated conservatively with splint/cast immobilization; this is ineffective when carpal instability is present, as they require opposite directions of movement to maintain reduction (scaphoid requires wrist extension, while lunate requires wrist flexion).
2. ***Chronic Tears:*** usually requires surgical intervention for symptomatic cases; degenerative soft tissue supporting structures are not commonly amenable to direct repair methods.

   - Without treatment, can lead to advanced SL collapse (SLAC wrist) and/or progressive, painful wrist arthritis.
   - Clenched fist view in ulnar deviation most effectively expands SL joint space, placing maximum stress on SL ligament; positive intercarpal widening is commonly referred to as "Terry Thomas" sign (>2 mm widening).

B. ***DRUJ instability:*** common cause of pain and limited ROM following distal radius fractures.

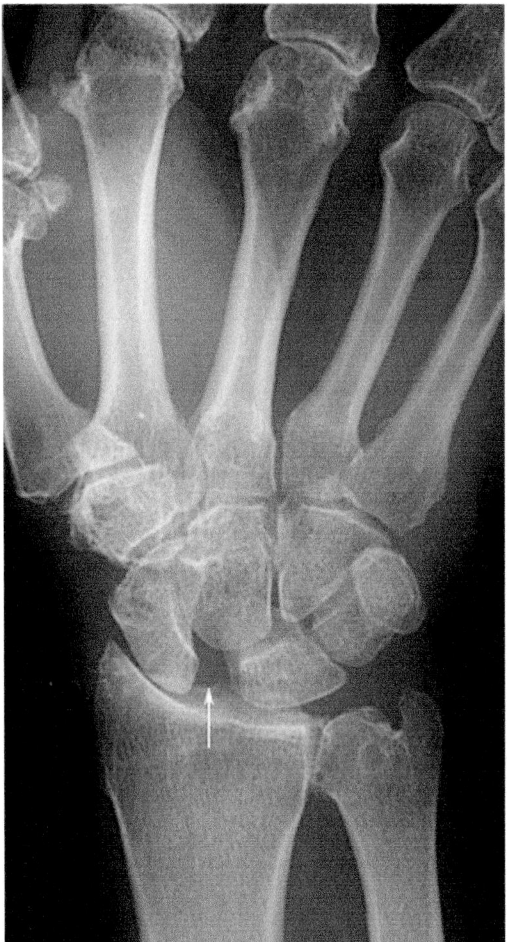

FIGURE 8.25 Scapho-lunate dissociation (arrow). (Used with permission from: http://www.wikiradiography.net/page/The+Terry-Thomas+Sign)

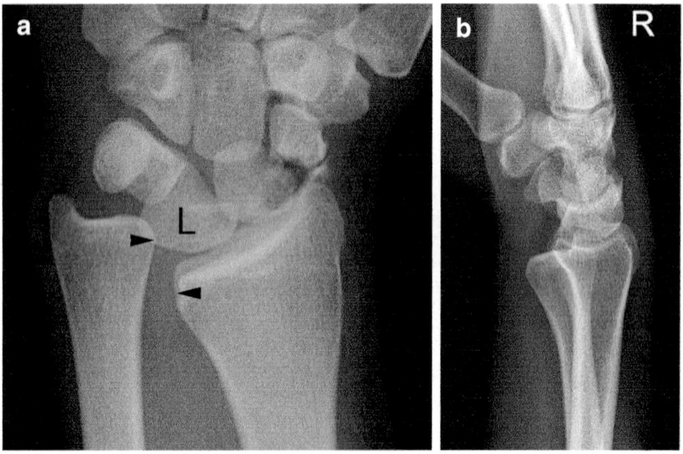

Figure 8.26 DRUJ injury: (**a**) PA view: distal radio-ulnar joint widening (arrowheads), (**b**) Lateral view: volar displacement of the distal ulna demonstrates subluxation of the DRUJ A. (Image reprinted with permission from Claire K Sandstrom, MD, University of Washington Medical Center and Harborview Medical Center, published by Medscape Drugs & Diseases (http://emedicine.medscape.com/), 2017, available at: http://emedicine.medscape.com/article/389069-overview; **b**: Used with permission from http://www.wikiradiography.net/page/Subluxation+of+the+distal+radioulnar+joint)

- Encountered as component of Galeazzi fractures, ulnar styloid fractures, TFCC injuries, and ulnar impaction syndrome (See Fig. 8.26a, b).
- Clinical findings suggestive of DRUJ instability:
  - Pain with pronation/supination of forearm (holding the wrist, not the hand).
  - Pain with lateral compression of radius against the ulna.
- **"Piano-key" test:** fully pronate hand and stabilize distal radius; apply an anterior-posterior force on the ulna with the other hand. If the ulna displaces with little

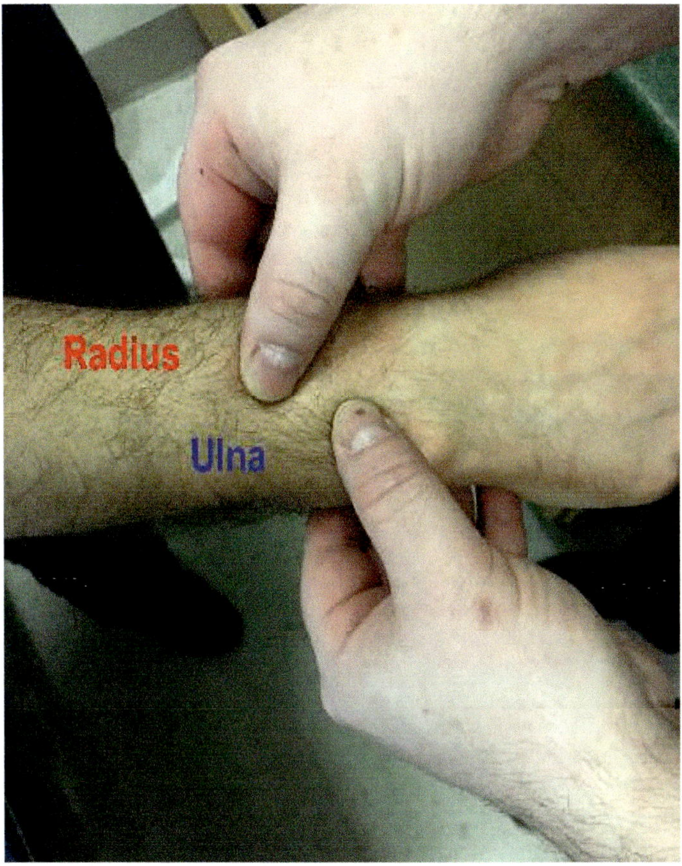

FIGURE 8.27 "Piano-key" test: stabilize the distal radius and apply an anterior-posterior force to the distal ulna

resistance ("like pressing a piano key"), DRUJ instability is present (See Fig. 8.27).

- ***Treatment/prognosis:*** primary method to prevent chronic disability is anatomic reduction of distal radius, which often results in an "anatomically reduced" DRUJ.

Suggested Reading

1. Adams JE, et al. Acute scaphoid fractures. Orthop Clin North Am. 2007;38(2):229.
2. Armbruster E, et al. Perilunate dislocation: case studies of a frequently missed diagnosis: delayed treatment adversely affects clinical results. J Musculoskelet Med. 2008;25:390–5.
3. Baratz ME, Dunn MJ. Ligament injuries and instability of the carpus: scapholunate joint. In: Berger RA, Weiss APC, editors. Hand surgery, vol. 1. Philadelphia: Lippincott Williams & Wilkins; 2004. p. 460–79.
4. Beeson M. Wrist dislocation in emergency medicine. February 13, 2015; Emedicine.com. Retrieved from: https://emedicine.medscape.com/article/823944-overview.
5. Berger RA. Lunotriquetral joint. In: Berger RA, Weiss APC, editors. Hand surgery, vol. 1. Philadelphia: Lippincott Williams & Wilkins; 2004. p. 495–509.
6. Bookman A, et al. Wrist and Hand. In: Fam's musculoskeletal examination and joint injection techniques. Mosby Elsevier: Philadelphia, PA 2nd ed; 2010. p. 29–43.
7. Breitenseher MJ, Gaebler C. Trauma of the wrist. Eur J Radiol. 1997;25:129–39.
8. Cardoso R, et al. Wrist anatomy and surgical approaches. Hand Clinics. 2010;26:1–19.
9. Cetti R, et al. Fracture of the lunate bone. Hand. 1982;14:80–4.
10. Compson JP. The anatomy of acute scaphoid fractures. A three-dimensional analysis of patterns. J Bone Joint Surg Br. 1998;80:218–24.
11. Cooney WP, et al. Fractures and dislocations of the wrist. In: Rockwood CA, Green DP, Bucholz RW, et al., editors. Rockwood and greens fractures in adults. Philadelphia: Lippincott Williams & Wilkins; 1996. p. 745–867.
12. Crosby EB, et al. Scaphotrapezial trapezoidal arthrosis. J Hand Surg. 1978;3:223.
13. Daniels JM, et al. Hand and wrist injuries: Part I. Nonemergent evaluation. Am Fam Physician. 2004;69(8):1941.
14. De Beer JD, Hudson DA. Fractures of the triquetrum. J Hand Surg. 1987;12-B:52–3.
15. Dias JJ, et al. Patterns of union in fractures of the waist of the scaphoid. J Bone Joint Surg Br. 1989;71:307–10.
16. DiGiovanni B, Shaffer J. Treatment of perilunate and transscaphoid perilunate dislocations of the wrist. Am J Orthop. 1995;24:818–26.

17. Foucher G, et al. Fractures of the hook of the hamate. J Hand Surg. 1985;10-B:205–210.57.
18. Fisk GR. The wrist. J Bone Joint Surg. 1984;66:396–407.
19. Gaebler C, et al. Magnetic resonance imaging of occult scaphoid fractures. J Trauma. 1996;41:73–6.
20. Garcia-Elias M. Carpal bone fractures (excluding scaphoid fractures). In: Watson HK, Weinberg J, editors. The wrist. Philadelphia: Lippincott Williams & Wilkins; 2001. p. 173–86.
21. Garcia-Elias M. Dorsal fractures of the triquetrum. Avulsion or compression fractures? J Hand Surg. 1987;12-A:266–8.
22. Gelberman RH, Menon J. The vascularity of the scaphoid bone. J Hand Surg. 1980;5:508–13.
23. Geissler W, Slade JF. Fractures of the carpal bones. In: Green DP, editor. Operative hand surgery. 6th ed. Philadelphia: Churchill Livingstone; 2011. p. 639.
24. Goldfarb C, et al. Wrist fractures: what the clinician wants to know. Radiology. 2001;219:11–28.
25. Hertzberg G, et al. Perilunate dislocations and fracture dislocations: a multicenter study. J Hand Surg. 1993;18-A:768–79.
26. Ilyas AM, Mudgal CS. Radiocarpal fracture-dislocations. J Am Acad Orthop Surg. 2008;16:647–55.
27. Innes L, et al. Systematic review of the treatment of Kienböck's disease in its early and late stages. J Hand Surg Am. 2010;35(5):713–7, 717.e1–4.
28. Kauer JMG. The mechanism of carpal joint. Clin Orthop Relat Res. 1986;202:16–26.
29. Kauer JMG. Functional anatomy of the wrist. Clin Orthop Relat Res. 1980;149:9–20.
30. Linscheid RL. Kinematic considerations of the wrist. Clin Orthop Relat Res. 1986;202:27–39.
31. Mann FA, et al. Radiographic evaluation of the wrist: what does the hand surgeon want to know? Radiology. 1992;184(1):15–24.
32. Mayfield JK, et al. Carpal dislocations: pathomechanics and progressive perilunate instability. J Hand Surg. 1980;5:226–41.
33. McCue FC, Bruce JF Jr, Koman JD. Wrist and hand. In: DeLee and Drez's orthopedic sports medicine principles. 2nd ed. Philadelphia: Saunders; 2003.
34. Moritomo H, et al. The scaphotrapezio-trapezoidal joint. Part I: an anatomic and radiographic study. J Hand Surg. 1999;25-A:899–910.
35. Nagle DJ. Evaluation of chronic wrist pain. J Am Acad Orthop Surg. 2000;8(1):45–55.

36. Perron A. Orthopedic pitfalls in the ED: lunate and perilunate injuries. Am J Emerg Med. 2001:157–62.
37. Rettig AC. Management of acute scaphoid fractures. Hand Clin. 2000;16(3):381–95.
38. Ruby LK. Carpal instability. J Bone Joint Surg. 1995;77-A:476–87.
39. Seitz WH Jr, Papandrea RF. Fractures and dislocations of the wrist. In: Bucholz RW, Heckman JD, editors. Rockwood and green's fractures in adults. 5th ed. Philadelphia: Lippincott Williams & Wilkins; 2002.
40. Shin AY, Battaglia MJ. Lunotriquetral instability: diagnosis and treatment. J Am Acad Orthop Surg. 2000;8:170–9.
41. Walsh JJ. Current status of scapholunate interosseous ligament injuries. J Am Acad Orthop Surg. 2002;10:32–42.
42. Watson HK, Weinzweig J. Physical examination of the wrist. Hand Clin. 1997;13(1):17–34.
43. Watson HK, Ryu J. Evolution of arthritis of the wrist. Clin Orthop. 1986;202:57–67.
44. Watson HK, Ballet FL. The SLAC wrist: scapholunate advanced collapse pattern of degenerative arthritis. J Hand Surg [Am]. 1984;9(3):358–65.
45. Wong K, et al. Delays and poor management of scaphoid fractures: factors contributing to nonunion. J Hand Surg Am. 2011;36(9):1471–4. Epub 2011 Jul 31.
46. Young D, et al. Physical examination of the wrist. Hand Clin. 2010;26:21–36.
47. Zoltie N. Fractures of the body of the hamate. Injury. 1991;22:459–62.
48. Berger RA, Weiss AP. "Ch 23: Carpal bone fractures other than scaphoid". In: Hand surgery. 1st ed. Philadelphia, PA: Lippincott & Williams; 2003. p. 410–23.
49. Berger RA, Weiss AP. "Ch 4: Basic vascular pathophysiology of the hand, wrist and forearm". In: Hand surgery. 1st ed. Philadelphia, PA: Lippincott & Williams; 2003.
50. Seiler JG. "Ch 21: Fractures of the carpus: scaphoid". In: Hand surgery. 1st ed. Lippincott & Williams; 2003. p. 382–409; Chronic carpal instability. In: Essentials of hand surgery. Philadelphia, PA Lippincott Williams & Wilkens; 2002. p. 87–89.

Chapter 9
The Hand

Daniel Purcell, Justin Chapman, and Bryan A. Terry

Introduction

- Injuries to the hand account for ~5–10% of emergency department visits.
- Failure of appropriate care during the acute injury period can lead to poor cosmetic, and more importantly, diminished functional results, that challenge even the most seasoned of hand specialists that ultimately assume care.
- Knowledge and experience breeds comfort, and this begins with an understanding of hand anatomy and the physiologic principles that comprise and regulate its function.

D. Purcell (✉)
Emergency Department, New York University Langone Medical Center Brooklyn, New York, NY, USA
e-mail: daniel.purcell@nyumc.org

J. Chapman
Department of Emergency Medicine, UMass Memorial Medical Center, Worcester, MA, USA

B. A. Terry
The Brooklyn Hospital Center, Brooklyn, NY, USA

D. Purcell et al. (eds.), *Emergency Orthopedics Handbook*,
https://doi.org/10.1007/978-3-030-00707-2_9

Anatomy

A. ***Structural:*** (See Fig. 9.1)

- The hand "proper" is composed of 5 metacarpals and 14 individual phalanges (4 lesser fingers have 3 phalanges each, while the thumb has only 2).
- Phalanges are designated as proximal, middle, and distal in consideration of their anatomic location; their respective articulations are described as metacarpal (MCPJ), proximal (PIPJ), and distal (DIPJ) phalangeal joints.

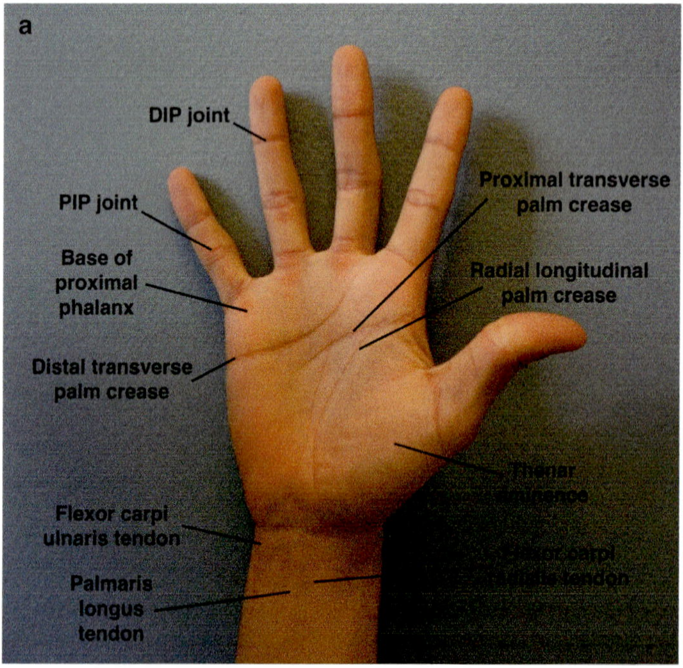

FIGURE 9.1 Surface anatomy of the hand: (**a**) volar view, (**b**) dorsal view

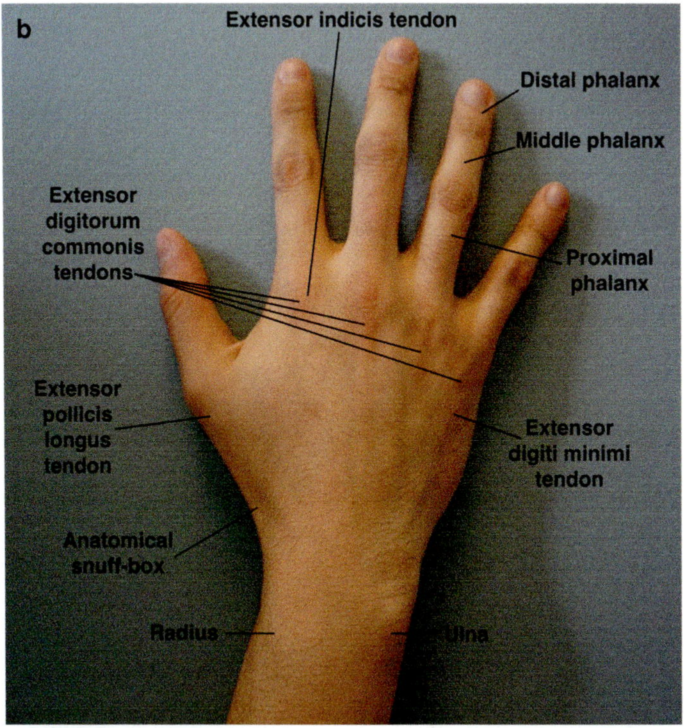

FIGURE 9.1 (continued)

- ***Intrinsic hand muscles*** originate and are contained entirely within the hand, while ***extrinsic muscles*** exert their action through distant tendinous attachments (See Fig. 9.2).
- ***Thenar region:*** fleshy muscle pad at the base of the thumb responsible for thumb abduction, opposition, and flexion at the metacarpophalangeal joint (MCPJ).
- ***Hypothenar region:*** reciprocal musculature at the base of the little finger ***(all innervated by the ulnar nerve)*** that performs fifth finger abduction, opposition, and flexion (See Fig. 9.3).

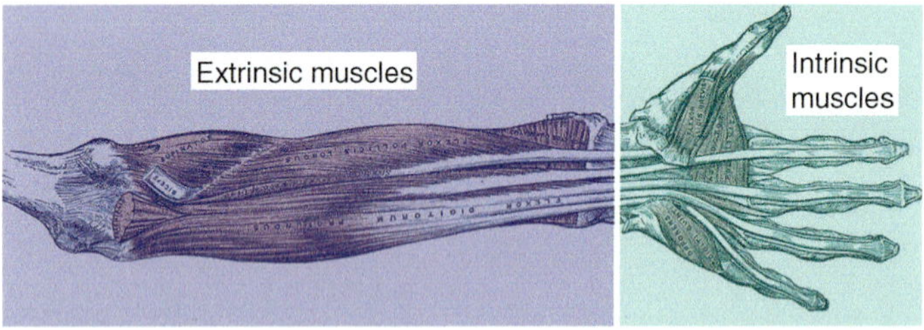

FIGURE 9.2 Origin of hand musculature. (Adapted from Wikipedia: https://commons.wikimedia.org/wiki/File:Gray415.png)

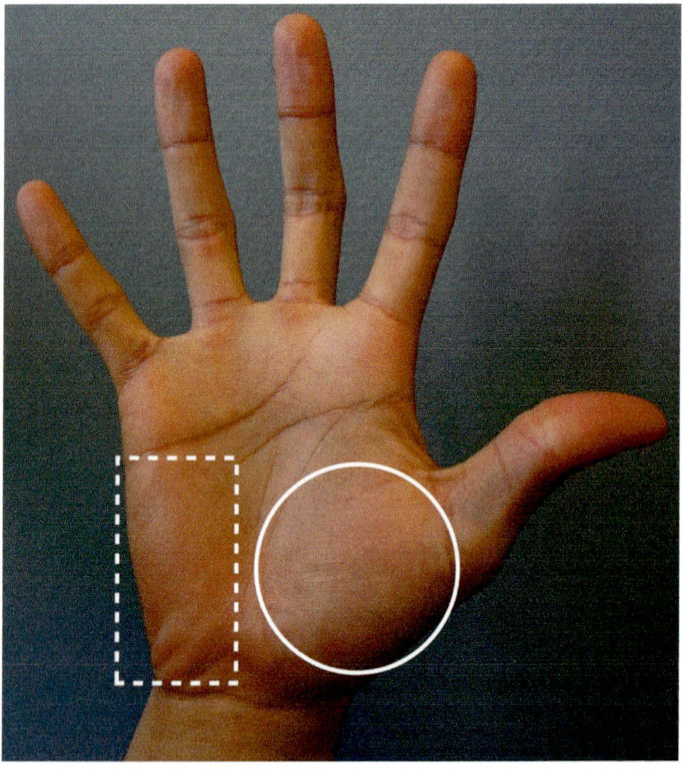

FIGURE 9.3 Hand: thenar region (circle) and hypothenar region (rectangle)

- ***Flexor Tendon Anatomy:***
  - The flexor tendon system is arranged by anatomic region and/or function (the lesser fingers are grouped independently from the thumb) (See Fig. 9.4).

1. ***Lesser Fingers:***

- ***Zone I*** consists of the FDP tendon only, bounded proximally by the FDS insertion.
- ***Zone II*** commonly referred to as Bunnell's "no man's land" secondary to poor outcomes following

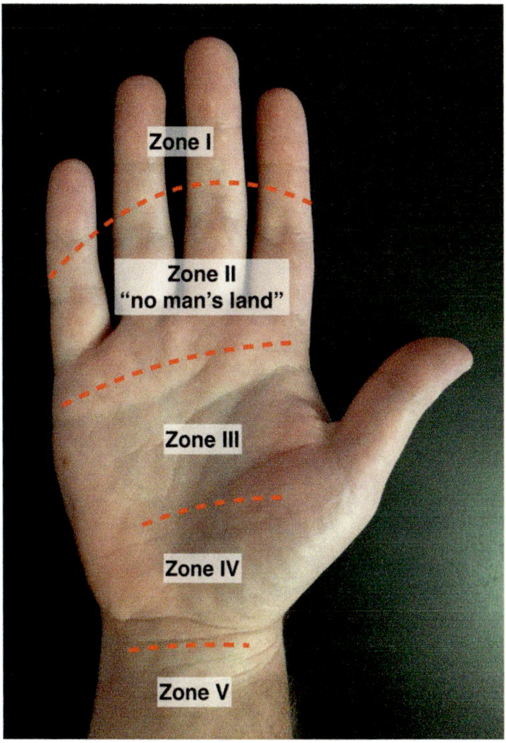

FIGURE 9.4 Flexor tendon anatomic zones

attempted injury repair; has the highest rate of adhesion formation leading to decreased tendon function ("gliding").

Within zone II the individual FDS tendons split into two separate tendinous slips, dividing around the FDP tendon and then reuniting to insert onto the middle phalanx *(Camper's chiasm).***

- ***Zone III*** extends from the carpal ligament to the initiation of the A1 pulley; the lumbricals take their origin from the FDP tendons within this zone; the distal palmar crease represents its distal margin.
- ***Zone IV*** includes the carpal tunnel and its respective contents.
- ***Zone V*** extends from the carpal tunnel proximally to the origin of the extrinsic flexor tendons.

  ****The location of tendon laceration/disruption DIRECTLY affects healing potential****

- ***Volar plate:*** fibrocartilagenous thickening of the joint capsule that separates the flexor tendons from the joint space; it protects the volar articular surface, while also preventing joint hyperextension (See Fig. 9.5).
- ***Flexor Pulley System:***
  Fibro-osseous pulley system designed to prevent tendon "bowstringing" and improve systematic function.
- ***Extensor Tendon Anatomy:*** (See Fig. 9.6)
  - The "extrinsic" finger extensors extend the MCPJ; they are maintained in a central position over the MCPJ by the encircling ***sagittal bands***.
  - They also help create the extensor hood, with extension of its central portion generating the ***central slip***.
  - The ***central slip*** inserts on the proximal aspect of the middle phalanx and extends the PIPJ.
  - The "intrinsic" tendons (lumbricals/interossei) coalesce distally along the borders of each digit to form the ***lateral bands*** and also contribute to formation of the central slip.
  - This divergent course allows the intrinsic musculature to flex the MCP joints, yet also extend the IP joints.

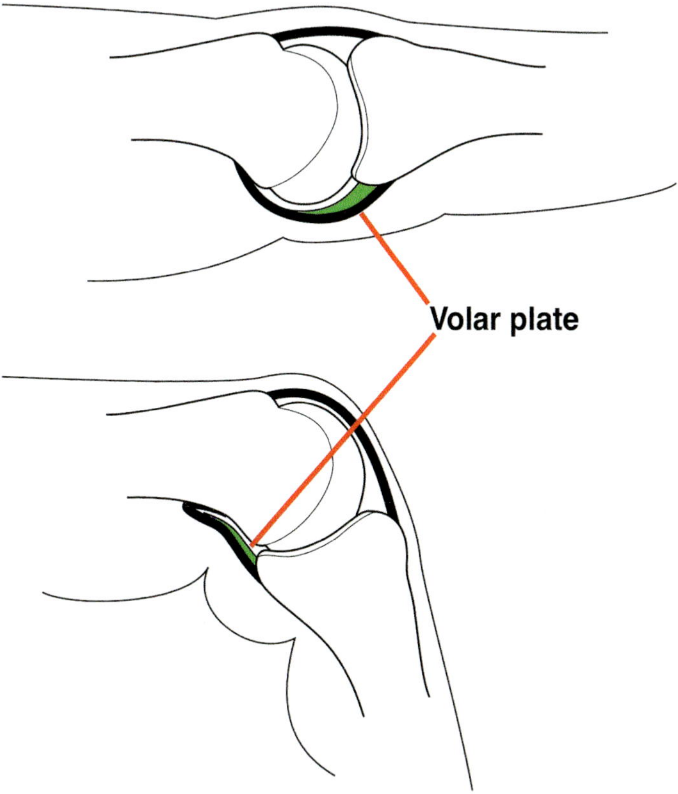

FIGURE 9.5 Volar plate anatomy. (Adapted from Fama Clamosa: https://commons.wikimedia.org/wiki/File:Metacarpophalangeal_joint_illustration.svg. With permission from Creative Commons Attribution: https://creativecommons.org/licenses/by-sa/3.0/deed.en)

- The lateral bands then continue distally to insert on the distal phalanx, forming the ***terminal extensor tendon,*** which helps extend the DIPJ.
- The "extrinsic" extensors to the thumb include the EPL (extensor pollicis longus) and EPB (extensor pollicis brevis) tendons. The EPL extends the thumb IPJ, while the EPB extends the MCPJ.

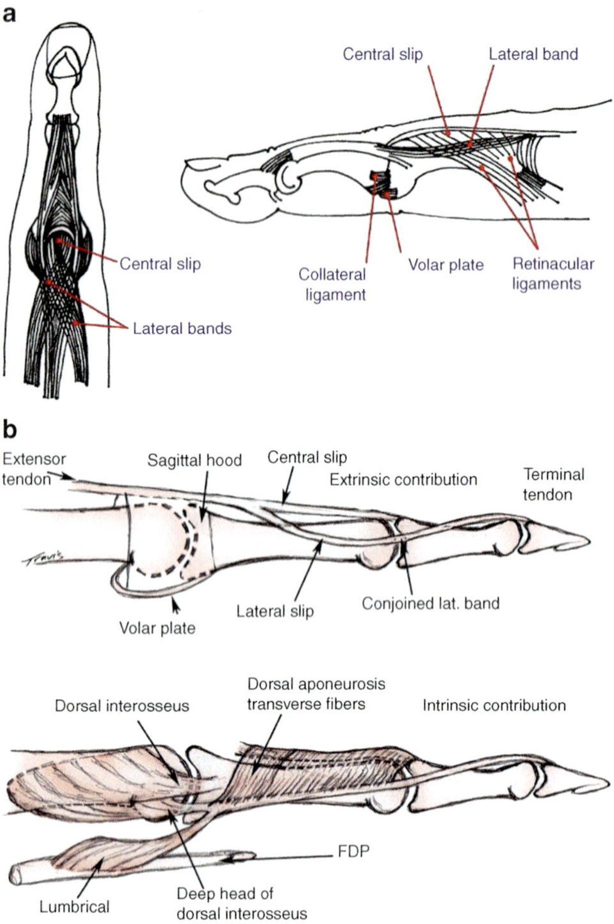

FIGURE 9.6 Extensor tendon anatomy: (**a**) Simplified diagram, (**b**) extrinsic and intrinsic contributions: note the central slip, volar plate, terminal extensor tendon, and FDP tendon, (**c**) Note the sagittal bands. (**a**: Image reprinted with permission from Medscape Drugs & Diseases (http://emedicine.medscape.com/), 2017, available at: http://emedicine.medscape.com/article/98081-overview#showall; **b**, **c**: Images reprinted with permission from Medscape Drugs & Diseases (http://emedicine.medscape.com/), 2017, available at: http://emedicine.medscape.com/article/1286225-overview)

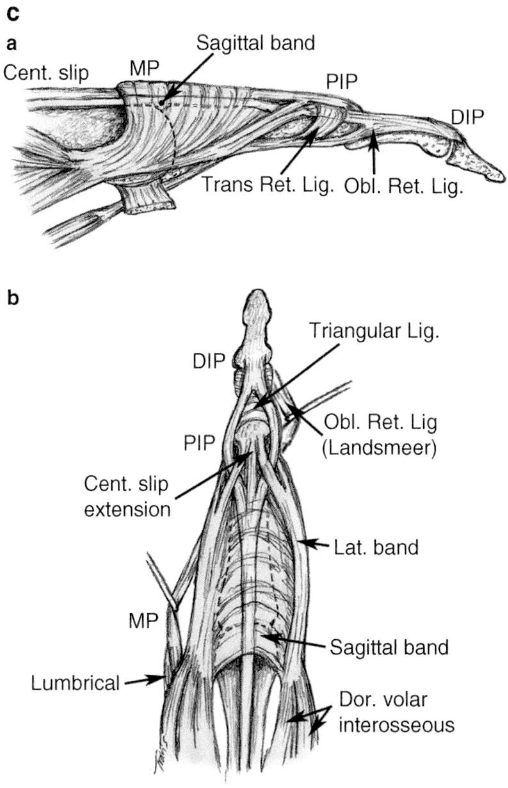

FIGURE 9.6 (continued)

- ***Metacarpals:*** tubular bones that help create the longitudinal/transverse arches of the hand; metacarpal heads exhibit a cam-like mechanism with respect to their corresponding collateral ligaments, predicated upon their origin being dorsal to the MCPJ axis of flexion.
- The collateral ligaments are thus lax with MCPJ extension (→ less bone surface area contact = less stable), but become increasingly taut with increasing flexion (→ more bone surface area contact = more stable); this permits finger adduction/abduction at ~70° of MCPJ flexion, while also providing stabilization for power grip/pinch (See Fig. 9.7).

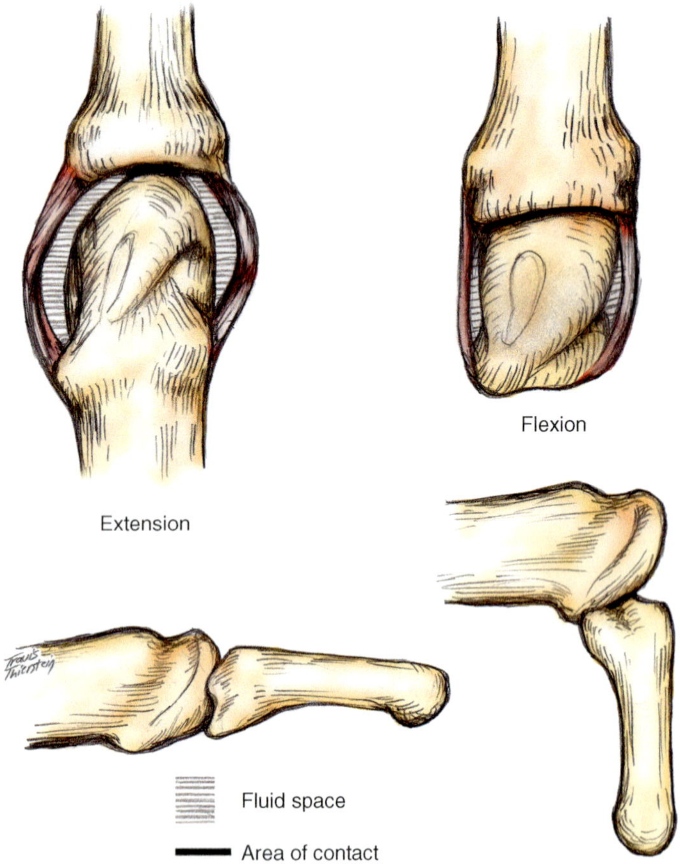

FIGURE 9.7 MCP joint: collateral ligaments are lax with extension and taut with flexion. (Image reprinted with permission from Medscape Drugs & Diseases (http://emedicine.medscape.com/), 2017, available at: http://emedicine.medscape.com/article/1243815-overview)

****MCP joints should be immobilized in at least 70° of flexion to maintain maximum stretch of the collateral ligaments, decreasing the risk of residual digital stiffness*****

- ***Proximal Phalanx:*** base (proximal end) receives a portion of its adjacent lumbrical attachment, while its bilateral edges provide an insertion point for the interosseous muscles. The ligamentous origin of the volar plate is derived from its distal end.
- ***Middle Phalanx:*** cartilaginous portion of the volar plate inserts at its base, while the central slip attaches on its dorsal aspect.
- ***Distal Phalanx:*** consists of the following regions (base, shaft, tuft). Possesses a volar tubercle for attachment of the FDP tendon, while the "terminal extensor tendon" inserts on its dorsal surface.
- ***Fingertip*** consists of the structures distal to insertion of the flexor/extensor tendons on the distal phalanx (nail plate, nail bed, and remaining distal phalanx) (See Fig. 9.8).
- ***Nail bed:*** soft tissue structure beneath the nail plate, bound to the underlying periosteum of the distal phalanx; it is comprised of the ***germinal and sterile matrices:***

1. ***Germinal matrix*** covers the proximal volar nail fold, ending at the level of the lunula; it is immediately distal to the extensor tendon attachment at the base of the distal phalanx ***(accounts for ~ 90% of nail growth)***.

   *****Damage/scar tissue development in this region leads to the characteristic defects associated with post-traumatic nail plate deformities (split or absent nail)*****
2. ***Sterile matrix*** comprises the majority of the nail bed and assists in maintaining the nail plate tightly affixed to the dorsal finger. The proximal nail fold is termed the ***eponychium***, while the distal junction of the nail bed/fingertip skin is delineated the ***hyponychium*** (contains large numbers of WBCs that protect the subungual tissue from potential infection). The ***paronychium*** contains the lateral nail fold and surrounding skin border.

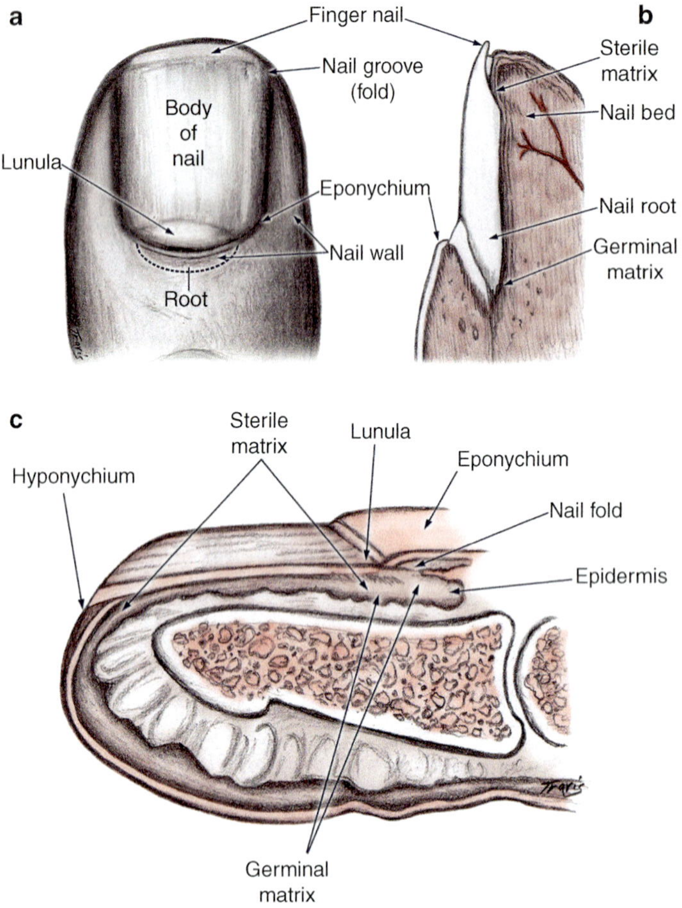

FIGURE 9.8 Fingertip anatomy: (**a**) gross, (**b**) note the germinal matrix and sterile matrix compose the nail bed, (**c**) midsagittal view. (**a**–**c**: Images reprinted with permission from Medscape Drugs & Diseases (http://emedicine.medscape.com/), 2017, available at: http://emedicine.medscape.com/article/82926-overview)

- The digital neurovascular structures arborize near the DIPJ of the lesser fingers, with the nerves traveling volar versus the arteries as they course toward the distal finger.

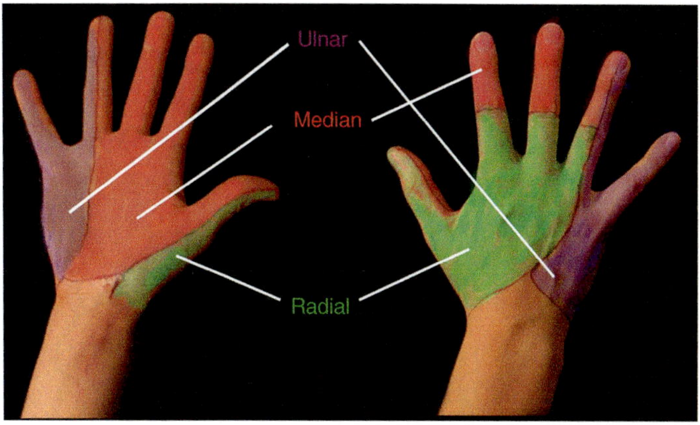

FIGURE 9.9 Hand cutaneous sensory distribution. (Adapted from Ailes D, Waseem M. Regional anesthesia (nerve blocks). In: Ganti L, editor. Atlas of emergency medicine procedures. New York, NY: Springer; 2016. p. 511–23. With permission from Springer Nature)

B. ***Functional***

1. ***Neurologic Innervation:***

A. ***Sensory*** (See Fig. 9.9)
B. ***Motor***

1. ***Median nerve*** innervates the superficial/intermediate muscles of the anterior forearm, except for the flexor carpi ulnaris (FCU). Distally, its extension supplies the thenar musculature, superficial head of the FPB and radial (2nd/3rd digit) lumbricals.

- ***Anterior interosseous nerve (AIN):*** branch off the median nerve proper that innervates the pronator quadratus (PQ), flexor pollicis longus (FPL), and radial half FDP musculature ***(no sensory component)***.
- Functional testing performed by observing patient ability to make an "OK" sign; requires intact thumb (FPL)/index finger IPJ flexion (FDP) (See Fig. 9.10).

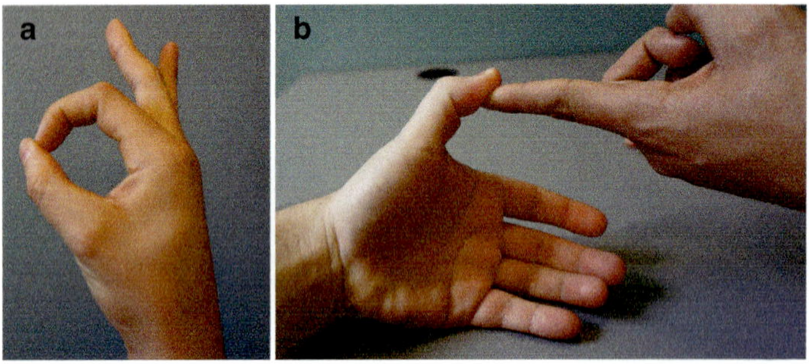

FIGURE 9.10 Testing median nerve/AIN function: (**a**) "OK" sign, (**b**) resisted IPJ flexion

2. ***Ulnar Nerve*** innervates the FCU/medial FDP forearm muscles (4th/5th digits), the hypothenar group, the adductor pollicis, the deep head of the FPB, and all the "intrinsic" hand musculature (except for the radial lumbricals).

   - Functional testing is performed by asking the patient to either cross their lesser fingers or demonstrate adduction/abduction against resistance to assess interossei muscle function (See Fig. 9.11).

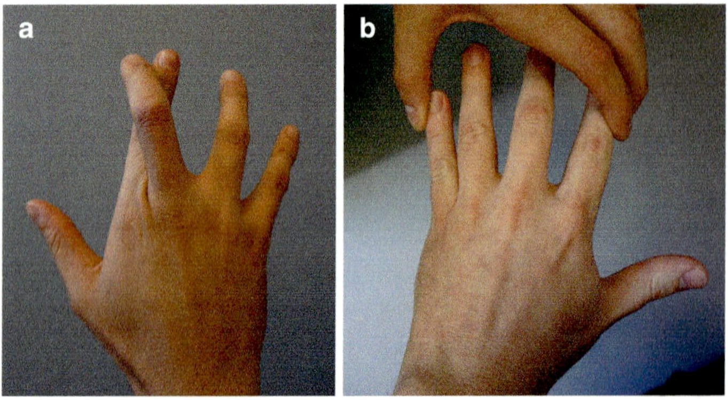

FIGURE 9.11 Ulnar nerve testing: (**a**) crossing fingers, (**b**) abduction against resistance

3. ***Radial Nerve*** innervates the extensor/supinator muscles of the forearm, wrist, and hand in combination with the deep branch of the superficial radial nerve (posterior interosseous nerve – PIN)

   - The radial nerve proper innervates the triceps surae to extend the forearm at the elbow, while the PIN is primarily responsible for extending the wrist and digits.
   - Functional testing of their continuity involves having the patient perform a "thumb's up" maneuver, which specifically evaluates extensor pollicis longus (EPL) function (See Fig. 9.12).

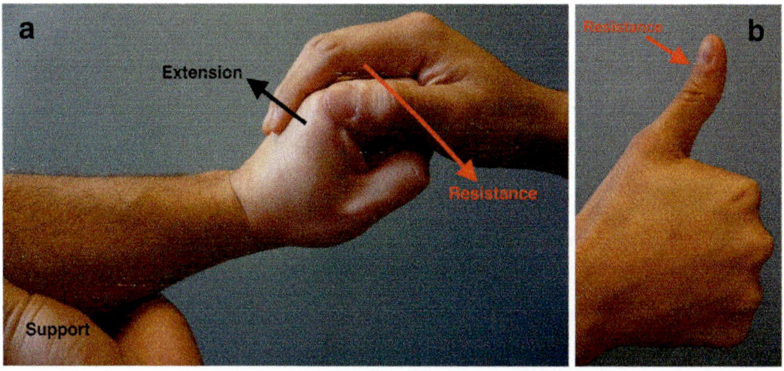

FIGURE 9.12 Radial nerve (PIN testing): (**a**) extension against resistance, (**b**) "thumbs up"

Clinical Evaluation

A. ***History:*** obtain information regarding age, hand dominance, prior injuries, occupation/hobbies, systemic illnesses (DM)/immune status, social history (tobacco use), time/mechanism of injury, and previous treatment prior to presentation (antibiotics, tetanus status, etc.).

B. ***Physical Examination***

   1. ***Inspection:*** note the resting posture of the extremity, any readily visible signs of injury (new or old), baseline appearance of the overlying skin, and evidence of any

muscular atrophy/gross trophic changes consistent with potential innervation/perfusion deficits.

2. ***Palpation:*** investigate all bony structures, protuberances, and/or soft tissue attachment sites.
3. ***Range of motion:*** monitor for any restrictions/deficits of motion (active and passive) and/or abnormal kinematic function.
4. ***Muscle/Tendon Testing:***

   - ***Lesser Digital Flexion:***

     (a) ***Flexor digitorum superficialis (FDS):*** flexes PIPJ of the lesser fingers.
       - ***Testing*** have the patient lay their hand flat, immobilize the remaining fingers in full extension, and stabilize the finger of concern just proximal to the PIPJ; observe for isolated active flexion at the PIPJ (See Fig. 9.13).

     (b) ***Flexor digitorum profundus (FDP)*** flexes the DIPJ of the lesser fingers; its function is independent of the other fingers, thus it is only necessary

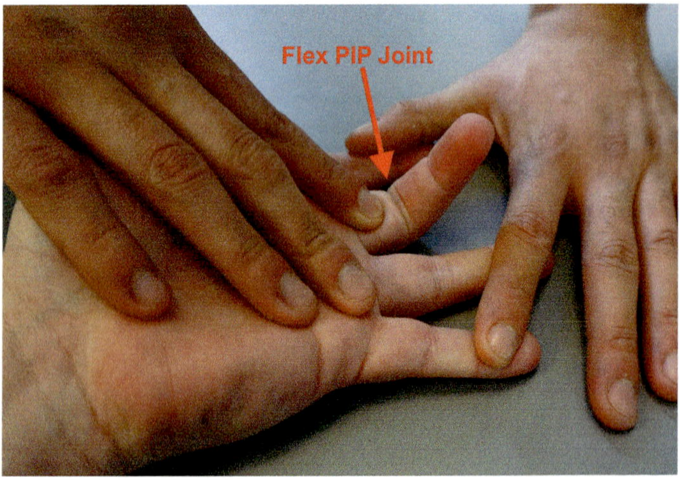

Figure 9.13 FDS testing

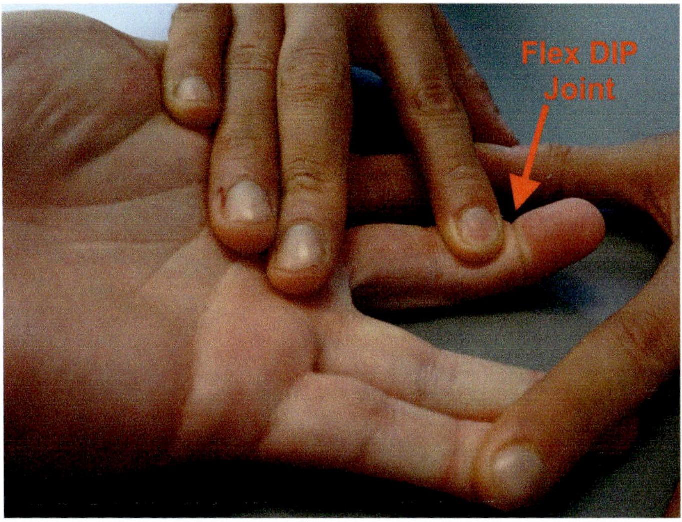

FIGURE 9.14 FDP testing

to immobilize just proximal to the DIPJ of the involved finger and examine for active DIPJ flexion (See Fig. 9.14).

- ***Lesser digit extension:*** more complicated versus determination of flexion deficits; injury can occur anywhere along an extended structural continuum from the "extrinsic" extensor tendon origin to the insertion of the "terminal extensor tendon" on the distal phalanx; all of which can cause loss of active functional extension and/or potential paradoxical motion.
- ***Thumb:*** in comparison to lesser finger examination, evaluation of thumb motion may be tested individually; ***flexion*** deficits at the IPJ indicate injury to the FPL tendon, while failure of MCPJ flexion signals an FPB injury; similarly, the EPL is responsible for ***extension*** at the IPJ, with the EPB at the MCPJ.
- ***Tenodesis effect:*** normally, passive wrist extension should produce digital flexion, and passive wrist flexion should produce digital extension. Tests for potential flexor/extensor tendon disruption (See Fig. 9.15).

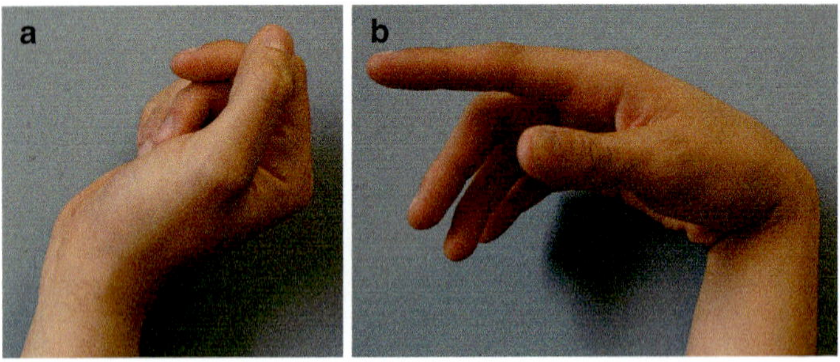

FIGURE 9.15 Normal tenodesis effect: (**a**) wrist extension yields digital flexion, (**b**) wrist flexion yields digital extension

- ***Digital rotation:*** assessment of proper rotation can be assessed by asking the patient to make a fist; all fingers (nail plates) should point toward the scaphoid, with no neighboring finger overlap ("scissoring"); clinical assessment should be made in consideration of the opposite hand for comparison and/or in consideration of previous injury (See Fig. 9.16).

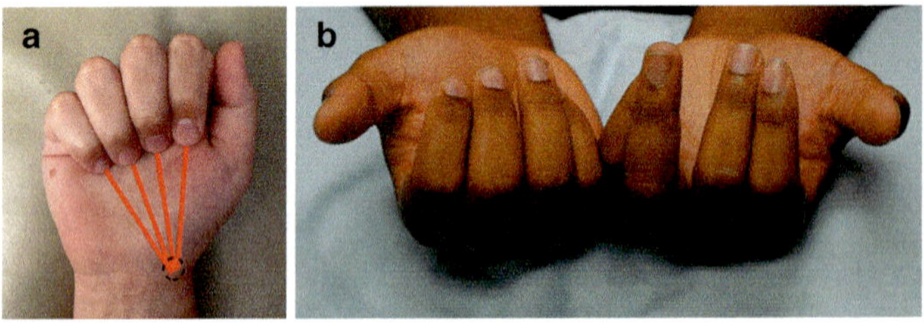

FIGURE 9.16 Digital rotation: (**a**) normal (**b**) left hand demonstrates "scissoring" of ring/little fingers (**b**: Reprinted from Lin IC. Hand injuries. In: Mattei P, Nichol P, Rollins II M, Muratore C, editor. Fundamentals of pediatric surgery. Cham, Switzerland: Springer International Publishing; 2017. p. 195–203. With permission from Springer Nature)

- ***Two-point discrimination:*** evaluates quality of sensory innervation by determining the minimum distance at which two points can be distinguished from one another.
  - It should be performed on both hands, with the non-injured hand generating baseline function. A

standard paperclip/manipulated tongue depressor can serve this purpose.

- Normal value is generally ***~3–5 mm*** at the volar fingertip.

Pathology

A. *Imaging:*

- PA and lateral views of the hand/digit should always be obtained, but 30-degree oblique views may be necessary to avoid superimposition of overlying structures.
- CT may be used for better elucidation of intra-articular fractures, non/malunion, while MRI may be helpful in cases of soft tissue complication(s) accompanying or distinct from bony pathology.
- Dislocations/subluxations are generally evident, but ***stress views*** may be necessary to better characterize suspected injuries (e.g., gamekeeper's/skier's thumb).

B. *Fractures*

1. *Metacarpal Fractures:*

- ***Shaft:*** fracture pattern often denotes the mechanism of injury:

  (a) Direct/axial force-transverse/oblique fractures
  (b) Torsional stress-spiral fracture

- Index/middle finger carpometacarpal articulations are more rigid versus ring/little fingers; acceptable angulation in consideration of potential nonoperative treatment therefore increases from 10–15 to 30–40 degrees progressing from the index to the small finger.
- ***Neck (boxer's fracture)*** results from direct trauma (e.g., bluntly striking object).
- Can generally be reduced "closed", but hard to maintain upon immobilization; ***no*** rotational deformity is acceptable, as grip strength/overall power can be significantly diminished.

Reduce displaced metacarpal shaft/neck fractures using the Jahss technique: Flex the MCPJ/PIPJs to 90 degrees and apply upward pressure on the middle phalanx and downward pressure over the dorsal apex of fracture (just proximal to fracture site).

- Flexing the MCPJ tightens the collateral ligaments, providing a rigid lever for reduction (See Fig. 9.17).

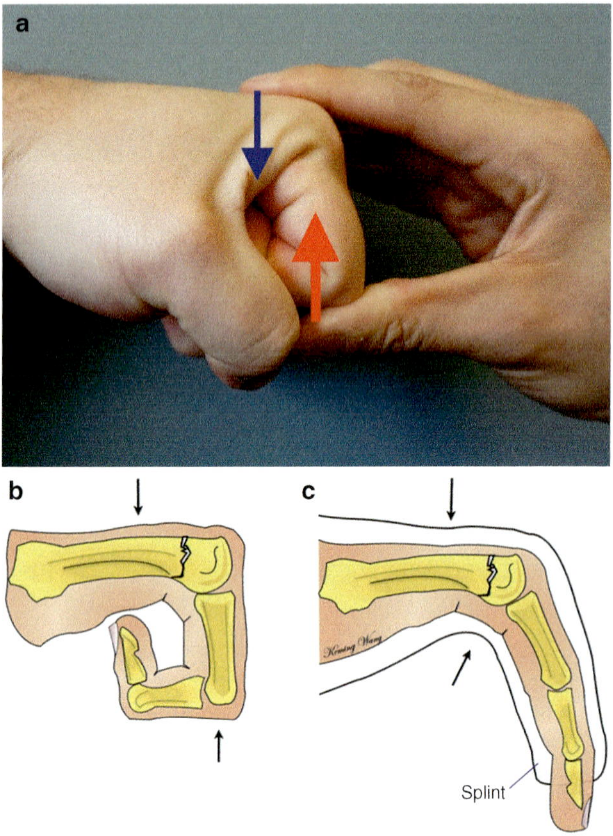

FIGURE 9.17 JAHSS (aka 90–90) technique for closed reduction of metacarpal neck fractures: (**a**) red arrow shows major force, blue arrow demonstrates counter stabilizing force (**b**) bone view, (**c**) arrows indicate line of force in cast/splint immobilization after reduction (**b**, **c**: Reprinted from Diaz-Garcia R, Waljee JF. Current management of metacarpal fractures. Hand Clin. 2013;29(4):507–18. With permission from Elsevier)

2. ***Proximal Phalanx Fractures:***

- Often unstable secondary to the opposing forces exerted on the fracture fragments by both the intrinsic and extrinsic hand muscles.
- Both the lumbricals and interossei (“intrinsic muscles”) insert at or near the proximal phalanx, while the extensor digitorum tendon runs along the dorsum. The FDP/FDS tendons navigate the volar aspect.
- Proximal phalanx fractures often present with apex volar angulation because the “intrinsics” pull the proximal fragment into a volar (palmar) position, while the distal fragment is translated dorsally (extended) by the central slip acting on the base of the middle phalanx (See Fig. 9.18).

3. ***Middle Phalanx Fractures:***

- Architecture of deformity depends upon where the bony disruption occurs.
- Fractures at or near the middle phalanx base tend to angulate in an apex dorsal direction secondary to the extensile force of the central slip and the flexion force provided by the FDS tendon.
- More distal fractures, at the neck region, angulate in an apex volar direction secondary to the isolated pull of the FDS tendon (See Fig. 9.19).

4. ***Distal Phalanx Fractures:***

- Accounts for ~ 50% of all hand fractures.
- Generally three types of patterns are observed: tuft, shaft, and intra-articular.

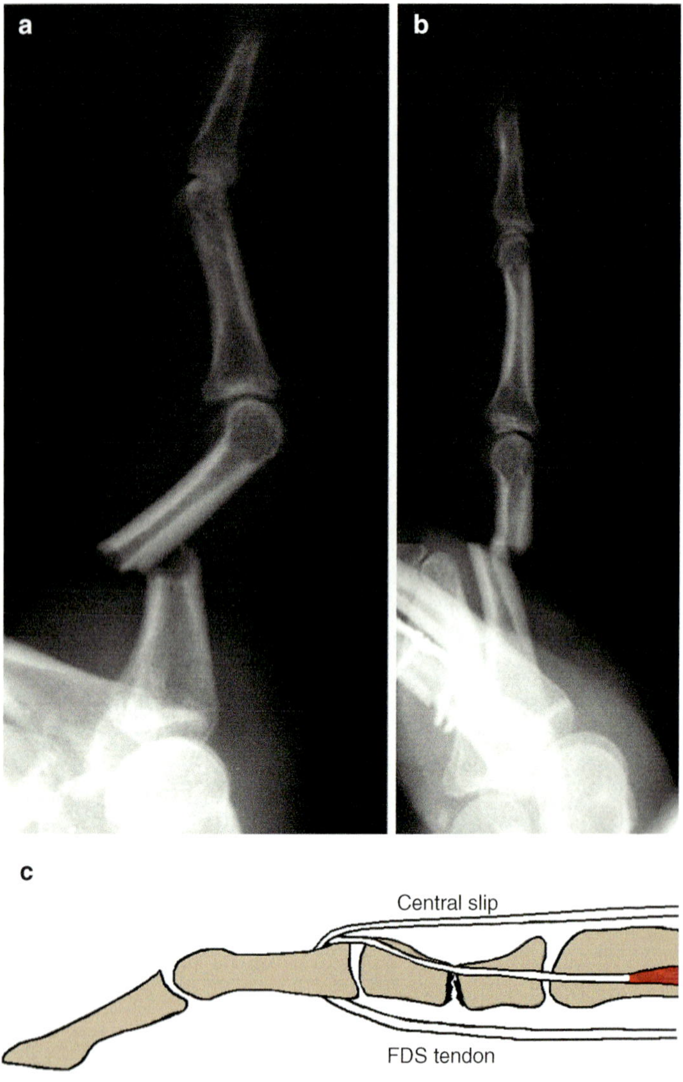

Figure 9.18 Proximal phalanx fracture: (**a**) lateral X-ray of second digit with angulation, (**b**) lateral X-ray of 4th digit, (**c**) drawing of tendons causing angulation. (**a**, **b**: Reprinted from Freeland AE, Orbay JL. Extra-articular hand fractures in adults: a review of new developments. Clin Orthop Relat Res. 2006;445:133–45. With permission from Wolters Kluwer Health, Inc.)

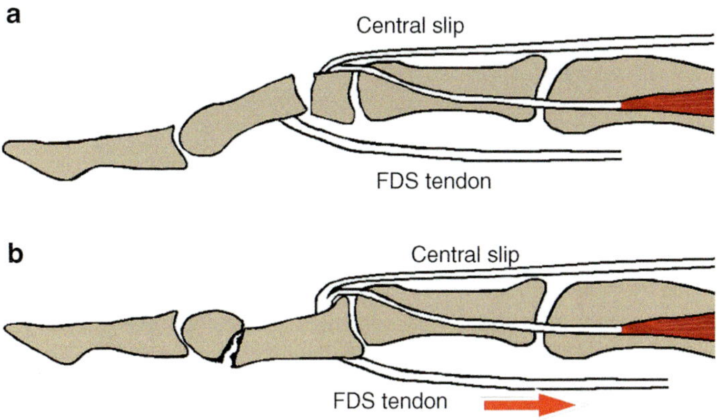

FIGURE 9.19 Middle phalanx fracture: (**a**) fracture proximal to FDS insertion yields apex dorsal angulation, (**b**) fracture distal to insertion will have apex volar angulation

- Extensive soft tissue damage to the pulp +/– associated nail bed laceration may occur.
- Examination should include evaluation of DIJP motion and two-point discrimination.
- Closed fractures are usually stable; however, reduction may be required if it is significantly angulated and/or displaced.
- "Alumafoam" can be used for injury protection and to help maintain reduction.
  ****Do not immobilize the PIPJ*****
- Intra-articular fractures involving >1/3rd of the articular surface warrant hand specialist consultation because operative treatment is often required.
- "Open" injuries generally require antibiotic prophylaxis even when obvious contamination does not exist.
- Inadequately treated injuries can progress to a painful nonunion, malunion, and/or osteomyelitis.

5. ***Thumb Fractures:***

   (a) ***Bennett/Rolando fracture:***

      1. ***Bennett fracture:*** two-part, intra-articular injury at the base of the first metacarpal.

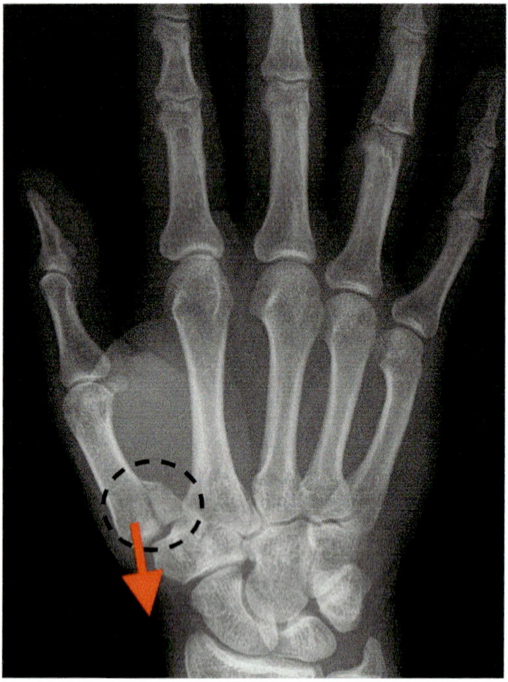

Figure 9.20 Bennett fracture: inherently unstable; volar-ulnar fragment remains attached to the trapezium, whereas the remainder of the metacarpal subluxates proximal, radial, and dorsal (red arrow). (Used with permission from: http://lifeinthefastlane.com/patella-dislocation/)

- Mechanism: sustained following an axial load on a flexed thumb.
- The smaller volar-ulnar fragment retains its ligamentous attachment to the trapezium at the 1st carpometacarpal (CMC) joint, whereas the rest of the metacarpal displaces proximally, radially, and dorsally due to pull of the abductor pollicis longus (APL) tendon (See Fig. 9.20).

2. ***Rolando fracture:*** comminuted, intra-articular 3-part injury through the base of the first metacarpal.

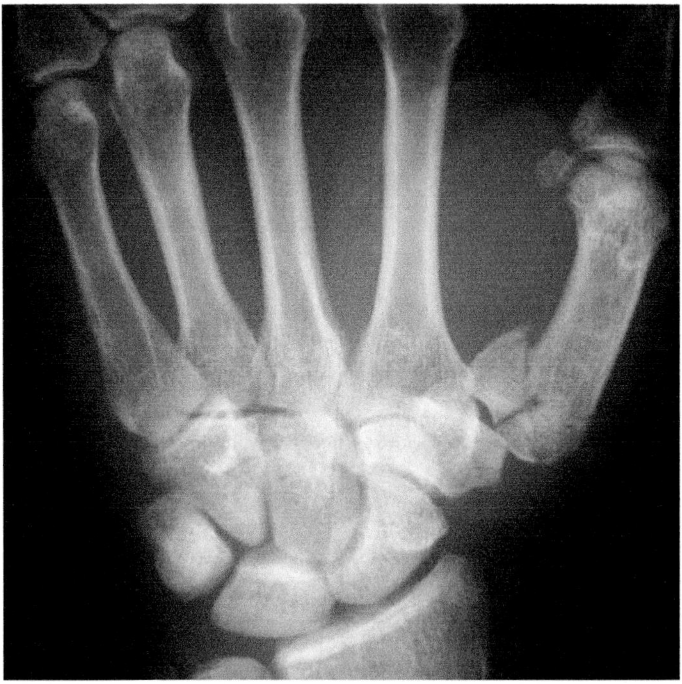

FIGURE 9.21 Rolando fracture. (Reprinted from: https://commons.wikimedia.org/wiki/File:Rolando_fracture.jpg. With permission from Creative Commons Attribution: https://creativecommons.org/licenses/by-sa/3.0/deed.en)

- In addition to a volar lip fracture (seen in Bennett's fracture), there is a large dorsal fragment resulting in a "Y-" or "T"-shaped fracture orientation (See Fig. 9.21)

6. ***Volar Plate Avulsion Fracture:*** failure to promptly recognize and treat can result in disabling pain, stiffness, and deformity attributable to accelerated osteoarthritis (See Figs. 9.22, 9.23 and 9.24).

- ***Injury mechanism:*** forced hyperextension of the involved finger (See Fig. 9.22).
- ***Presentation:*** pain over palmar aspect, swelling, and/or decreased active ROM.

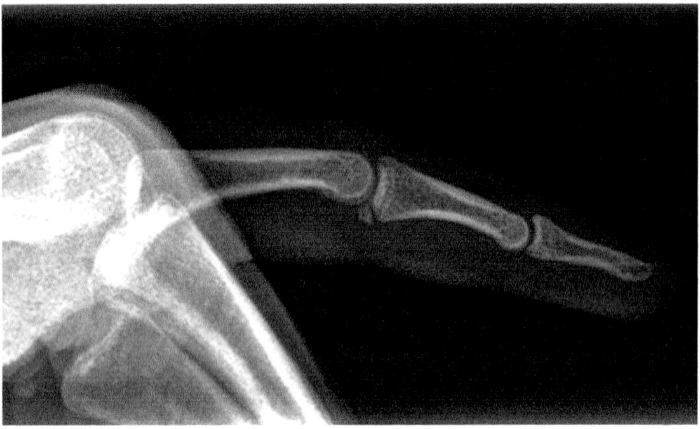

FIGURE 9.22 Volar plate avulsion fracture. (Reprinted from Pattni A, Jones M, Gujral S. Volar plate avulsion injury. Eplasty. 2016;16:ic22. With permission from The Author(s))

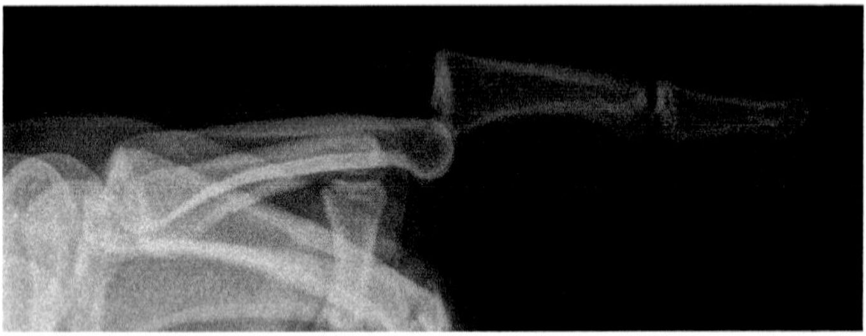

FIGURE 9.23 PIPJ dorsal dislocation. (Reprinted from Haase SC, Chung KC. Current concepts in treatment of fracture-dislocations of the proximal interphalangeal joint. Plast Reconstr Surg. 2014;134(6):1246–57. With permission from Wolters Kluwer Health, Inc.)

Involvement of >40% of the articular surface implies joint instability, best treated with surgical stabilization; PIPJ will otherwise remain dorsally displaced despite repeated attempts at reduction.

Obtaining a true lateral of the affected digit is essential; volar plate injury is most apparent in the sagittal plane.

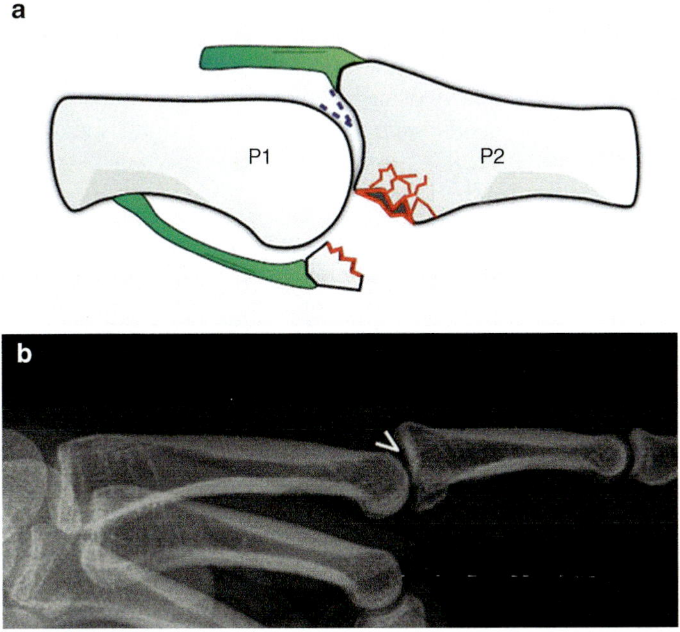

FIGURE 9.24 PIPJ fracture-dislocation: (**a**) Lateral schematic of the PIPJ shows a volar lip avulsion fracture and dorsal subluxation of the joint. The V-shaped gap shown in blue emphasizes the non-congruency of the dorsal portion of the joint, often referred to as a "V-sign." P1 = proximal phalanx. P2 = middle phalanx. (**b**) This lateral radiograph demonstrates the "V-sign" due to PIPJ subluxation. (Reprinted from Haase SC, Chung KC. Current concepts in treatment of fracture-dislocations of the proximal interphalangeal joint. Plast Reconstr Surg. 2014;134(6):1246–57. With permission from Wolters Kluwer Health, Inc.)

C. ***Soft Tissue Injuries:***

1. ***Ulnar collateral ligament (UCL):*** courses from the head of the thumb metacarpal to the inner aspect of the proximal phalanx base; its primary function is to provide support against valgus stress and volar subluxation of the MCPJ. Insufficiency results in volar-radial subluxation of the proximal phalanx at the MCPJ.

- Contains two distinct portions: the proper and accessory ligaments.
- Injury can result in loss of thumb pinch grip, power→early osteoarthritis if left untreated.
- ***Injury mechanism:*** sudden forceful abduction of the thumb; can occur during trauma/contact sports/ chronic stress.

  (a) ***Skier's thumb:*** attempting to brace oneself while firmly holding a ski pole/associated strap can place immense torque on the UCL (See Fig. 9.25).
  (b) ***"Gamekeeper's thumb":*** repetitive stress injury eventually results in chronic UCL laxity.

  - Complete rupture involves both accessory and proper collateral ligaments.

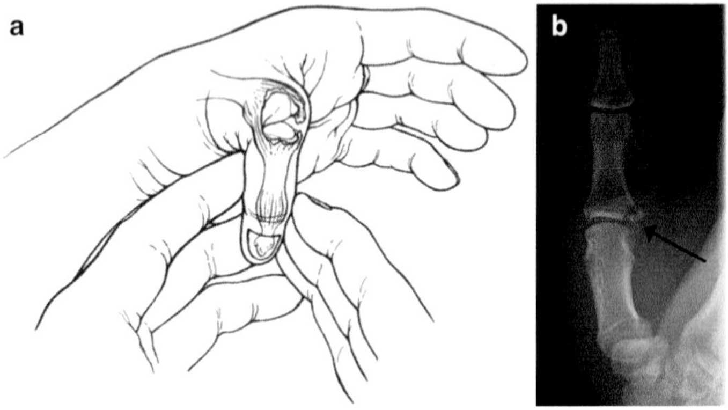

FIGURE 9.25 UCL injury: (**a**) application of valgus force reveals UCL disruption (**b**) imaging reveals avulsion fracture at the base of the proximal phalanx. (**a**: Reprinted from Phelps DB. Hand surgery. In: Kassity KJ, McKittrick JE, Preston FW, editors. Manual of ambulatory surgery. Comprehensive manuals of surgical specialties. New York: Springer; 1982. p. 180–222. With permission from Springer Nature; **b**: Reprinted from James Heilman, MD: https://commons.wikimedia.org/wiki/File:Game_keepers.png. With permission from Creative Commons Attribution: https://creativecommons.org/licenses/by-sa/3.0/deed.en)

- Injury may be associated with a ***Stener lesion*** (interposition of the adductor aponeurosis between the torn UCL and the MCPJ) which disrupts anatomic healing.

  *****Avulsion fracture from the base of the proximal phalanx is generally pathognomonic of a UCL injury.*****

  – ***Testing:*** valgus stress-testing should be performed in both extension and flexion to determine the status of the accessory and proper collateral ligaments, respectively.

  (a) ***UCL proper:*** have patient hold hand with the thumb extended and apply valgus (ulnar) stress, observing for a firm endpoint of translation (it is important that the thumb of the investigator is placed on the radial side of the MCPJ to apply counter pressure to prevent possible rotational effects); also compare to contralateral side noting restriction of movement versus a heightened degree of laxity).

  (b) ***UCL accessory:*** repeat the above maneuver with the thumb maintained in 30 degrees of flexion and again observe for a firm endpoint and compare to the opposite side (See Fig. 9.26).

2. ***Flexor digitorum profundus (FDP):*** *aka "jersey finger" avulsion of FDP tendon.*

   - Inserts at the volar surface of the distal phalanx, flexing the DIPJ.
   - ***Injury mechanism:*** forced hyperextension of a flexed DIPJ (See Fig. 9.27).
   - Examination of the affected finger usually demonstrates a bruised, swollen digit with the inability to flex at the DIPJ.

   *****Because of the risk of tendon retraction/need for surgical treatment, patients should receive early referral to a hand specialist.*****

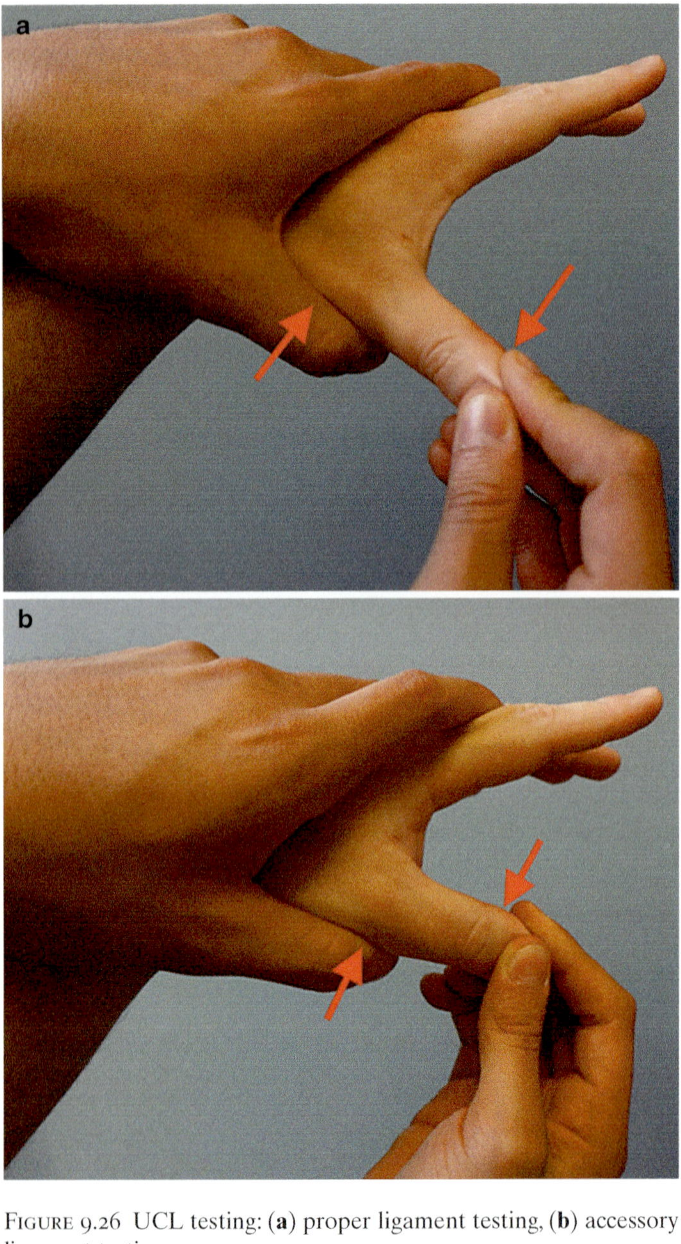

FIGURE 9.26 UCL testing: (**a**) proper ligament testing, (**b**) accessory ligament testing

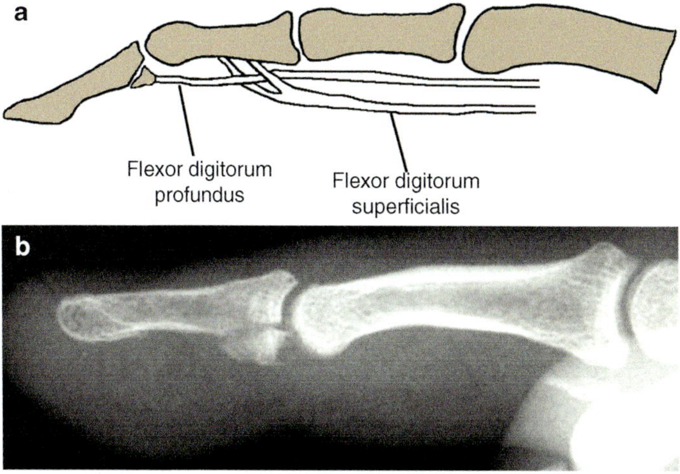

FIGURE 9.27 FDP Avulsion fracture: (**a**) schematic, (**b**) Note the bony fragment at the volar surface of the proximal distal phalanx. (**b**: Courtesy of Mr. Kanthan Theivendran)

3. ***Mallet finger:***

   - Injury occurs at the insertion of the "terminal extensor tendon" on the distal phalanx. The tendon can be torn without or with an attached avulsion fragment "bony mallet."
   - ***Injury mechanism:*** axial load to the tip of an extended finger; this leads to forced flexion at the DIPJ, causing an avulsion of the extensor tendon attached to the dorsal base of distal phalanx.
   - Typically includes a bony fragment that remains attached to the terminal extensor mechanism.
   - Treatment involves full-time DIPJ splinting in extension for 6–8 weeks (studies have shown no difference in outcomes among various splint types as long as DIP extension maintained) (See Fig. 9.28).

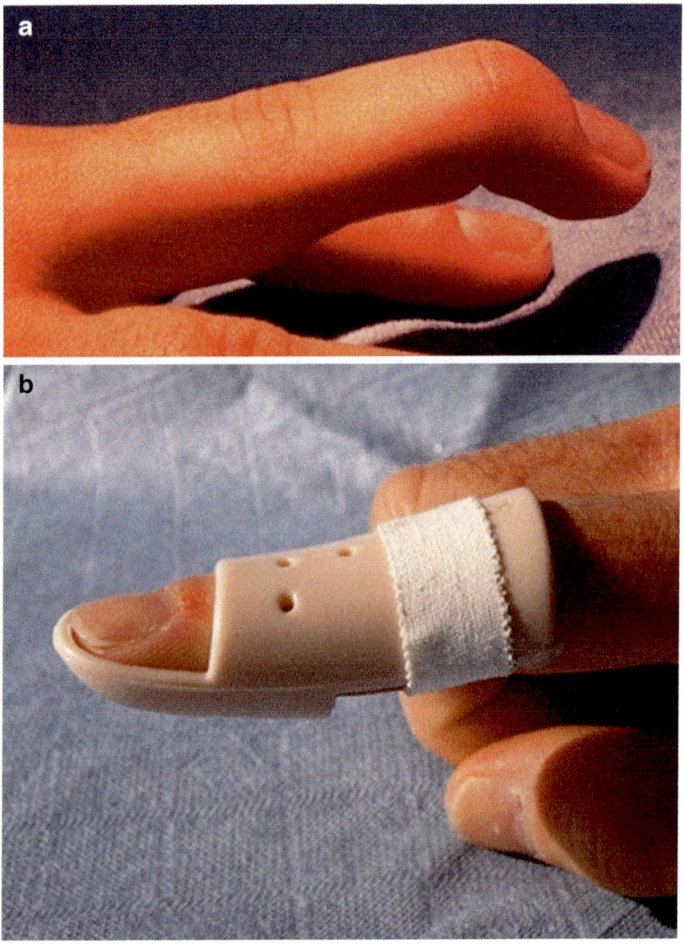

FIGURE 9.28 Mallet finger: (**a**) typical presentation, (**b**) example of a stack splint. (**a**, **b**: Images reprinted with permission from Medscape Drugs & Diseases (http://emedicine.medscape.com/), 2017, available at: http://emedicine.medscape.com/article/1242305-treatment.)

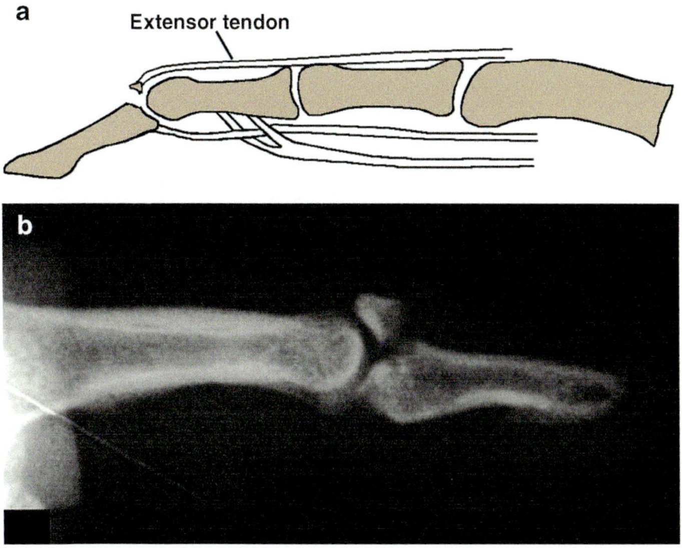

FIGURE 9.29 "Bony" mallet: (**a**) schematic avulsion fracture (**b**) note bony fragment at the dorsal surface of the proximal distal phalanx. (Courtesy of Mr. Kanthan Theivendran)

Imperative that DIPJ extension is maintained at all times during the treatment period; any flexion movement may affect healing, demanding the mandatory treatment period be initiated again*
If >1/3rd of the joint space is involved, surgical repair may be indicated* (See Fig. 9.29)

D. ***Tendon Disruption:***

1. ***General:***

- Tendon disruption is often indicated by a change in the resting posture of the hand/fingers, but should be clearly evident upon functional tendon testing (See Fig. 9.30).

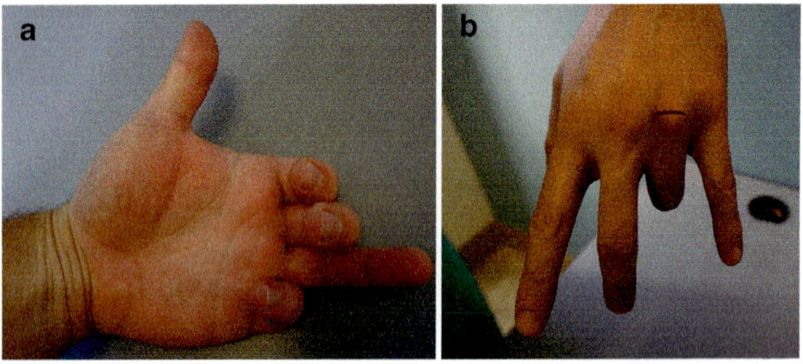

FIGURE 9.30 Typical presentation: (**a**) flexor tendon disruption, (**b**) extensor tendon injury

- ***Treatment:*** irrigation, "loose" skin closure, tetanus as indicated, antibiotics for contaminated wounds, and splint in a position that keeps the tendon ends approximated/decreases risk of tendon retraction.
  ****If tendon ends are clearly visible, delineate ("mark") tendon ends or consider repair depending upon comfort/experience level.****
- Implement a Bunnell-/Kessler-type tendon core repair technique with 5-0 nonabsorbable suture material (See Fig. 9.31).
  *****Immobilize flexor tendon injuries/repairs on the dorsal wrist/hand*****
  *****Tendons should be repaired within 2 weeks of injury to optimize results*****
- Hand surgery should be consulted and expedited follow-up care arranged.

– ***Extensor tendon disruption:***

- If injury occurs over the PIPJ, it can lead to a Boutonniere deformity, versus over the DIPJ, whereby a Mallet deformity may result.
- Treatment follows the algorithm for flexor tendon injuries, but splinting should occur on the volar wrist/hand.

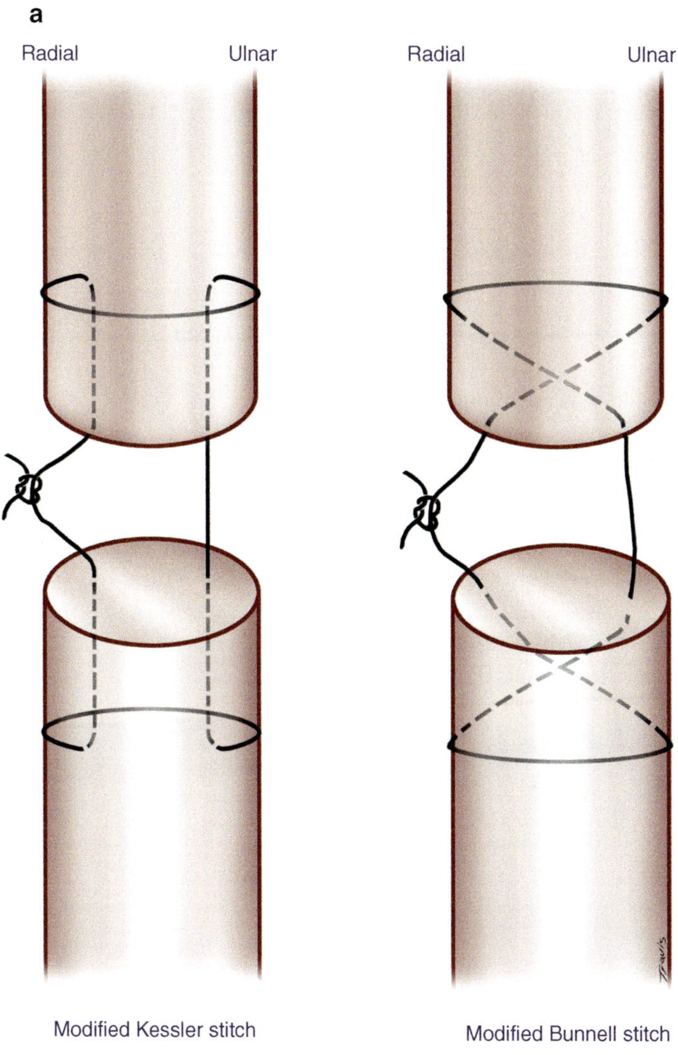

FIGURE 9.31 Tendon repair: (**a**) Modified Kessler and Bunnell stitch, (**b**) Pennington-modified Kessler stitch. (**a**: Image reprinted with permission from Medscape Drugs & Diseases (http://emedicine.medscape.com/), 2017, available at: http://emedicine.medscape.com/article/109111-technique.)

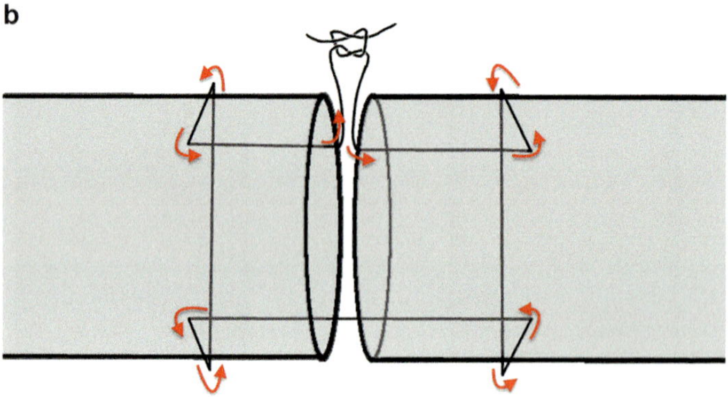

FIGURE 9.31 (continued)

E. *Nail Bed Injuries:*

- Nail bed injuries are often accompanied by significant soft tissue injuries (subungual hematomas, lacerations to the surrounding skin, crush/avulsion injuries) and/or associated distal phalanx fractures (present in ~50% of nail bed injuries, most commonly involving the distal tuft) (See Fig. 9.32).

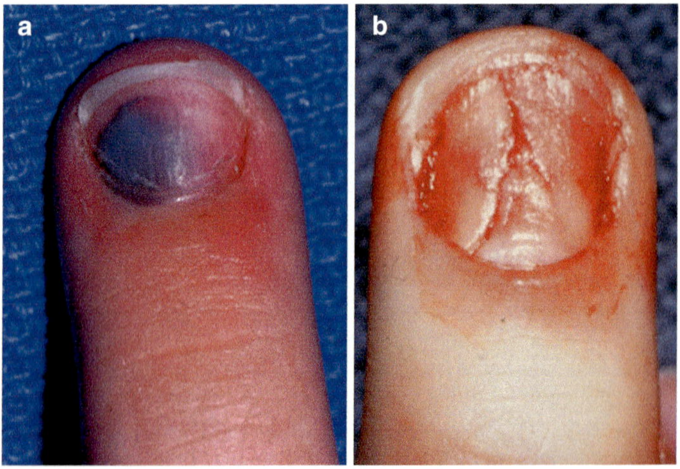

FIGURE 9.32 Subungual hematoma: (**a**) gross appearance (**b**) nail plate removal reveals nail bed laceration. (**a**, **b**: Published with kind permission of © Nicole Z. Sommer, MD)

- Fracture reduction/healing is extremely important to final nail plate formation, with poor bony "reduction" directly translating into increased risk of cosmetic irregularities and poor functional outcomes.
- Nail bed lacerations generally require realignment of affected segments with definitive reduction of accompanying fracture performed following completion of nail bed reconstruction.
  ****However, recent studies have demonstrated that nail bed injuries with no/negligible accompanying bony pathology that are allowed to heal by "secondary intention" +/− skin adhesives (Ex: Dermabond) alone, may yield potentially similar results*****

1. ***Procedure:***
   *****Perform a complete neurovascular examination prior to commencement*****
   - The involved hand should be thoroughly cleansed, prepared, and associated sterile field constructed.
   - Perform a digital block of the affected finger; consider exsanguination with a Penrose drain or finger unit removed from a sterile glove placed around the base of the finger to serve as a tourniquet (can help provide a blood-free field to improve visualization).
     *****Note tourniquet time*****
   - Elevate the nail plate using the blades of a fine/curved scissors instrument, small elevator, or Kelly/Hemostat clamp; use a blunt dissecting technique as the chosen instrument is advanced underneath the nail plate toward the nail fold.
     *****Care must be taken to avoid further damage to underlying nail bed/nail fold; minimal to no debridement should be performed (aggressive debridement can cause undue tension on the subsequent repair, resulting in scarring and accompanying long-term deformity)*****
   - Once the nail plate is sufficiently separated from the nail bed, it is gently removed by applying slow, firm, and steady distal traction.
   - The nail bed is then re-approximated using 6-0/7-0 absorbable sutures (chromic gut), with any associated

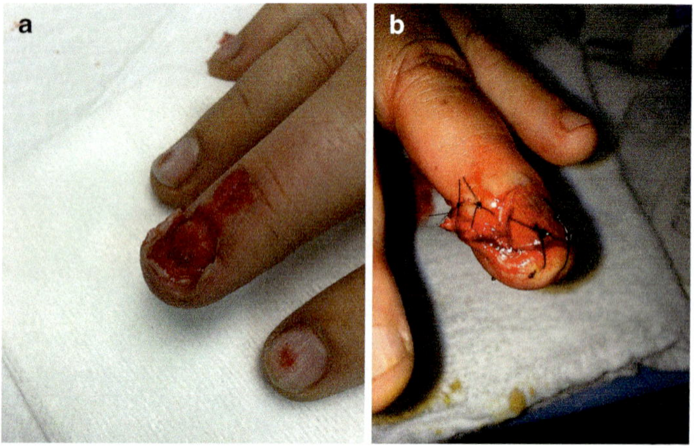

FIGURE 9.33 (**a**) Nail bed/fold injury. (**b**) Nail bed/fold repair. (**a**: Reprinted from https://lacerationrepair.com/anatomic-regions/nailbed-injuries-part-i/. with permission from Brian Lin, MD; **b**: Reprinted from https://lacerationrepair.com/anatomic-regions/nailbed-injuries-part-ii/. with permission from Brian Lin, MD)

lacerations repaired with monofilament-type suture material (e.g., Prolene) (See Fig. 9.33).

- Following repair, the nail plate, if salvageable, should be replaced into the proximal nail fold and secured to serve as protection/biologic dressing, allowing for optimal growth opportunity of the new nail.
  ****If the nail plate is irreversibly damaged, petroleum gauze or a carefully constructed portion of a sterile suture packet** can be inserted into nail bed to serve as a temporary nail plate; suture in place to ensure its continued adherence.***
- Full growth of the nail plate can take approximately 4–6 months.

F. ***Infection:***

- Many hand infections improve with early splinting, elevation, appropriate antibiotics, +/– tetanus prophylaxis and/or I&D if an associated abscess is present.
- Pyogenic flexor tenosynovitis and clenched fist injuries are more serious infections and often require surgical intervention.

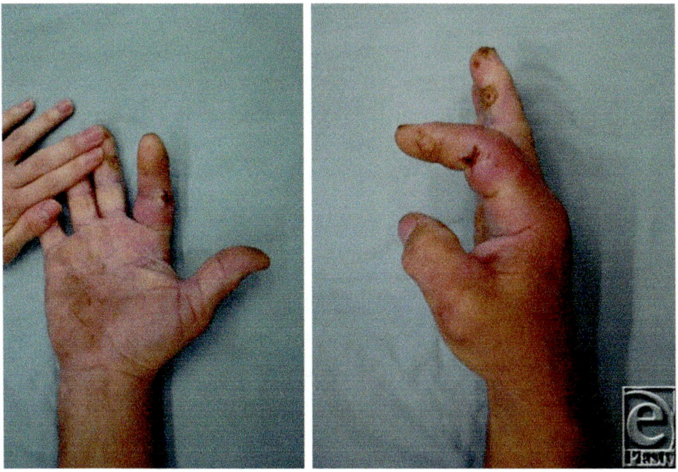

FIGURE 9.34 Flexor tenosynovitis index finger. (Reprinted from Barry RL, Adams NS, Martin MD. Pyogenic (suppurative) flexor tenosynovitis: assessment and management. Eplasty. 2016;16:ic7. With permission from Nick Adams, MD)

1. ***Pyogenic Flexor Tenosynovitis (PTFS):*** acute synovial space infection involving the flexor tendon sheath (See Fig. 9.34)
   *****Can present with four cardinal examination findings (KANAVEL signs)*****
   1. Uniform, symmetric (fusiform) digital swelling.
   2. Affected digit held in partial flexion.
   3. Excessive tenderness elicited upon palpation of the flexor tendon sheath course.
   4. Pain along the flexor tendon sheath with passive digital extension ***(most clinically reproducible of the four potential signs)***.

   *****Hand service consultation for surgical assessment should be obtained immediately with any suspicion of PTFS.*****
   - Patients may not recall any antecedent trauma/portal of entry mechanism.
   - Injury often occurs at the region of the flexor crease where the tendon sheath is most superficial.

- Early diagnosis and treatment are required to prevent tendon necrosis, adhesion formation, and/or spread to deep fascial spaces.
- Infections discovered in its early stages may respond to non-operative treatment: splinting, elevation, and IV antibiotics; however, many patients require admission and formal surgical intervention despite a relatively inert mechanism/level of inoculation (DM, immunocompromised patients).
- No improvement within 12–24 hrs warrants formal surgical intervention that involves full tendon exposure and copious irrigation, and/or debridement.

2. ***Clenched Fist Injury:***

- Human bite injuries to the hand result from either a direct bite or a "fight bite" mechanism (fist striking an object-another person's face/mouth leading to inoculation) (See Fig. 9.35).

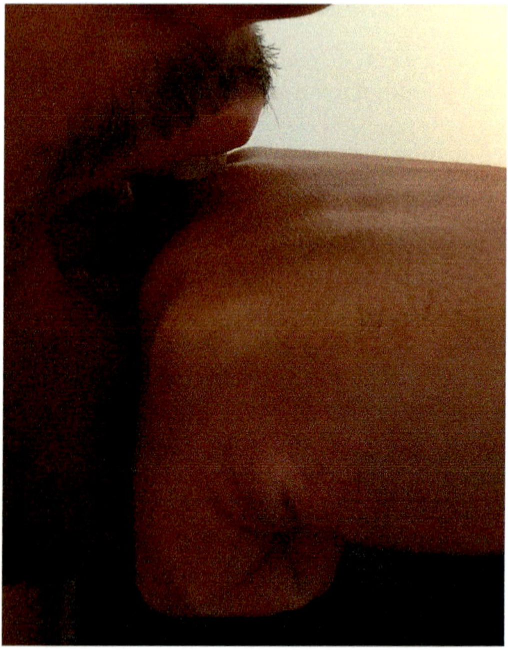

FIGURE 9.35 Classic "fight bite" injury

- Striking a tooth can penetrate an extensor tendon/MCP joint capsule and even cause a metacarpal/phalangeal fracture.
- The injury is generally characterized by a small (3–5 mm) laceration on the dorsum of the hand, overlying and/or adjacent to the MCPJ.

  The extensor tendon injury is usually proximal to the skin laceration because the MCP joint is flexed at the time of impact (tendon injury moves proximal to the skin damage as the extensor muscle contracts during MCP extension); the skin wound is thus distal to the zone of the underlying injury**
- ***Overall Treatment Approach:***
  - Most important therapeutic intervention: aggressive I&D to remove all devitalized tissue (wounds may need to be extended to facilitate exposure of all injured tissue).
  - All contaminated wounds should be left open to heal by secondary intention.
  - Tetanus status should be evaluated.
  - Patients may be splinted in a position of function, with the limb strictly elevated to help diminish swelling.

    Prophylactic antibiotics should be initiated in all but the most superficial of wounds**
  - **Recommended regimens:** amoxicillin/clavulanic acid (Augmentin), doxycycline, or clindamycin for 7–10 days.

    First-generation cephalosporins are not effective for outpatient monotherapy; they possess potential for resistance by Eikenella corrodens.**

    In patients allergic to penicillin and/or in patients with a heightened MRSA potential, clindamycin or similar extended spectrum coverage should be considered.**
  - Radiographs can be obtained to evaluate for fracture/early signs of osteomyelitis, foreign body deposition, and/or potential gas in the soft tissue if clinically appropriate.

- ***Temporal Approach:***

  1. ***Early Presentation: (<24 hrs from the Event)***
     - ***Uncomplicated Versus Complicated***

       A. ***Uncomplicated*** – patients with uncomplicated wounds (no joint capsule penetration/tendon injury) can generally avoid extensive I&D/wound extension. May be given prophylactic antimicrobial therapy, tetanus status updated, and closely followed as outpatients (Repeat wound check in 24–48 hrs).

       B. ***Complicated*** – patients that despite presenting early, possess appreciable signs of infection, extensor tendon injury, have a history of non-compliance and/or some associated clinically worrisome feature, generally requires admission, IV antibiotics (e.g. ampicillin/sulbactam (Unasyn) and hand consultation/intervention).

  2. ***Late Presentation***

     - Treatment is straightforward for delayed evaluations/obviously infected wounds: *****Hand consultation, OR for formal I&D, IV antibiotics, and extended monitoring*****

  *****Some clinicians believe any presentation of this injury requires inpatient admission/formal surgical exploration.*****

G. ***Animal Bite Wounds (Dog and Cat)***

- Dog bite wounds are generally a crushing-type injury based upon their round teeth/crushing jaws, versus the discrete puncture wounds/lacerations that more closely resemble the sharp, pointed teeth of the feline species.

- Hand injuries tend to generate higher rates of infection versus other anatomic regions (e.g., face) based upon a diminished blood supply/difficulty in maintaining proper hygiene.
  - Most common bacterium is ***Pasteurella multocida***.
- ***Evaluation/Treatment***
  - History should invariably include the time/location of the event, type of animal/health status (e.g., rabies vaccination status), pre-hospital treatment, and patient health history.
  - Physical examination should always document neurovascular status, bony/soft tissue involvement, and/or joint space violation.
  - If concern exists for bony involvement, deep structure penetration, FB deposition, etc., imaging should be obtained.
  - Copious irrigation and debridement of devitalized tissue is highly effective in preventing subsequent infection.
  - "Primary closure" may be considered in thoroughly cleansed "fresh" bite wounds that involve certain anatomical regions (e.g., face) or gaping wounds, versus delayed presentations (> ~8–12 hrs) of extremity injuries, that should be generally left open to heal by secondary intention.
  - Puncture wounds may require extension of the affected area to allow for adequate irrigation/debridement.
  - Implement prophylactic antibiotics based upon individual cases/type of animal involved (Augmentin is generally the first-line prophylactic agent unless MRSA coverage required).
  - Consider tetanus prophylaxis and rabies vaccine/immunoglobulin as required.

    "*Cat-scratch disease*": *(Bartonella species) – for those with severe local/systemic involvement +/− immunosuppression, treat with Azithromycin (e.g., Z-pack)*

H. ***Felon***

- Abscess of the distal pulp and/or fingertip pad.
- Closed-space infection (pulp of fingertip divided into numerous smaller compartments by fibrous septa that run from the distal phalanx periosteum to the skin). Pressure accumulation in these non-compliant compartments can lead to significant pain, swelling, and/or tissue necrosis. In addition, septal attachments to the periosteum also provide access to the bony architecture, and a potential for the development of osteomyelitis.
- Generally caused by bacterial inoculation via penetrating trauma (e.g., splinters, abrasions, puncture wounds, contiguous spread of an untreated/undertreated paronychia, etc.)
- Time course of injury generally follows one of two paths:

  1. Initial injury→cellulitis, confined by the fibrous septa; infection may still resolve spontaneously, particularly with antibiotics.
  2. Most patients present at later stages of infection, with severe, throbbing pain, erythema, and swelling of the fingertip.

- ***Treatment:***
  - If diagnosed early, may be amenable to elevation, PO antibiotics (if surrounding cellulitis present), and warm soaks.
  - Radiographs may be considered to evaluate for foreign body/bony involvement, and tetanus status should also be considered.
  - If an area of fluid collection is present, formal I&D should be initiated

- ***Procedure:***
  - Preferred techniques are the ***volar longitudinal or high-lateral incision*** methods.
  - Performed under sterile conditions, digital anesthesia, +/– digital tourniquet.

1. ***Volar longitudinal technique:***

   - Incision starts ~3–5 mm distal to the DIPJ flexor crease and extends to the end of the distal phalanx; depth of incision is to the level of the dermis.

- Gently dissect/explore the SQ tissues with a small hemostat; excise any necrotic skin edges, copiously irrigate, and decompress the abscess.
- Evacuate pus using a blunt instrument in order to decrease the chance of injuring neurovascular structures and/or entering the flexor tendon sheath.

2. ***High lateral technique:***

- Incision is made on the ***non-oppositional side*** of the appropriate digit ***(ulnar side of index, middle, and ring fingers, versus radial aspect of the thumb and little finger)***.
- It begins ~5 mm distal to flexor DIPJ crease and continues parallel to the lateral border of the nail plate, maintaining approximately 5 mm between the incision and the border of the nail plate ***(distance should allow for avoidance of the more volar neurovascular structures)***.
- Subcutaneous tissue should be dissected just volar to the volar cortex of distal phalanx.

  *****Regardless of the technique implemented, consider packing the wound with sterile gauze to allow for continued drainage and healing by secondary intention.*****

  *****Incision should not cross the DIPJ to prevent formation of a flexion contracture.***** (See Fig. 9.36)

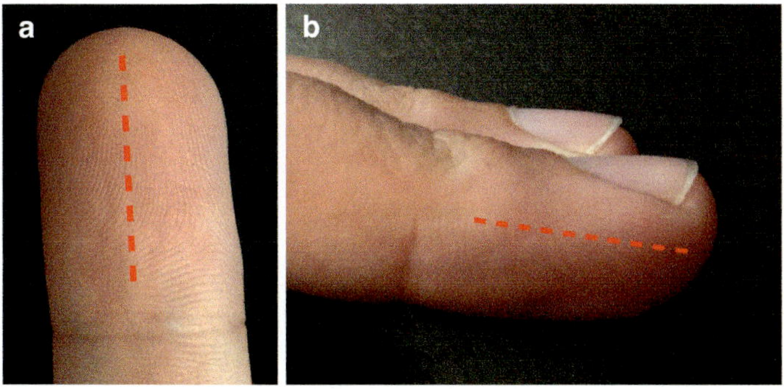

FIGURE 9.36 Felon drainage techniques: (**a**) volar longitudinal, (**b**) high lateral

I. ***Paronychia:***

- Most common infection of the hand, representing ~35% of all hand infections in the US.
- It is a painful, superficial infection of the epithelium lateral to the nail plate.
- Commonly precipitated by localized trauma, with a break in the soft tissue seal on the dorsal periphery of the nail plate a frequent portal of entry (See Fig. 9.37).

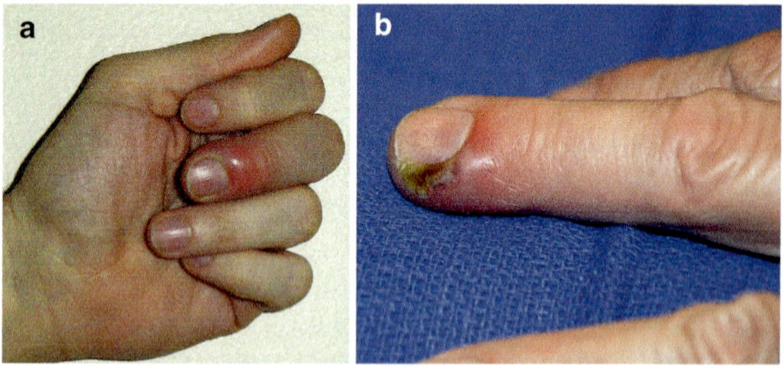

FIGURE 9.37 (**a**, **b**) Examples of paronychia. (**a**: Reprinted from https://commons.wikimedia.org/wiki/File:Paronychia.jpg. With permission from Chris Craig. **b**: Image reprinted with permission from Medscape Drugs & Diseases (http://emedicine.medscape.com/), 2017, available at: http://emedicine.medscape.com/article/1106062-overview#showall.)

- ***Treatment:*** warm water soaks + PO antibiotics may be effective in the early stages; however, if spontaneous drainage does not occur or an abscess is present, formal I&D is warranted.
- ***Procedure:***
  - Thoroughly cleanse the affected finger and perform a digital block.
  - Dissect with a sharp instrument/surgical blade to elevate the lateral nail fold; attempt to enter the sulcus between the lateral aspect of the nail plate and the adjacent lateral epithelium (purulent drainage generally erupts upon entering the sulcus) (See Fig. 9.38).

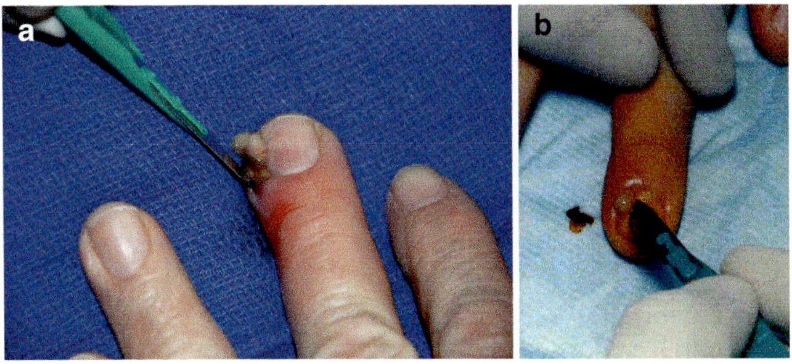

FIGURE 9.38 (**a**, **b**) I&D of paronychia. (**a**: Image reprinted with permission from Medscape Drugs & Diseases (http://emedicine.medscape.com/), 2017, available at: http://emedicine.medscape.com/article/1106062-overview#showall; **b**: Image reprinted with permission from Medscape Drugs & Diseases (http://emedicine.medscape.com/), 2017, available at: http://emedicine.medscape.com/article/782537-treatment.)

- The lateral skin fold should also be slightly elevated and copiously irrigated.
  Care must be taken to direct the sharp edge of the dissection instrument toward the paronychial fold and away from the nail bed to avoid injury to nail matrix, which can result in scarring and/or nail growth deformities
- If there is any involvement of nail bed, remove the affected side of the nail plate, gently separating the lateral third of the nail plate from the nail bed to optimize results and help prevent recurrence.
  Infection can spread to the eponychium (proximal nail fold), eventually forming a "horseshoe" that includes the opposite nail fold and/or digital pulp space, leading to felon formation; it can also spread to the deep spaces of the hand/distal forearm with potential systemic consequences.
- Chronic/recurrent paronychial infections should be scrutinized to rule out malignancy and/or potential fungal infections (***Candida albicans***).

J. ***Herpetic Whitlow:*** (See Fig. 9.39)

- Caused by HSV via an interrupted skin barrier, most commonly a disrupted cuticle.
- It invades the dermal subcutaneous tissue, most commonly at the terminal phalanx.
- Healthcare workers (e.g., dentists) are commonly infected via a heightened exposure to oral body fluids.
- Symptoms may include an abrupt onset of edema, erythema, and significant localized tenderness; fever, lymphadenitis, and epitrochlear/axillary lymphadenopathy may also be present.

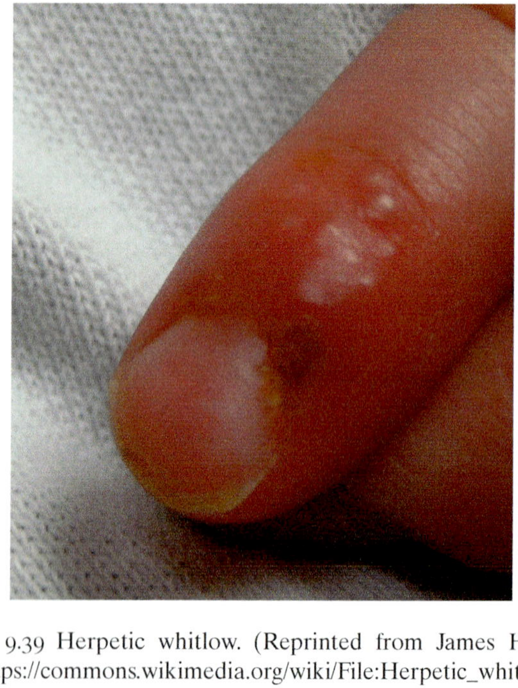

FIGURE 9.39 Herpetic whitlow. (Reprinted from James Heilman, MD: https://commons.wikimedia.org/wiki/File:Herpetic_whitlow_in_young_child.jpg. With permission from Creative Commons Attribution: https://creativecommons.org/licenses/by-sa/3.0/deed.en)

- ***Treatment:*** directed toward symptomatic relief, as it is a self-limited disease process.
- Suppressive therapy (antivirals, e.g., Acyclovir) may be prescribed if the infection is present <48 hrs and they may also be helpful to prevent recurrence.

  ****Irrigation and debridement is contraindicated: can lead to delayed resolution, bacterial superinfection, or systemic spread (can seed the joint space)****

  ****Pulp of the finger pad will be soft in cases of herpetic whitlow versus extremely tense in those patients with a felon.****

  ****Pain out of proportion to its appearance usually suggests an alternative diagnosis (e.g., felon).****
- Uncomplicated cases generally resolve 3–4 weeks.
- Healthcare workers should use gloves, practice strict handwashing, and scrupulously observe universal fluid precautions to prevent contracting and/or spread of infection.

K. ***High-Pressure Injuries:***

- Can occur following mishap with paint/grease guns, diesel injectors, etc.
- Common injury mechanism: unexpected discharge following an attempt(s) to clear a "blocked" tool with the non-dominant hand.
- Leads to deposition of foreign debris deep into tissues, tendon sheath(s), and/or between fascial planes.
- Injuries to the thumb and little finger are more problematic because their tendon sheaths are contiguous with the radial/ulnar bursae, permitting potential spread proximally to the forearm.
- The initial injury often looks benign; thus, delayed presentations are quite common; however within hours, the affected finger starts to become painful secondary to vasoconstriction and associated local inflammatory response; as tissue pressure rises, development of compartment syndrome becomes a potential complication.

- **Treatment:**
  - Measures may include prophylactic antibiotics, tetanus assessment, and/or surgical decompression to remove the inciting foreign material.
    ****Digital blocks are contraindicated because they further increase tissue pressure and the risk of necrosis upon anesthetic infiltration.*****

Pearls:

- ***Intrinsic Plus position: safe position for hand/wrist immobilization***; flexion of the MCPJs allows the collateral ligaments to remain taut and avoids the potential development of subsequent contractures following immobilization (See Fig. 9.40).
- ***General Indications for Replantation of Amputated Structures:***
  - Thumb
  - Multiple digits
  - Almost all parts in children
  - Injuries at the wrist or more proximal forearm
  - Individual digits *distal* to insertion of FDS (Zone II)

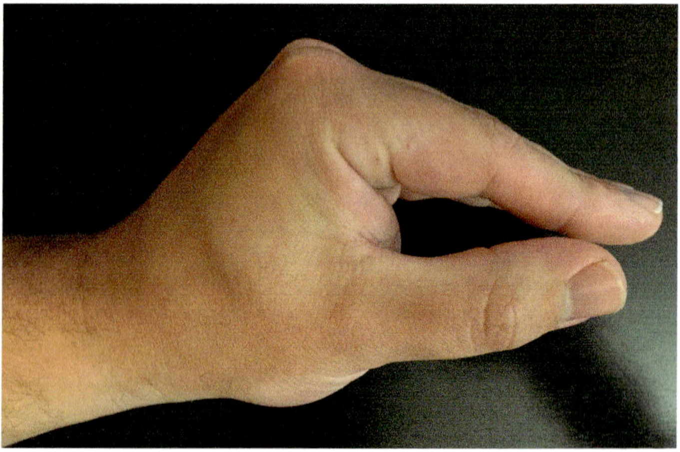

FIGURE 9.40 "Intrinsic plus position": MCP joints in 90° flexion, DIP, and PIP joints in full extension

- ***General Contraindications for Replantation:***
  - Single digit *proximal* to FDS insertion (Zone II)
  - Mangled parts, multiple levels
  - Prolonged ischemia time
  - ?Tobacco usage
- ***Optimal handling of amputated tissue involves the affected component being wrapped in moist gauze, placed in normal saline or LR solution, and transported in a sealed plastic bag containing ice.***

Suggested Reading

1. Perron A. Orthopedic pitfalls in the ED: lunate and perilunate injuries. Am J Emerg Med. 2001;19:157–62.
2. Yoong P. Four hand injuries not to miss: avoiding pitfalls in the emergency department. Eur J Emerg Med. 2011:1–6.
3. Duncan S, Weiland A. Hand surgery. 1st ed: Lippincott, PA: Williams & Wilkens; 2004.
4. Clark D. Common acute hand infections. Am Fam Physician. 2003;(11):68, 2167–2176.
5. Perron A. Orthopedic pitfalls in the ED: Galeazzi and Monteggia fracture-dislocation. Am J Emerg Med. 2001;19:225–08.
6. Murray PM, et al. Perilunate Fracture Dislocations. Medscape. https://emedicine.medscape.com/article/1240108.
7. Beeson M. Wrist dislocation in emergency medicine. Emedicine. com.
8. Perron A. Orthopedic pitfalls in the ED: fight bite. Am J Emerg Med. 20:114–7.
9. Jebson PJL. Infections of the fingertip. Hand Clin. 1998;14: 547–55.
10. Abrams RA, Botte MJ. Hand infections: treatment recommendations for specific types. J Am Acad Orthop Surg. 1996;4: 219–30.
11. Nagano A. Spontaneous anterior interosseous nerve palsy. J Bone Joint Surg Br. 2003;85(3):313–8.
12. Dang AC, Rodner CM. Unusual compression neuropathies of the forearm, part II: median nerve. J Hand Surg Am. 2009;34(10):1915–20.
13. Chi Y, Harness NG. Anterior interosseous nerve syndrome. J Hand Surg Am. 2010;35(12):2078–80.

14. Wang Q, et al. Fingertip injuries. Am Fam Physician. 2001; 63(10):1961–6.
15. Van Beek AL, Kassan MA, Adson MH, Dale V. Management of acute fingernail injuries. Hand Clin. 1990;6:23–38.
16. Lubahn JD, Koeneman J, Kosar K. The digital tourniquet: how safe is it? J Hand Surg [Am]. 1985;10:664–9.
17. Lubahn JD, Hood JM. Fractures of the distal inter phalangeal joint. Clin Orthop. 1996;(327):12–20. https://www.ncbi.nlm.nih.gov/pubmed/8641055
18. Armbruster E, et al. Perilunate dislocation: case studies of a frequently missed diagnosis: delayed treatment adversely affects clinical results. J Musculoskeletal Med. 2008;
19. Cardoso R, et al. Wrist anatomy and surgical approaches. Hand Clinics. 2010;26:1–19.
20. Young D, et al. Physical examination of the wrist. Hand Clinics. 2010;26:21–36.
21. Bookman A, et al. Wrist and hand. In: Fam's musculoskeletal examination and joint injection techniques. 2nd ed. Philadelphia: Mosby; 2010. p. 29–43.
22. Dye M. et al. Metacarpal fractures: treatment & management. Emedicine.com.
23. Alke J. et al. Hand fracture treatment & management. Emedicine.com.
24. Tintinalli JE, Ruiz E, Krome RL. Injuries to the hand and digits. In: Emergency medicine: a comprehensive study guide. 6th ed. New York: McGraw Hill; 2004. p. 1665–74.
25. Bates S, et al. Flexor tendon anatomy. Mescape. https://emedicine.medscape.com/article/1245236-overview.

Index

D. Purcell et al. (eds.), *Emergency Orthopedics Handbook*,
https://doi.org/10.1007/978-3-030-00707-2

Printed by Printforce, the Netherlands